HERBAL HOME APOTHECARY BOOK

350+ Medicinal Plants & Herbal Remedies for Natural Healing & Wellness

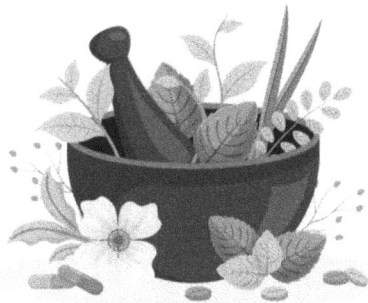

DR. TINA M. PENHOLLOW

TIMELESS PERSPECTIVES
— P U B L I S H I N G —

Timeless Perspectives Publishing
An imprint of Timeless Perspectives, LLC

Paperback Full Color Edition ISBN: 978-1-966018-13-1
Paperback Black and White Edition ISBN: 978-1-966018-11-7

TABLE OF CONTENTS

TABLE OF CONTENTS

5 Herbal Recipes for Common Ailments

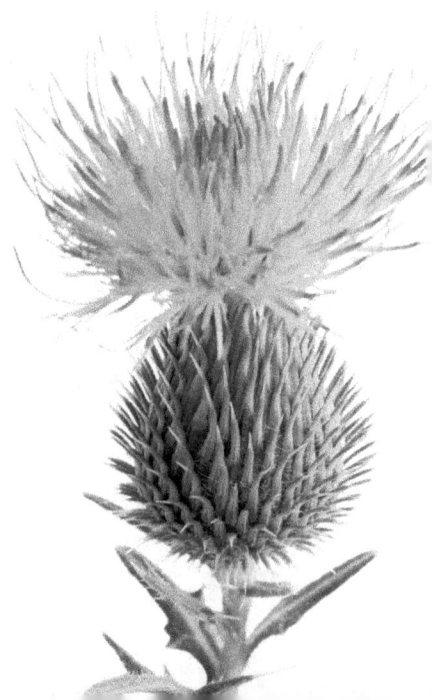

INTRODUCTION

"The physician treats, but nature heals."
— Hippocrates, Ancient Greek Physician

Imagine walking into your home and being greeted by the soothing scents of lavender, the warmth of ginger, and the golden hue of turmeric—each herb offering its healing power, ready to ease your mind, body, and spirit. This is the vision of *Herbal Home Apothecary*, a transformative guide designed to bring the ancient practice of herbal medicine into your modern life with ease and accessibility.

Long before synthetic pharmaceuticals dominated healthcare, our ancestors turned to plants for healing, nourishment, and prevention. These herbs were not just remedies; they were essential parts of daily life, deeply connected to the rhythms of nature and the cycles of the body. In ancient Egypt, scrolls recorded healing formulas made from aloe and frankincense, while in India, Ayurveda harnessed the anti-inflammatory powers of turmeric thousands of years ago. Across continents, indigenous cultures passed down their sacred knowledge of plant-based healing, teaching us that herbs could restore balance, nurture vitality, and elevate wellness.

In *Herbal Home Apothecary*, you'll embark on a journey to reclaim this ancient wisdom. Within these pages, you'll unlock the secrets of 100 essential medicinal herbs—each with its unique properties and profound healing potential. From the soothing leaves of chamomile to the immune-strengthening flowers of echinacea. These plants are more than mere ingredients—they are timeless allies in the pursuit of well-being. With carefully crafted, step-by-step instructions, you will learn to create over 250 remedies—teas, tinctures, salves, poultices, and more—that transform your home into a sanctuary of natural healing. Whether you're a curious beginner or an experienced herbalist, this book provides the tools and inspiration you need to create remedies tailored to your specific health needs.

This book offers more than just recipes—it invites you to experience herbal medicine as a transformative path. As you delve into the healing properties of these plants and hone the art of remedy-making, you will embrace a new paradigm of wellness—one that honors the wisdom of our ancestors while meeting the challenges of the modern world. Embracing the ancient practice of herbal medicine will not only enhance your well-being but also reconnect you with nature's wisdom, paving the way for a future of health and vitality.

WELCOME TO THE WORLD OF HERBAL WISDOM!

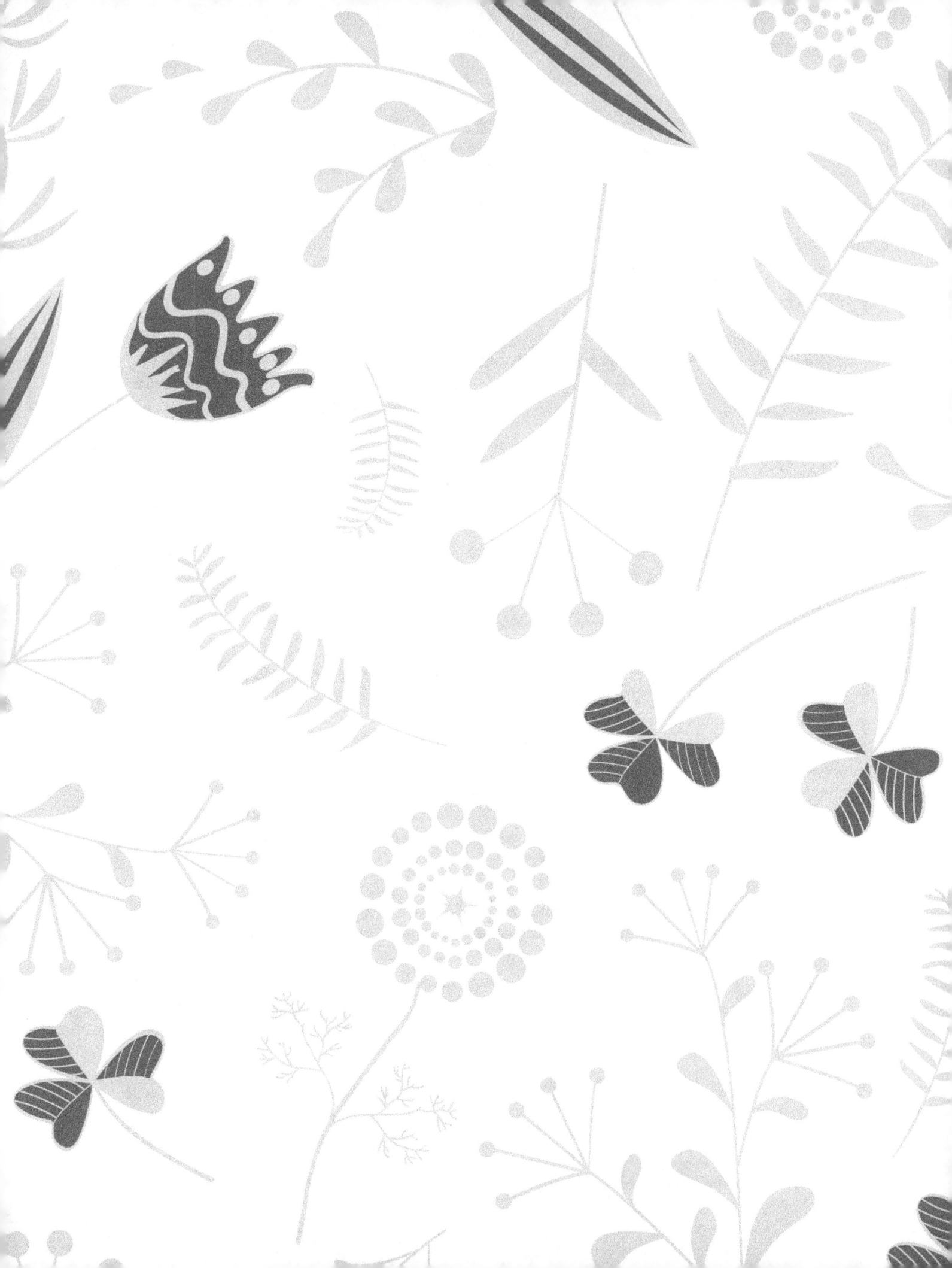

Chapter One

HERBOLOGY 101

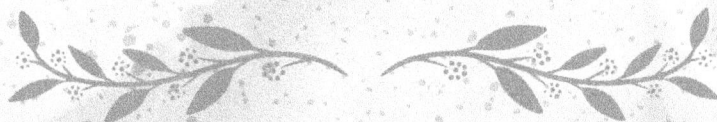

"*The use of plants for healing is not a matter of belief; it is a matter of history.*"
— Steven Foster, American Herbalist

HERBALISM

Herbal medicine is one of the world's oldest and most enduring health practices, deeply rooted in human history. Across cultures and centuries, plants have been sought out for their ability to nourish, heal, and promote spiritual well-being. Before modern pharmaceuticals, plants provided essential remedies, offering natural solutions to common ailments based on careful observation and a profound understanding of nature's power.

Ancient healers recognized the healing potential in nature's offerings—leaves soothed fevers, roots alleviated pain, and flowers calmed anxious minds. In ancient Egypt, fennel and aloe were cherished for their medicinal benefits. Traditional Chinese Medicine (TCM) developed sophisticated herbal formulas, still used today. Native American healers regarded plants as sacred tools, addressing physical, mental, and spiritual health, emphasizing the interconnectedness between body and nature. In Europe, apothecaries preserved these ancient herbal traditions, ensuring their survival into modern times.

This wealth of knowledge, passed down through generations, forms the foundation of herbalism—a practice that blends ancient wisdom with contemporary research. At its heart, herbology is the study of plants and their medicinal properties, focusing on how different plant parts—leaves, roots, flowers, and seeds—can be used to heal and restore balance. Herbalism is more than a body of knowledge; it's a living tradition that connects cultures worldwide.

Today, herbalism is experiencing a resurgence, merging age-old practices with modern science. Contemporary medicine is finally catching up with what ancient healers instinctively understood: plants hold remarkable powers to restore balance and vitality to the body. As you delve into herbalism, you'll find it's not just about remedies—it's a philosophy of life that fosters harmony between body, mind, and the natural world.

In today's hectic world, many of us feel disconnected—from our bodies, our communities, and even the Earth. Quick-fix solutions and synthetic medications often focus only on symptoms, leaving underlying imbalances unaddressed. Herbalism offers a path to reconnect with nature's wisdom, take control of your health, and embrace sustainable practices that promote lasting well-being. Herbs offer gentle, yet potent remedies for common modern-day concerns: alleviating anxiety, boosting immunity, supporting digestion, and detoxifying the body from environmental toxins. By integrating herbs into your routine, you cultivate a lifestyle that values holistic health, fostering a deeper, more enduring sense of wellness.

Herbalism offers a variety of methods to tap into the healing power of plants, including teas, tinctures, syrups, salves, and essential oils. Each approach provides distinct benefits, allowing you to choose the best form for your needs. Understanding the energetic properties of herbs—such as warming, cooling, moistening, or drying—helps you restore balance to your body. Warming herbs like cinnamon and cayenne encourage circulation, while cooling herbs like mint and lemon balm reduce inflammation and ease stress.

More than just a healing practice, herbalism is a transformative journey. It empowers you to actively care for your health, shifting from a passive recipient of medical treatment to an engaged participant in your well-being. Learning to identify plants and understand their medicinal properties gives you the tools to nurture your health and foster a deep connection with nature. Herbalism invites you to become a steward of the Earth's healing gifts, cultivating a balanced relationship between mind, body, and spirit.

NATUROPATHY

Imagine a world where nature provides all the healing you need—a world where your body's inherent ability to heal itself is nurtured and supported. This is the essence of naturopathy, a holistic system of medicine that emphasizes the body's natural healing power. While it may not be widely known, naturopathy is gaining recognition for its comprehensive approach to health, one that focuses not just on physical symptoms, but also on mental, emotional, and spiritual well-being. At its heart, naturopathy combines modern medical knowledge with traditional natural therapies like herbal medicine, nutrition, exercise, and stress management. This approach prioritizes prevention and empowers you to take charge of your health.

When you embrace naturopathy, you become an active participant in your own healing. Rather than simply masking symptoms with medication, you address the root causes of illness. Naturopathic practitioners look at your lifestyle, environment, and genetic predispositions to offer personalized care. Treatments may include detoxification, acupuncture, or hydrotherapy to restore balance and support your body's natural functions.

Why should naturopathy matter to you and those you love? As chronic conditions like diabetes, heart disease, and anxiety continue to rise, conventional treatments often focus on managing these diseases rather than preventing them. Naturopathy, however, works to prevent illness before it starts. By embracing natural therapies and promoting a healthy lifestyle, you can reduce your reliance on pharmaceuticals, improve your overall quality of life, and maintain long-term well-being.

Naturopathy also fosters a deeper connection to both your body and the natural world. In today's fast-paced, stress-filled environment, it's easy to neglect self-care. Naturopathy serves as a reminder that true health is not simply the absence of disease, but a vibrant state of balance that touches every aspect of your life.

ASTROLOGICAL HERBALISM

Astrological herbalism, also known as botanical astrology or astro-herbalism, is the art of using herbs in harmony with astrology to promote healing and restore balance. This practice has ancient roots, tracing back to the wisdom of figures like Hippocrates, Paracelsus, and Culpeper, who believed that celestial bodies influence all life on Earth, including the growth and energetic properties of plants. By integrating astrological knowledge—such as zodiac signs, planetary influences, and the elements—practitioners select herbs that align with an individual's unique physical and energetic needs. Each herb is carefully matched with its planetary ruler and corresponding zodiac sign, creating personalized remedies that resonate with a person's astrological chart to bring about holistic healing and well-being.

Planetary Rulerships in Herbalism

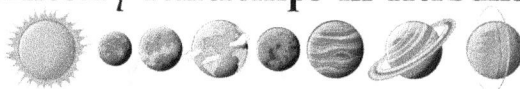

In astrological herbalism, plants are classified based on the energetic influences of the seven classical planets. Each planet is thought to govern specific plants, shaping their appearance, energetic qualities, and healing properties. Aligning herbal remedies with planetary energies can promote physical and emotional healing in tune with the natural rhythms of the cosmos. Below is a guide to the planetary rulerships and their corresponding herbs:

Sun (Vitality, Heart, Leadership)
The Sun represents life force, vitality, and warmth. Herbs ruled by the Sun often have bright, solar-like qualities that energize and promote overall well-being. These herbs strengthen the heart, boost immunity, and enhance self-confidence.
- Examples: St. John's Wort, Rosemary, Calendula.
- Uses: Often used for energy depletion, low self-esteem, and physical weakness.

Moon (Emotions, Intuition, Fluids)
The Moon governs emotions, cycles, intuition, and bodily fluids. Herbs ruled by the Moon tend to be calming, nurturing, and supportive of emotional balance. These plants are often associated with sleep, digestion, and reproductive health.
- Examples: Chamomile, Willow, Lemon Balm.
- Uses: Ideal for addressing stress, hormonal imbalances, and fluid retention.

Mercury (Communication, Mental Agility, Nervous System)
Mercury influences communication, intellect, and the nervous system. Herbs under this planet enhance mental clarity, adaptability, and neural function. They often support cognitive processes and improve respiratory or digestive health.
- Examples: Lavender, Fennel, Peppermint.
- Uses: Useful for conditions like mental fatigue, anxiety, and digestive issues.

Venus (Love, Beauty, Harmony, Kidneys)

Venus rules over beauty, love, sensuality, and balance. Herbs aligned with Venus are often aromatic, gentle, and nourishing, promoting emotional healing and physical beauty. These plants are used for skin health, fertility, and emotional well-being.

- Examples: Rose, Yarrow, Hawthorn.
- Uses: Applied in skin care, emotional healing, and heart-centered practices.

Mars (Action, Energy, Protection, Blood)

Mars governs physical strength, courage, and protection. Mars herbs are typically stimulating, spicy, and energizing. They are known for boosting stamina, circulation, and immunity, as well as offering protection against infections and harmful influences.

- Examples: Cayenne Pepper, Garlic, Nettle.
- Uses: Ideal for enhancing physical endurance, managing inflammation, and increasing overall vitality.

Jupiter (Expansion, Growth, Abundance, Liver)

Jupiter is associated with growth, optimism, and abundance. Herbs under Jupiter's influence are often expansive in nature, promoting physical and spiritual growth. They support liver function, digestion, and a sense of well-being.

- Examples: Dandelion, Sage, Licorice Root.
- Uses: Often used to support detoxification, digestion, and a positive mindset.

Saturn (Structure, Boundaries, Endurance, Bones)

Saturn rules discipline, structure, and long-term health. Saturnian herbs are often grounding, promoting bone health, resilience, and endurance. They support conditions requiring long-term healing and promote the stability of body systems.

- Examples: Comfrey, Horsetail, and Ashwagandha.
- Uses: Effective for strengthening bones, improving stamina, and supporting chronic conditions.

ELEMENTAL BALANCE

Astrology's four elements—earth, air, fire, and water—are mirrored in the energetic qualities of herbs.
- **Earth Signs (Taurus, Virgo, Capricorn):** Benefit from grounding, nourishing herbs like dandelion and nettle.
- **Air Signs (Gemini, Libra, Aquarius):** Thrive on herbs that support mental focus and creativity, such as gotu kola.
- **Fire Signs (Aries, Leo, Sagittarius):** May need cooling herbs, like chamomile, to balance their fiery energy.
- **Water Signs (Cancer, Scorpio, Pisces):** Align with herbs that support emotional well-being, such as lavender.

Zodiac Signs and Herbal Correspondences

Zodiac herbalism is the practice of associating herbs with the 12 zodiac signs. It blends astrology and herbalism, using the principles of the zodiac to enhance the medicinal, spiritual, and energetic power of plants. Each zodiac sign is intricately connected to specific herbs that align with its elemental nature (fire, earth, air, or water) and energetic qualities. These herbs reflect the sign's core characteristics, supporting physical and emotional balance. By working with zodiac-specific herbs, you can harmonize their strengths, address imbalances, and enhance their potential for growth and healing.

♈ Aries (March 21 - April 19) | Element: Fire | Planet: Mars
- Energetic, bold, and often prone to inflammation or tension
- Herbs: Cayenne pepper, ephedra, garlic, ginger, ginseng, maca root, onion
- Properties: Warming, circulation-boosting, and anti-inflammatory

★ ARIES

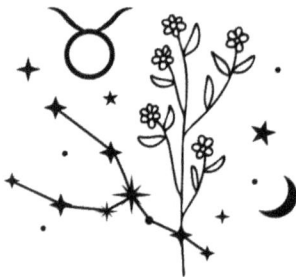

♉ Taurus (April 20 - May 20) | Element: Earth | Planet: Venus
- Grounded, sensual, and prone to, throat or neck issues
- Herbs: Violet, wild yam, red clover, plantain, licorice, coltsfoot
- Properties: Soothing, nourishing, and balancing

★ TAURUS

♊ Gemini (May 21 - June 20) | Element: Air | Planet: Mercury
- Communicative, curious, and sensitive to respiratory issues
- Herbs: Fenugreek, ginkgo biloba, horehound, lavender, parsley, peppermint
- Properties: Respiratory tonics, calming, and focus-enhancing

★ GEMINI

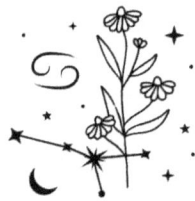

♋ Cancer (June 21 - July 22) | Element: Water | Planet: Moon
- Nurturing, emotional, and sensitive to digestive and emotional imbalances
- Herbs: Willow, thyme, slippery elm, chamomile, lemon balm, kava kava, evening primrose, marshmallow root
- Properties: Soothing, digestive support, and emotional balance

★ CANCER

♌ Leo (July 23 - August 22) | Element: Fire | Planet: Sun
• Confident, vibrant, and often prone to heart or circulatory issues
• Herbs: Angelica, cinnamon, dandelion, firebush, St. John's Wort
• Properties: Heart tonics, energy-boosting, and mood-enhancing

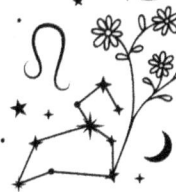

★ LEO

♍ Virgo (August 23 - September 22) | Element: Earth | Planet: Mercury
• Analytical, health-conscious, and sensitive to digestive issues
• Herbs: Anise, bilberry, fennel, caraway, cumin, gentian, hyssop, milk thistle
• Properties: Digestive aids, calming, and grounding

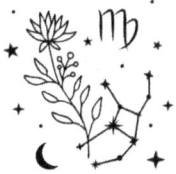

★ VIRGO

♎ Libra (September 23 - October 22) | Element: Air | Planet: Venus
• Harmonious, beauty-loving, and prone to kidney or hormonal imbalances
• Herbs: Wild rose, yarrow, hibiscus, meadowsweet, linden, lady's mantle
• Properties: Hormonal balancing, beautifying, and calming

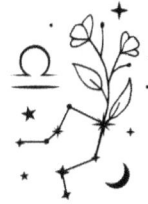

★ LIBRA

♏ Scorpio (October 23 - November 21) | Element: Water | Planet: Mars & Pluto
• Intense, transformative, and prone to reproductive or detox needs
• Herbs: Black cohosh, false unicorn, nettle, oregano, pomegranate
• Properties: Reproductive support, detoxifying, and stimulating

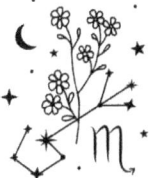

★ SCORPIO

♐ Sagittarius (November 22 - December 21) | Element: Fire | Planet: Jupiter
• Adventurous, optimistic, and sensitive to liver or hip issues
• Herbs: Turmeric, sage, myrrh, juniper, clove, chicory, cardamom
• Properties: Liver-supportive, warming, and grounding

★ SAGITTARIUS

♑ Capricorn (December 22 - January 19) | Element: Earth | Planet: Saturn
• Disciplined, practical, and prone to bone, skin, or joint issues
• Herbs: Arnica, ashwagandha, bay leaf, black walnut, burdock, comfrey, frankincense
• Properties: Bone-strengthening, anti-inflammatory, and skin-supportive

★ CAPRICORN

♒ Aquarius (January 20 - February 18) | Element: Air | Planet: Uranus
• Innovative, independent, and sensitive to circulatory or nervous issues
• Herbs: Blue vervain and eucalyptus
• Properties: Nervous system tonics, calming, and circulatory support

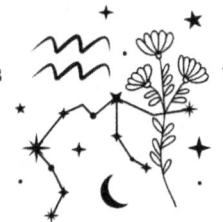

★ AQUARIUS

♓ Pisces (February 19 - March 20) | Element: Water | Planet: Neptune
• Dreamy, compassionate, and prone to emotional or lymphatic imbalances
• Herbs: Cowslip, holy basil, passionflower, valerian
• Properties: Nervous system support, immune-boosting, and detoxifying

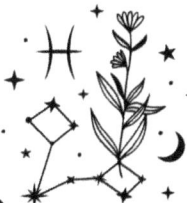

★ PISCES

Lunar Gardening and Herbal Harvesting

Throughout the medieval and Renaissance eras in Europe, alchemists blended astrology with herbalism to create "spagyric" tinctures, believing that aligning plant remedies with celestial forces would amplify their healing properties. They understood that the cosmic rhythms—governed by the stars and planets—could enhance the potency of herbal treatments. Like astrology, herbalism has long adhered to the natural cycles of the Earth, from lunar phases to seasonal shifts. This deep connection between celestial movements and plant growth has shaped traditional practices such as planting, harvesting, and preparing remedies according to the phases of the moon. Experienced herbalists carefully observed these astrological rhythms, selecting the most auspicious times to cultivate, gather, and craft remedies, ensuring the herbs harnessed their fullest energetic potential.

- **New Moon:** A time for planting leafy herbs and beginning new herbal remedies, fostering fresh growth and vitality.
- **Waxing Moon:** Ideal for encouraging plant growth; it's the perfect phase for harvesting above-ground herbs, as they are at their most vibrant.
- **Full Moon:** The peak of potency, making it the optimal time to harvest herbs, when their energy is believed to be at its fullest and most powerful.
- **Waning Moon:** Best suited for harvesting roots and preparing long-lasting remedies such as tinctures, as this phase encourages deeper, more enduring healing properties.

HOLISTIC HEALING

Astrology and herbalism both embrace a profound understanding of health as a holistic system, recognizing the deep connection between mind, body, and spirit. By examining an individual's astrological chart, herbalists can create personalized remedies that address imbalances influenced by planetary and elemental forces present at birth. This alignment of astrology and herbalism enhances healing on physical and energetic levels, combining the wisdom of the cosmos with the healing power of nature's plant-based remedies to restore balance and vitality.

Now that you've explored the fundamentals of herbal medicine, the next chapter will guide you through the transformative process of creating your own home apothecary. This space will become your personal sanctuary for natural healing, where you can blend ancient wisdom with contemporary practices. Whether you have a dedicated room for your herbal work or simply a small shelf tucked away in a corner, this chapter will provide you with the knowledge and tools to design a functional and inspiring space that reflects your unique lifestyle.

Chapter Two

BUILDING YOUR HOME APOTHECARY

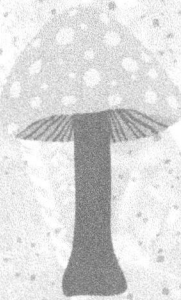

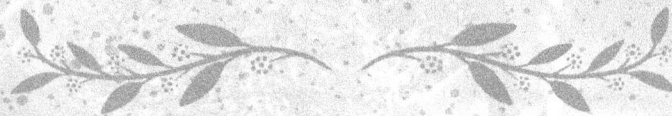

"Healing through plants is the most ancient form of medicine and the most reliable for the treatment of many ailments. "
- Sebastian Kneipp, Founder of Naturopathic Medicine

The Essentials of a Home Apothecary

Since the dawn of humanity, plants have played a vital role in our pursuit of health and healing. Long before synthetic medications were introduced, our ancestors turned to the natural world to treat wounds, alleviate pain, and restore balance to both body and mind. The tradition of plant-based healing is woven into the very fabric of human history, and it is the foundation of the home apothecary—a sacred space where nature's gifts converge with the time-honored art of herbal medicine.

The practice of creating a home apothecary dates back to ancient times, where herbalists and healers would gather plants from the earth to craft remedies that addressed physical and spiritual well-being. In medieval Europe, apothecaries were the cornerstone of community health, blending the wisdom of herbalism with the emerging practices of alchemy and medicine. These early apothecaries were often more than just stores of herbs— they were sacred spaces, often found in homes or small workshops, where plants were prepared, preserved, and transformed into healing potions, tinctures, and balms. In many cultures, the home apothecary was passed down through generations, a symbol of familial knowledge and a deep connection to the natural world.

In this chapter, you'll learn how to build and organize your own home apothecary to preserve the potency and quality of your ingredients. You'll discover the importance of choosing the right containers, understanding the shelf life of dried herbs and oils, and getting familiar with essential tools such as mortar and pestles for grinding herbs and amber bottles for tinctures. With this knowledge, you'll create an apothecary that is more than just a collection of supplies—it will be a bridge to ancient healing traditions and a powerful tool to nourish your mind, body, and spirit.

A home apothecary is more than just a few jars and bottles lining a shelf; it is a sanctuary of healing, a reflection of your self-reliance and connection to nature's rhythms. It transforms a simple corner of your home into a space where dried herbs, tinctures, salves, and syrups are always within reach. Whether you are easing the discomfort of a cold, supporting digestion, or calming the nervous system, your apothecary becomes an indispensable resource for empowering your health and caring for loved ones.

Modern science continues to validate the ancient wisdom of herbal medicine, uncovering the wide-reaching benefits of plants in treating a variety of ailments. Lavender soothes the mind, elderberries strengthen immunity, chamomile aids digestion, and peppermint revitalizes the senses. Each herb holds a wealth of knowledge passed down through generations, waiting for you to integrate it into your daily life. A home apothecary invites you into a more mindful relationship with the natural world. You'll establish a practice that nurtures your body, mind, and spirit, all while honoring the healing traditions passed down for centuries.

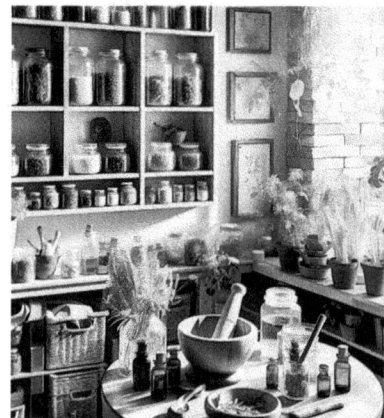

ESSENTIAL TOOLS

Building a home apothecary involves equipping yourself with the essential tools that will allow you to craft remedies efficiently and effectively. In this section, you will learn about the key tools that form the foundation of your herbal practice. From mortar and pestles for grinding dried herbs to amber bottles for preserving tinctures, each tool serves a unique purpose in helping you create the highest quality remedies. With the right tools at your disposal, you'll be able to craft everything from soothing salves to potent tinctures with confidence, knowing that each step is supported by the tools that enhance your connection to the healing powers of plants.

Scales

A precise scale is an essential tool in herbalism, particularly for ensuring accurate measurements of herbs and ingredients. Whether you're making tinctures, teas, or capsules, a scale allows you to measure herbs by weight, which is more reliable than volume measurements. This ensures that your remedies are consistent and potent, helping you maintain the right dosage. Scales also provide precision when creating complex formulations, ensuring that each herb is properly balanced for optimal effectiveness and accuracy.

Airtight Glass Jars

Glass jars in varying sizes are indispensable for storing dried herbs, powders, and salves. Their airtight seals keep your ingredients fresh and potent, while the transparency allows for easy identification. These jars also lend a polished and organized look to your apothecary, ensuring every ingredient is within reach and protected from moisture or contamination.

Tincture Bottles

Amber and cobalt blue glass bottles with droppers are a cornerstone for storing and dispensing tinctures and herbal extracts. The dark glass shields contents from light exposure, preserving potency and extending shelf life. These bottles also allow for precise dosing, making them ideal for daily use and a polished way to share your creations.

Mortar and Pestle

This timeless tool is perfect for grinding fresh or dried herbs, unlocking their active compounds, and preparing them for teas, salves, or infusions. The tactile nature of using a mortar and pestle connects you to your ingredients, adding a layer of authenticity and intention to your remedies.

Measuring Tools

Precision is key when crafting safe and effective remedies. Measuring spoons and cups ensure consistent ratios of herbs, oils, and other components, giving you confidence in your creations. These tools are invaluable for both beginners and experienced herbalists seeking consistent results.

Muslin or Cheesecloth

These fine straining cloths are essential for separating plant material from liquids when preparing tinctures, infusions, or oils. They ensure your final product is smooth, free from debris, and visually appealing. Keep several on hand to accommodate multiple projects.

Double Boiler

A double boiler is critical for crafting salves, balms, and lotions, allowing you to gently melt oils and waxes without scorching their delicate properties. If you don't have one, you can improvise by placing a heatproof bowl over a pot of simmering water, ensuring your ingredients heat evenly and retain their therapeutic benefits. If you don't have a boiler, you can heat the mixture directly in a saucepan on low heat or place a heatproof bowl over a pot of simmering water to create a makeshift double boiler effect. This allows you to gently melt the ingredients without overheating them.

Herb Drying Rack

Preserving freshly harvested herbs is vital for maintaining their medicinal qualities. A drying rack provides the perfect environment for air-drying herbs while retaining their aroma, color, and potency. Properly dried herbs are a ready resource for teas, tinctures, and powders year-round.

Labeling Supplies

Accurate labeling is the key to staying organized. Use labels and markers to document each remedy's ingredients, preparation date, and intended use. Thoughtful labeling ensures you can track freshness, monitor effectiveness, and recreate successful recipes with ease.

Essential Oil Diffuser

A diffuser is a must-have for enjoying the benefits of essential oils through aromatherapy. By releasing calming, uplifting, or purifying scents into the air, a diffuser helps create a soothing and wellness-focused atmosphere. Whether you want to unwind, boost your energy, or enhance focus, this tool seamlessly integrates essential oils into your everyday routine. As you immerse yourself in the art of herbalism, you'll embody the role of a modern-day alchemist, turning simple ingredients into powerful solutions that promote health, harmony, and self-sufficiency.

ADVANCED TOOLS

If you're looking to elevate your home apothecary, investing in a few advanced tools can revolutionize the way you craft, store, and personalize your remedies. These optional additions are perfect for passionate herbalists ready to refine their skills and create high-quality preparations with greater ease and precision. By incorporating these advanced tools, you'll streamline your workflow, expand your creative possibilities, and ensure the utmost quality in your herbal practice.

Salve Tins

Compact, durable, and aesthetically pleasing, salve tins are indispensable for storing your handcrafted balms and ointments. Designed to shield your creations from air, light, and moisture, these tins help maintain the potency and freshness of your remedies over time. The smooth, flat lids are perfect for labeling, allowing you to easily track ingredients, uses, and preparation dates.

Dehydrator

A dehydrator is a game-changer for herbalists dealing with fresh harvests, enabling you to dry herbs, flowers, and roots efficiently while preserving their vibrant color, aroma, and therapeutic properties. Unlike traditional air-drying methods, which can be inconsistent and vulnerable to humidity, a dehydrator ensures optimal drying conditions for superior results in a fraction of the time. This tool is especially valuable for gardeners and wildcrafters, turning each harvest into a long-lasting resource without waste. With precise temperature control, a dehydrator preserves the delicate compounds in your herbs, ensuring their maximum effectiveness in teas, tinctures, or powders.

Capsule Machine

A capsule machine is a must-have for creating personalized herbal supplements. This user-friendly device simplifies the process of filling capsules, allowing you to create custom blends tailored to your specific health needs. From immunity boosters to digestive aids, the machine empowers you to control the ingredients, ensuring purity and eliminating the additives or fillers often found in commercial products. The ability to craft remedies with precise dosages deepens your connection to the herbal practice, fostering confidence in the quality of your creations.

KEY SUPPLIES

Building a versatile home apothecary begins with a selection of essential ingredients. These staples are the foundation of countless remedies, allowing you to craft everything from nourishing skincare products to health-boosting tonics. Each ingredient has unique properties, making them indispensable for your natural creations.

Carrier Oils

Carrier oils are a cornerstone of natural remedies, providing a safe and nourishing base for essential oils and other herbal infusions. They dilute concentrated essential oils for safe application and enhance the absorption of active compounds into the skin. Herbalist use three main types of carrier oils:

- **Coconut Oil:** Renowned for its intense moisturizing properties, coconut oil is perfect for dry or sensitive skin and forms the base for rich, nourishing balms and salves.
- **Jojoba Oil:** This lightweight, non-greasy oil closely mimics the skin's natural sebum, making it ideal for facial serums and remedies suitable for all skin types.
- **Olive Oil:** A classic carrier oil, olive oil is packed with antioxidants and fatty acids, offering deep nourishment and supporting anti-inflammatory treatments..

Beeswax

Beeswax is an essential ingredient for creating salves, lotions, and balms, offering both structure and nourishment to your formulations. As a natural thickener, beeswax solidifies your blends, providing them with a silky, spreadable consistency that is easy to apply. Its unique ability to form a breathable, protective barrier on the skin helps lock in moisture while shielding against external irritants, making it particularly beneficial for dry or sensitive skin. With a subtle honey-like aroma, beeswax enhances the sensory appeal of your creations and complements a variety of herbal ingredients. Its natural emollient properties hydrate the skin and aid in soothing minor irritations, making it a cornerstone of any apothecary.

Apple Cider Vinegar

Apple cider vinegar is a cornerstone ingredient in natural health and beauty practices. Its rich profile of enzymes and beneficial acids serves as a base for herbal infusions and tonics that promote digestive health, aid detoxification, and support pH balance. This versatile elixir extends beyond internal remedies, offering clarifying properties for hair care. It effectively removes buildup, strengthens strands, and restores vitality to dull hair. Apple cider vinegar's ability to balance oil production also makes it a useful addition to skincare routines, where it can be used as a toner to calm and rejuvenate the complexion. Equally effective for internal and topical applications, apple cider vinegar is a must-have for anyone seeking holistic wellness solutions.

Honey

Honey is a timeless ingredient cherished for its remarkable healing and hydrating properties. As a natural antibacterial agent, it is effective for treating minor wounds, calming cuts, scrapes, and burns, while promoting faster healing. Its humectant qualities draw moisture into the skin, making it a standout ingredient in nourishing masks, balms, and serums that leave the skin soft, glowing, and rejuvenated. In herbal teas and tonics, honey provides a delicate sweetness and also supports immune health and soothes sore throats, offering comfort during colds and seasonal ailments.

Alcohol (such as Vodka or Brandy)

Alcohol is a key ingredient for making herbal tinctures, where it acts as a solvent to extract and preserve the medicinal properties of herbs. The high alcohol content ensures the herbs' active compounds are concentrated, creating potent, long-lasting extracts that can be used for a variety of therapeutic purposes. Alcohol also acts as an excellent preservative, extending the shelf life of your homemade remedies. Beyond tinctures, alcohol can be used for herbal extractions or as a base for cleansing tonics, offering an effective way to harness the healing power of plants in a concentrated form.

Glycerin

Glycerin is a plant-based, alcohol-free alternative to alcohol-based tinctures. It has a sweet, thick consistency and is ideal for creating glycerites, which are gentle, sweetened herbal extracts that are especially useful for children or individuals sensitive to alcohol. Glycerin has hydrating properties, making it a common addition to skincare formulations such as creams, lotions, and serums. It draws moisture into the skin, helping to soothe irritated or dry skin. As an ingredient for internal use, glycerin works as a mild digestive aid and is commonly included in remedies that target the throat or digestive tract.

Aloe Vera Gel

Aloe vera gel is a powerful, soothing ingredient widely used in both skincare and internal remedies. Known for its anti-inflammatory and healing properties, it is especially beneficial for treating sunburns, skin irritations, burns, and cuts, providing immediate cooling relief and promoting faster healing. Aloe vera gel is rich in vitamins and minerals that nourish the skin, making it a popular addition to moisturizing lotions, balms, and facial masks. Internally, aloe vera is known for its gentle detoxifying effects and its ability to promote digestive health, particularly for soothing the stomach and relieving constipation. Its versatility makes aloe vera a staple in your herbal medicine cabinet and skincare regimen.

SOURCING INGREDIENTS

Building a home apothecary begins with selecting or sourcing the highest quality ingredients to create safe and effective remedies. Opting for sustainably grown, organic, and ethically harvested materials enhances the quality of your creations and supports the environment and the communities that cultivate these natural resources. Thoughtful choices like these help you care for your health while positively impacting the planet. The efficacy and safety of your natural remedies are deeply tied to the quality of the ingredients you use. High-quality herbs, oils, and other raw materials deliver superior therapeutic benefits while safeguarding against harmful contaminants. By prioritizing quality, you elevate the integrity of your remedies, transforming your apothecary into a space of mindful, sustainable healing.

Where to Source Ingredients

- **Reputable Suppliers:** Partnering with trusted suppliers is key to ensuring that your ingredients meet the highest standards of quality and purity. Seek out companies that are transparent about their sourcing practices, offering information about where their herbs, oils, and other products are grown and how they are harvested. Certifications such as USDA Organic, Fair Trade, and cruelty-free serve as reliable markers of ethical and sustainable practices. Many reputable suppliers also conduct third-party purity testing, ensuring their products are free from contaminants and meet stringent quality standards.

- **Local Farmers and Co-ops:** Local farmers' markets and co-ops are excellent sources of fresh, pesticide-free herbs and natural ingredients. Purchasing directly from local growers ensures peak freshness, reduces your carbon footprint, and supports eco-friendly agriculture. Many small-scale farms use sustainable farming methods that prioritize soil health and biodiversity, resulting in higher-quality herbs.

- **Your Own Herb Garden:** Cultivating your own herbs is one of the most sustainable and rewarding ways to source ingredients for your apothecary. Even with limited space, you can grow staples like basil, mint, lavender, or chamomile in pots, containers, or small garden beds. By growing your herbs, you gain complete control over their care, ensuring they are free from synthetic chemicals and harvested at their peak potency. Tending your garden fosters a deeper connection to the healing power of plants and offers a meditative practice that complements your herbal craft. Homegrown ingredients also reduce dependency on commercial suppliers and enhance the personal touch in every remedy you create.

- **Sustainably Sourced Oils:** When selecting essential and carrier oils, prioritize brands that emphasize sustainability and eco-friendly extraction methods. Certifications such as organic, non-GMO, and third-party purity testing are essential indicators of quality. Supporting companies that value environmental stewardship and ethical labor practices ensures that your oils are as beneficial to the planet as they are to your apothecary.

Building a Sustainable Practice

Crafting effective remedies begins with choosing high-quality ingredients and embracing a practice rooted in sustainability and mindfulness. By sourcing herbs from local farmers, working with trusted suppliers, or cultivating your own garden, you contribute to a wellness approach that honors the environment and strengthens your community.

Safety Precautions in Herbal Medicine

While herbal remedies offer natural healing, they can still pose risks if not used correctly. Follow these guidelines to minimize potential harm:

- **Proper Identification:** Ensure that all herbs are accurately identified, especially when foraging or purchasing from local sources. Misidentification can lead to the use of toxic plants.
- **Allergies and Sensitivities:** Be aware of individual allergies and sensitivities. Test new herbs on a small area of skin or start with a low dose to gauge reactions.
- **Dosage Awareness:** Herbal remedies vary in potency. Follow recommended dosages and consult reputable sources to avoid under- or over-dosing.
- **Interactions with Medications:** Some herbs can interact with prescription medications. Consult a healthcare provider if you or others are taking medications.
- **Storage and Shelf Life:** Store herbs and oils in a cool, dry place away from direct sunlight. Proper storage prevents contamination and preserves potency.
- **Pregnancy and Children:** Certain herbs are unsafe for pregnant individuals or young children. Always verify the safety of herbs before use in these cases.

The next chapter will guide you into the hands-on world of herbal preparation, where you'll learn how to transform the raw potential of your herbs into powerful, practical remedies. Step-by-step, you will explore how to create soothing teas, aromatic infusions, and concentrated decoctions that extract the full healing properties of plants. You'll also discover how to craft healing syrups, nourishing salves, and soothing balms that can be tailored to address specific health needs. Whether you're looking to ease a cold, soothe dry skin, or promote overall well-being, this chapter will provide you with the techniques and recipes to confidently prepare a variety of herbal remedies in your own apothecary.

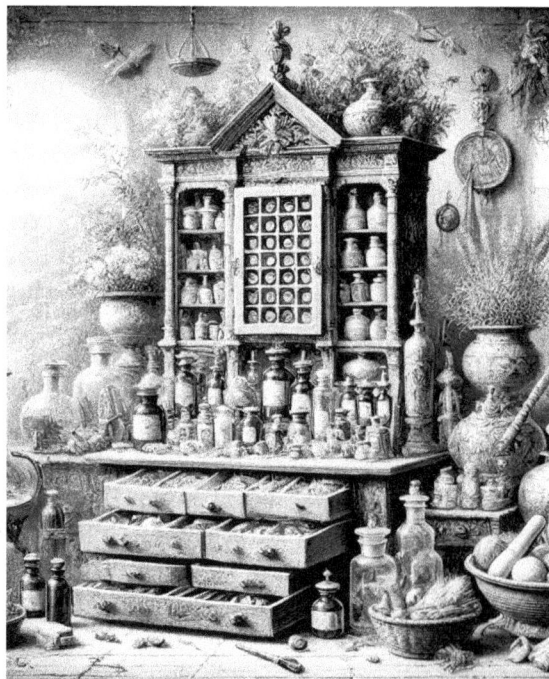

Chapter Three

THE ART OF HERBAL PREPARATION

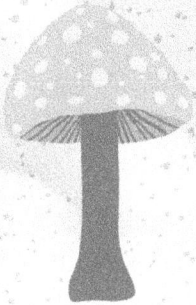

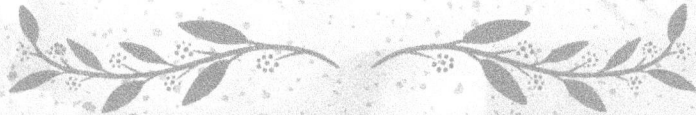

"*A weed is a plant whose virtues have not yet been discovered.*"
— Ralph Waldo Emerson, American Philosopher

Crafting Herbal Remedies

This chapter delves into the art and science of creating herbal remedies, from soothing teas to potent tinctures, nourishing infusions, sweet syrups, and versatile salves. Each method brings out the unique qualities of the herbs, catering to diverse needs and health goals.

Herbal teas, for instance, are one of the simplest and most accessible ways to experience the benefits of nature. With just a handful of herbs and hot water, you can create a calming, aromatic drink that supports relaxation, digestion, and gentle healing. On the other hand, tinctures offer a more concentrated approach, relying on alcohol to extract the deeper medicinal compounds of plants. These are perfect for individuals seeking long-term benefits in a compact, stable form.

Infusions take the concept of tea a step further. By steeping herbs for hours or even overnight, infusions provide a nutrient-dense, highly concentrated remedy, ideal for addressing more persistent health concerns or replenishing the body. Meanwhile, with their soothing and protective qualities, salves focus on external applications, harnessing the healing power of herbs and essential oils to care for the skin. This chapter provides an accessible guide to crafting these timeless remedies, blending straightforward steps with helpful tips for their use. Now it's time to explore the timeless art of herbal preparation and discover how these techniques can bring healing, nourishment, and balance into your life.

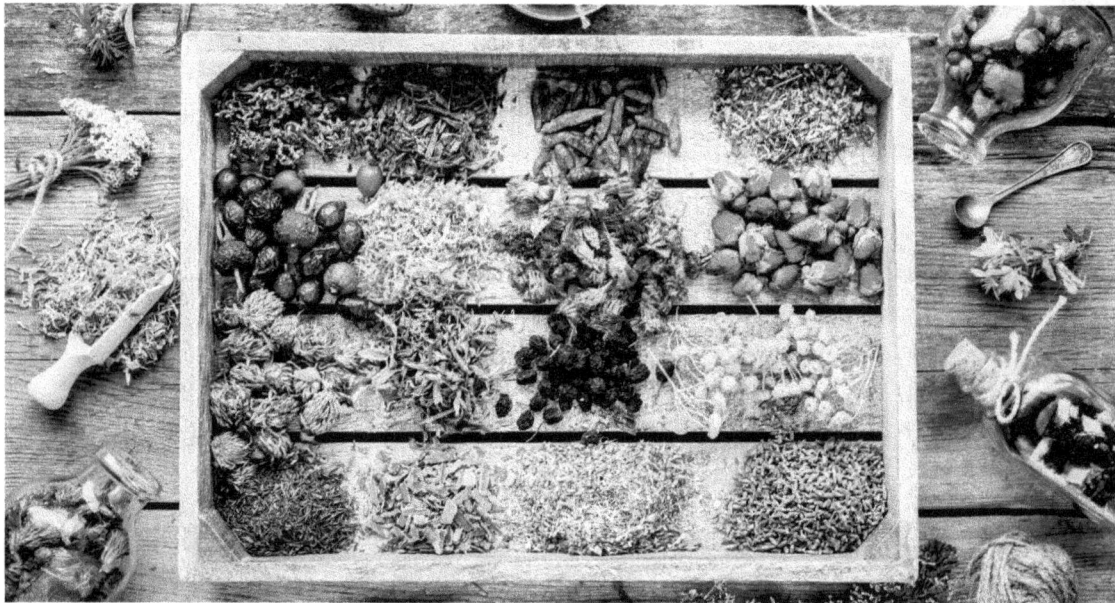

How to Make a Medicinal TEA

Tea is a simple and enjoyable way to experience the benefits of herbs. Easy to prepare by steeping fresh or dried herbs in hot water, herbal teas offer gentle relief for everyday concerns. With a rich history in ancient healing traditions, they have long been used to promote relaxation, digestion, and immune support. Herbal teas continue to serve as natural, time-honored remedies for the mind, body, and soul.

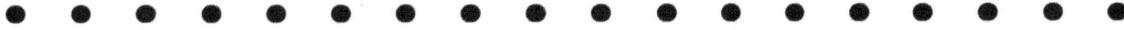

● ● ● ● ● ● ● ● ● ● ● ● ● ● ● ● ●

DIRECTIONS

1. **Measure Your Herbs:** Start by selecting your herbs. Use about 1 teaspoon to 1 tablespoon of dried or fresh herbs for each cup of hot water. The amount can be adjusted depending on the strength of flavor or desired therapeutic effects. Herbs like chamomile, peppermint, or lavender are popular choices, each offering its unique benefits. Feel free to experiment to find your ideal balance.

2. **Steep:** Pour freshly boiled water over the herbs and allow them to steep. For delicate, milder flavors, steep for 3–5 minutes. For a more potent brew with deeper medicinal properties, let the herbs steep for up to 10 minutes. The longer the steeping time, the more concentrated the flavors and benefits will be.

3. **Strain and Enjoy:** After the herbs have steeped to your liking, strain the tea using a fine mesh strainer or tea infuser to remove the plant material. Pour the fragrant, warm liquid into your favorite mug, and take a moment to savor the soothing experience.

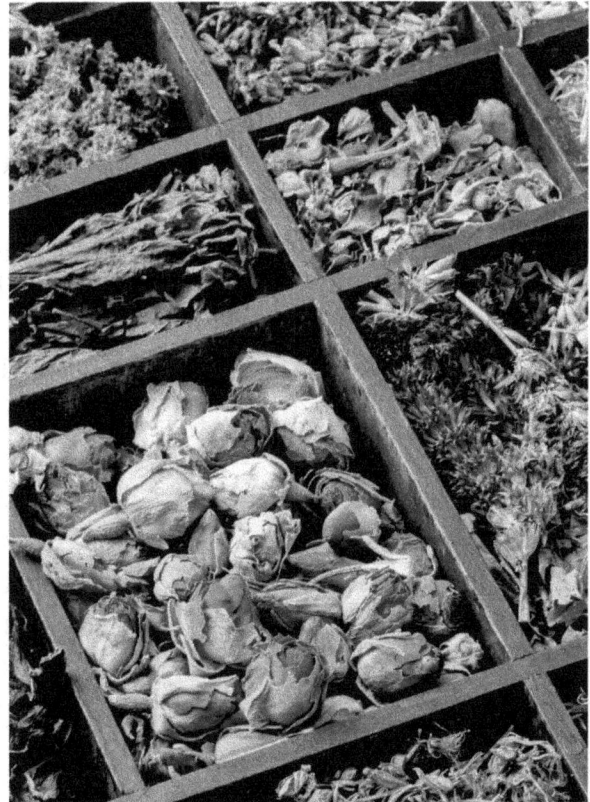

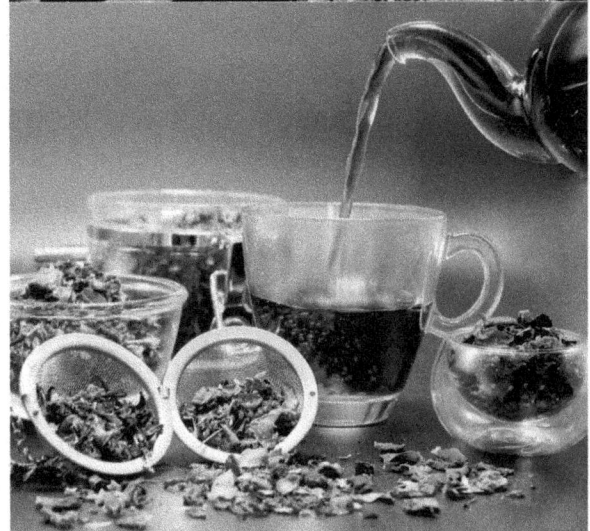

25

How to Make a Medicinal INFUSION

Infusions elevate the art of herbal tea by extending the brewing time, which allows the active nutrients and medicinal compounds to be extracted more fully from the plant material. This method offers a deeper, more potent experience compared to traditional teas. Infusions provide a richer, more concentrated form of herbal medicine, making them an excellent choice for addressing specific health concerns or offering profound nourishment to the body, mind, and spirit.

DIRECTIONS

1. **Select Your Herbs:** Choose your herbs based on the health benefits you seek. For infusions, opt for nutrient-rich or medicinal herbs like chamomile, nettle, peppermint, or elderflower. Roots such as ginger, turmeric, or licorice root also work well for infusions, as they contain potent compounds that require longer steeping times to be fully extracted.

2. **Measure Your Herbs:** For most herbs, use 1 to 2 tablespoons of dried plant material per cup of water. For roots or seeds, you may wish to use a little more to ensure a stronger, more concentrated infusion. Fresh herbs can be used as well, though you'll need to adjust the quantity depending on their potency.

3. **Boil and Steep:** Bring water to a boil and pour it over the herbs, ensuring they are fully submerged. Then, cover the vessel with a lid to keep the oils and compounds from escaping in the steam. Let the herbs steep for 15–60 minutes. The longer the infusion, the stronger and more medicinal it will be. For roots or tougher herbs, aim for at least 30 minutes to an hour.

4. **Strain and Sip:** Once the herbs have steeped to your satisfaction, strain out the plant material using a fine mesh strainer or cheesecloth. The remaining liquid is your infusion—rich in nutrients, minerals, and healing compounds. Enjoy it while it's warm, or refrigerate it for later use.

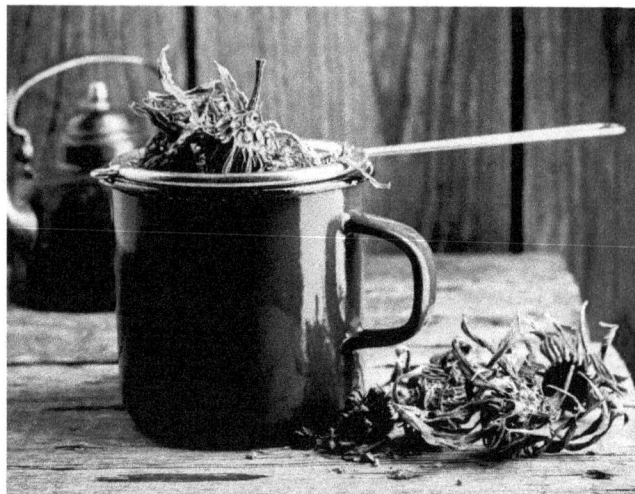

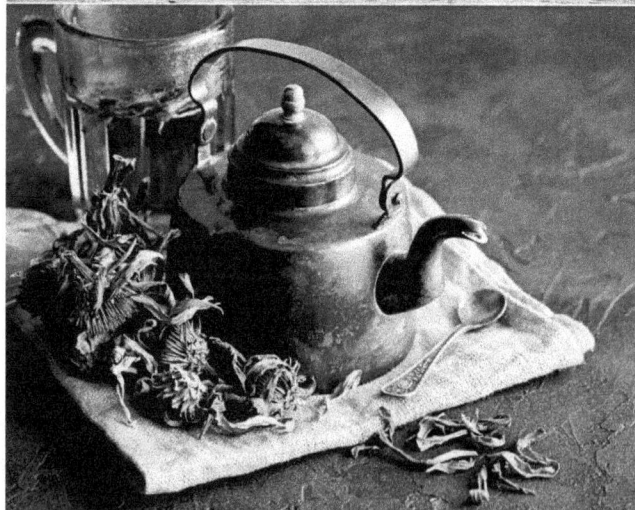

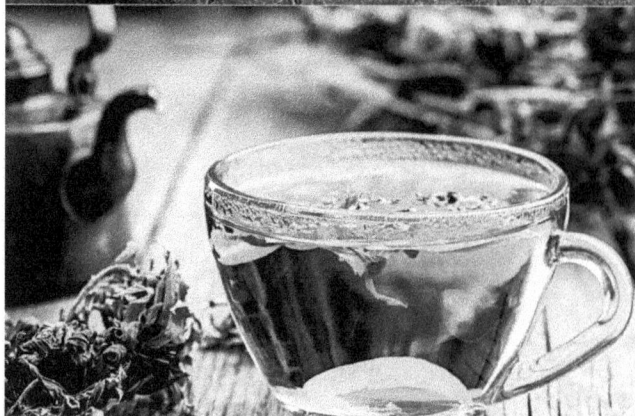

How to Make a SOLAR & LUNAR INFUSION

Solar and lunar infusions are created utilizing the energy of the sun or the moon, which infuse your remedies with the elemental power of nature, enhancing their therapeutic effects. A solar infusion captures the vibrant, life-giving energy of the sun, making it ideal for uplifting and energizing remedies. This method gently warms the herbs, preserving delicate compounds that may degrade under intense heat. A lunar infusion harnesses the soothing, introspective energy of the moon, making it ideal for calming, restorative remedies. It is particularly effective for promoting sleep, relaxation, and emotional balance.

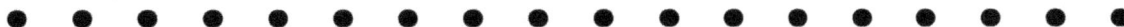

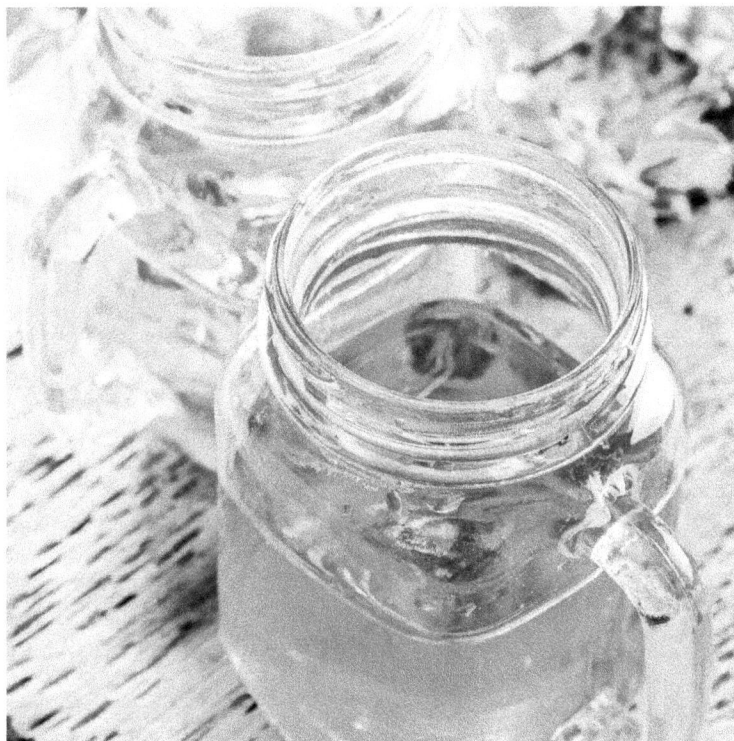

● ●

Solar Infusion

Purpose: Excellent for promoting joy, energy, and clarity.

INGREDIENTS

- 1–2 tablespoons of dried herbs (or fresh herbs)
- 1 quart of filtered water
- A clear glass jar with a lid

DIRECTIONS

1. Add your herbs to the glass jar.
2. Pour filtered water over the herbs, filling the jar.
3. Seal the jar with a lid and place it in direct sunlight for 4–6 hours. Choose a location that will receive consistent sunlight during this time.
4. After infusion, strain the herbs and transfer the liquid to a clean container.
5. Enjoy the infusion immediately or store it in the refrigerator for up to 24 hours.

Lunar Infusion

Purpose: Lunar Infusions are perfect for rituals promoting introspection, healing, and deep relaxation.

INGREDIENTS

- 1–2 tablespoons of dried herbs (or fresh herbs)
- 1 quart of filtered water
- A clear glass jar with a lid

DIRECTIONS

1. Place your herbs in a glass jar.
2. Pour filtered water over the herbs, filling the jar.
3. Seal the jar with a lid and set it outside under the moonlight. For best results, perform this infusion during a full moon or new moon to maximize its energy.
4. Allow the jar to sit overnight (approximately 8–12 hours).
5. In the morning, strain the herbs and transfer the liquid to a clean container.
6. Drink the infusion fresh or store it in the refrigerator for up to 24 hours.

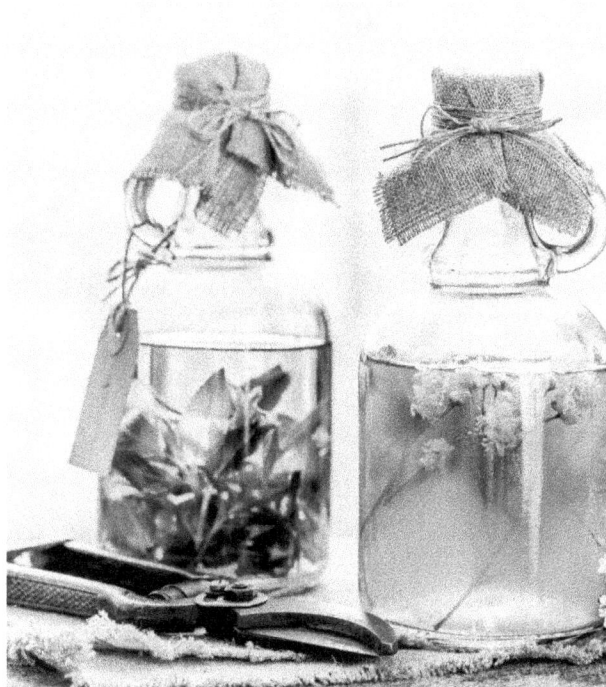

How to Make a Medicinal DECOCTION

Decoctions are a time-honored method for extracting potent healing compounds from tough plant materials like roots, bark, seeds, and woody stems. These parts are dense and rich in nutrients, minerals, and therapeutic compounds, which cannot be easily extracted through steeping methods like teas or infusions. Instead, decoctions involve boiling and simmering the herbs for an extended time, breaking down the plant's fibrous structure to release its active constituents. The result is a highly concentrated and powerful herbal remedy, packed with bioactive compounds that enhance the plant's medicinal benefits.

● ● ● ● ● ● ● ● ● ● ● ● ● ● ● ● ● ●

DIRECTIONS

1. **Select Your Herbs:** Choose your herbs based on your health needs. Roots, bark, and seeds are often the most suitable for decoction, as they tend to have hard, dense structures that require boiling to release their active compounds.

2. **Measure Your Herbs:** For decoctions, a general rule of thumb is to use 1–2 tablespoons of dried herbs per cup of water. Adjust the amount depending on the strength you desire and the specific plant material being used. Tougher materials like roots may require slightly more.

3. **Boil and Simmer:** Place your herbs in a pot with cold water and bring it to a boil. Once boiling, reduce the heat to a simmer and allow the herbs to steep for 20–30 minutes, or even longer for denser materials like bark or roots. During this time, the tough plant fibers begin to break down, releasing their beneficial compounds into the liquid.

4. **Strain and Enjoy:** After simmering, strain out the plant material using a fine mesh strainer or cheesecloth. The remaining liquid is a concentrated decoction filled with the plant's medicinal properties. This can be consumed as a strong herbal tea, or used as an ingredient in other herbal preparations.

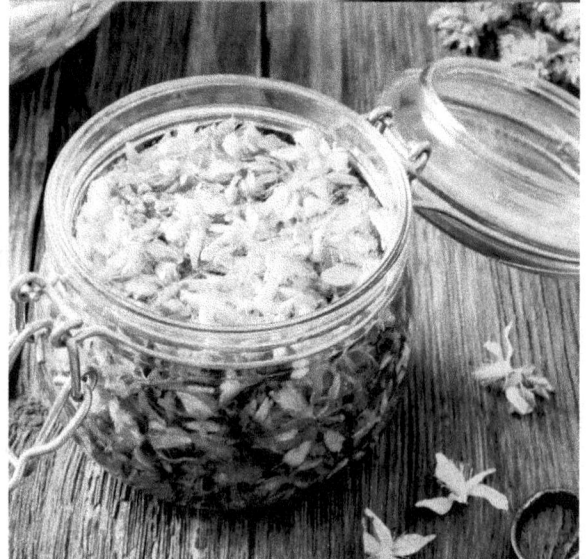

How to Make a Medicinal SYRUP

Herbal syrups offer a flavorful and comforting way to experience the healing power of herbs, combining their medicinal properties with the sweet allure of honey, sugar, or glycerin. This preparation method softens the often bitter or earthy flavors of herbs and transforms them into a remedy that appeals to both children and adults who favor a gentler, sweeter taste. Highly versatile and simple to prepare, herbal syrups are perfect for soothing common ailments such as coughs, sore throats, and seasonal immune challenges. Their ease of use and broad appeal make them an essential addition to any herbalist's repertoire.

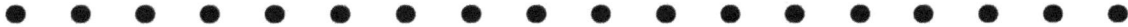

● ● ● ● ● ● ● ● ● ● ● ● ● ● ● ● ● ● ●

DIRECTIONS

1. **Prepare the Herbal Base:** Start by making a strong infusion or decoction using your chosen herbs. For a decoction, simmer roots, bark, or seeds for 15–45 minutes. For an infusion, steep leaves or flowers for 15–30 minutes. Strain the liquid to remove solids, ensuring only the concentrated herbal liquid remains.

2. **Reduce the Liquid:** Pour the strained herbal liquid back into the pot and gently simmer until it reduces by about one-third. This concentrates the flavors and medicinal compounds.

3. **Add a Sweetener:** Mix the reduced liquid with your sweetener of choice, using a ratio of 2 parts liquid to 1 part sweetener (e.g., 2 cups herbal liquid to 1 cup honey or sugar). Stir thoroughly to combine. If using honey, add it after the liquid has cooled slightly to preserve its natural enzymes and nutrients.

4. **Store Your Syrup:** Pour the syrup into a sterilized, airtight glass bottle or jar. Label it with the date and ingredients. Store in the refrigerator, where it will keep for up to 2–3 months.

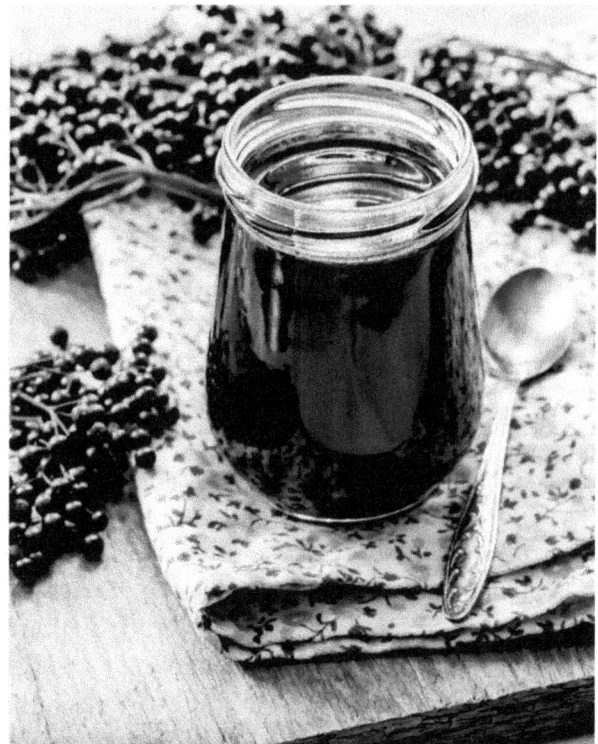

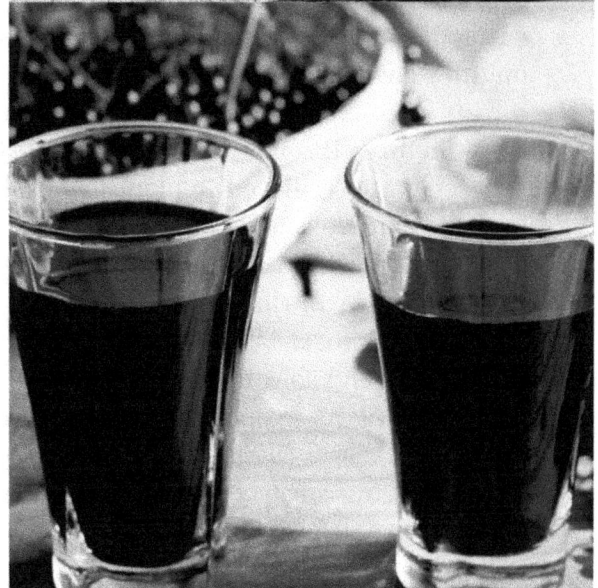

How to Make a Medicinal TINCTURE

Tinctures provide a potent and long-lasting way to harness the healing properties of herbs by extracting their active compounds using alcohol, glycerin, or vinegar. This preparation method offers a highly concentrated form of herbal medicine that is easy to store and convenient to use. A few drops of tincture can deliver powerful therapeutic effects, making it ideal for those seeking quick and effective remedies.

DIRECTIONS

1. **Prepare the Herbs:** Select your herbs based on the intended purpose of the tincture. Use fresh or dried herbs. Chop fresh herbs into small pieces to maximize surface area and ensure optimal extraction.

2. **Choose a Solvent:** Alcohol-based tinctures: Use a high-proof alcohol (such as vodka or brandy) for strong extractions. Aim for 40-60% alcohol by volume.

3. **Non-alcohol Alternatives:** For alcohol-free tinctures, use vegetable glycerin or apple cider vinegar. Note that these may not extract all compounds as effectively as alcohol.

4. **Combine Herbs and Solvent:** Fill a clean, sterilized glass jar with your herbs. Pour your solvent over the herbs until they are fully submerged, leaving about an inch of space at the top. Use a ratio of about 1 part dried herbs to 4 parts solvent or 1 part fresh herbs to 2 parts solvent. Seal the jar tightly with a lid.

5. **Macerate and Infuse:** Shake the jar gently and store it in a cool, dark place for 4–6 weeks. Shake the jar every few days to agitate the mixture and encourage extraction. This process allows the solvent to draw out the active compounds from the herbs.

6. **Strain and Bottle:** After the infusion period, strain the tincture through a fine mesh strainer or cheesecloth to remove the plant material. Press the herbs to extract as much liquid as possible. Pour the strained liquid into a sterilized amber glass bottle with a dropper for easy use.

7. **Label and Store:** Label the bottle with the date, herbs used, and solvent type. Store the tincture in a cool, dark place. Properly made tinctures can last for several years. Tinctures are highly concentrated and taken in small doses—usually 1–2 droppers (about 30–60 drops) diluted in water or tea.

How to Make a Medicinal POULTICE

Poultices are one of the oldest and most accessible methods for delivering the healing power of herbs directly to the skin. Rooted in centuries of traditional medicine, this time-honored practice involves applying a moist, paste-like mixture of herbs to a specific area of the body to target localized discomfort and support the body's natural healing processes. Simple yet highly effective, poultices are a versatile remedy for soothing inflammation, alleviating pain, drawing out toxins, and accelerating recovery.

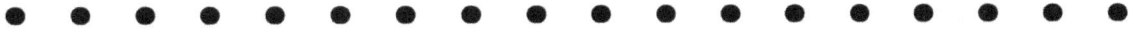

DIRECTIONS

1. **Prepare the Herbs:** For fresh herbs, finely chop or mash them using a mortar and pestle to release their natural juices. For dried herbs, grind them into a fine powder using a blender or spice grinder.

2. **Mix the Herbs:** Combine the prepared herbs with a liquid, such as warm water, herbal tea, apple cider vinegar, or carrier oil, to create a thick paste. For added potency, warm the liquid slightly to help the herbs release their active compounds.

3. **Apply the Poultice:** Spread the mixture directly onto the skin or onto a clean cloth. Place the cloth over the affected area and secure it with another layer of fabric, bandage, or wrap.

4. **Leave in Place:** Allow the poultice to remain for 20–30 minutes or longer, depending on the desired effect. After removal, gently clean the area with warm water.

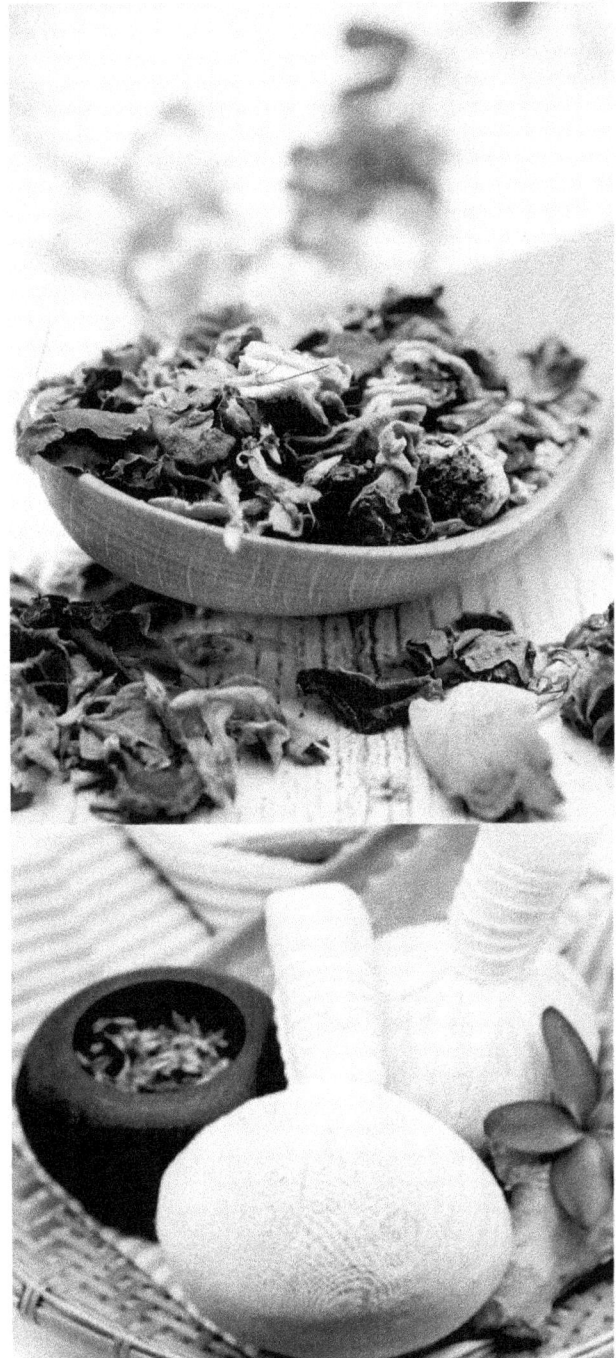

How to Make Medicinal SALVES & BALMS

Salves and balms are among the most effective and versatile herbal preparations for topical use, offering concentrated healing directly to the skin. These ointment-like remedies combine the therapeutic properties of herbs with nourishing oils and protective waxes to soothe, repair, and protect the skin. Unlike creams or lotions, salves are thicker and create a moisture-locking barrier, making them ideal for delivering long-lasting relief. Salves and balms are semi-solid herbal preparations made by infusing oils with medicinal herbs and thickening them with beeswax or a plant-based alternative.

● ● ● ● ● ● ● ● ● ● ● ● ● ● ● ●

DIRECTIONS

1. **Infuse Your Oil:** Choose a carrier oil such as olive, sunflower, coconut, or jojoba oil. Add your chosen herbs (e.g., calendula for soothing, comfrey for healing, or arnica for pain relief) to the oil. Infuse the oil using one of these methods:

   a. **Slow Heating:** Gently warm the oil and herbs in a double boiler or slow cooker for 2–4 hours.

   b. **Solar Infusion:** Place the herbs and oil in a sealed jar and let it sit in the sun for 2–6 weeks, shaking it occasionally. Strain the infused oil through a fine mesh or cheesecloth to remove plant material.

2. **Prepare the Base:** For every cup of infused oil, use approximately 1 ounce of beeswax or a plant-based alternative (like candelilla or carnauba wax for a vegan option). Heat the strained oil and beeswax in a double boiler until fully melted.

3. **Add Essential Oils:** Remove the mixture from heat and add a few drops of essential oils for added benefits. For example: lavender for calming and soothing, tea tree for antimicrobial properties and peppermint for cooling relief.

4. **Pour and Cool:** Pour the mixture into sterilized jars or tins while still liquid. ·Allow it to cool completely before sealing.

How to Make Medicinal ESSENTIAL OILS

Essential oils are potent, aromatic plant extracts offering various therapeutic and practical applications. These concentrated oils are carefully extracted from specific parts of plants, such as flowers, leaves, bark, roots, or fruit—preserving their unique fragrance and beneficial properties. Extraction methods like steam distillation and cold pressing ensure the oils retain their natural essence and efficacy. Renowned for their versatility, essential oils play a prominent role in aromatherapy, helping to promote relaxation, balance emotions, and support mental well-being.

● ● ● ● ● ● ● ● ● ● ● ● ● ● ● ● ● ● ● ●

DIRECTIONS

1. **Identify the Purpose of the Blend:** Determine the specific health goal for the blend (e.g., improving sleep, boosting immunity, relieving stress).
2. **Choose Your Herbs:** Select herbs with properties that align with your goal. Adjust proportions based on the strength and taste of the herbs. Use a balance of the following types:
   a. **Primary Herbs:** The main therapeutic ingredient (e.g., chamomile for relaxation).
   b. **Supporting Herbs:** Herbs that enhance or complement the primary herb (e.g., lavender for calming).
   c. **Balancing Herbs:** Herbs that round out the formula, often improving flavor or easing digestion (e.g., peppermint or licorice).
3. **Determine Proportions:** Use ratios to create a balanced blend. A common guideline is:
   a. **Primary Herbs:** 60% of the blend
   b. **Supporting Herbs:** 30% of the blend
   c. **Balancing Herbs:** 10% of the blend
4. **Measure the Herbs:** Measure each herb according to your formula. For example, in a 10-cup blend:
   a. 6 cups of the primary herb(s)
   b. 3 cups of the supporting herb(s)
   c. 1 cup of the balancing herb(s)
5. **Blend the Herbs:** Gently mix the herbs in a large, clean bowl. Use your hands or a wooden spoon to combine them thoroughly, ensuring even distribution.
6. **Store the Blend:** Transfer the blend to an airtight glass jar or container. Store it in a cool, dark, dry place to preserve potency. Label the jar with the blend name, ingredients, and date.
7. **Prepare a Test Serving:** Before regular use, test your blend by preparing a cup of tea or infusion. Adjust the ratio of herbs as needed to balance flavor and effectiveness.
8. **Use Your Herbal Blend:** A general guideline is 1–2 teaspoons of the blend per cup of hot water, steeped for 10–15 minutes.

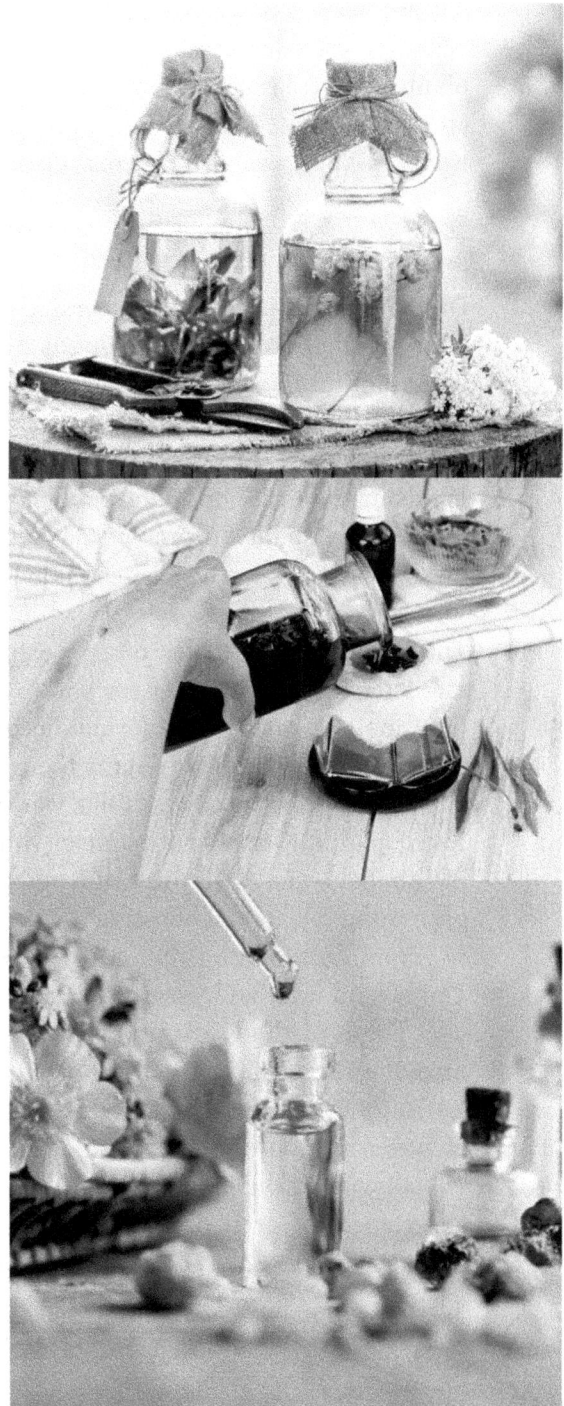

AROMATHERAPY

Aromatherapy is a holistic healing practice that utilizes the therapeutic properties of essential oils extracted from plants to promote physical, emotional, and mental well-being. Through inhalation or topical application, the scents and active compounds in essential oils can stimulate the body's natural healing processes, improve mood, reduce stress, alleviate pain, and support overall health. Whether used in massage, diffusers, baths, or skincare, aromatherapy harnesses the power of plant-based fragrances to create a balanced, calming environment and enhance one's physical and emotional state. This ancient practice is gaining renewed popularity as a natural, non-invasive way to support wellness and restore harmony to the body, mind, and spirit.

Diffusion

Diffusion is the process of dispersing essential oils into the air to create a therapeutic atmosphere, allowing their aromatic compounds to be inhaled for various health benefits. This is typically done using a diffuser, a device that breaks down the oils into tiny molecules and disperses them into the room. As the essential oils fill the space, they interact with the olfactory system, sending signals to the brain's limbic system, which can influence emotions, mood, and even physical well-being. Diffusing essential oils is a popular method in aromatherapy, as it provides a natural way to improve air quality, promote relaxation, enhance focus, and reduce stress, depending on the oils used. It's a simple, effective technique for incorporating the healing power of scent into daily life.

The following two tables offer a comprehensive guide to the most popular herbal preparation methods, making it easier for you to craft remedies that suit your personal wellness needs. The first table focuses on internal herbal preparations, including teas & infusions, decoctions, tinctures, and syrups. It details the specific plant parts to use—whether flowers, roots, or bark—and the appropriate solvents like water, alcohol, or glycerin to extract their beneficial compounds. Each method is further explained with preparation times, dosage guidelines, and estimated shelf life to help you determine the most effective approach for addressing your needs, such as promoting relaxation, boosting immunity, or aiding digestion.

The second table addresses external preparations, featuring salves, balms, poultices, and essential oils. These methods are primarily used for addressing skin conditions, inflammation, or wound care. It offers clear instructions on which plant parts and solvents to use, such as oils for salves or water for poultices. The table also includes preparation times and shelf-life recommendations, empowering you to create soothing, healing products that nurture your skin. Both tables provide a holistic view of herbal crafting, covering common uses, recommended strength, and the sensory experiences of each preparation. These resources are designed to help you confidently create herbal remedies tailored to your wellness journey.

HERBAL PREPARATIONS FOR INTERNAL USE

	TEA & INFUSION	DECOCTION	TINCTURE	SYRUP
VITAL PARTS	Leaves, Flowers	Roots, Bark, Seeds, or Woody Stems	Dried or fresh herbs: Leaves, flowers, roots, bark, or seeds	Any Plant Part (fresh or dried)
SOLVENT	Hot/Boiling Water	Warm Water	Alcohol (40–60% ABV), Glycerin, or Apple Cider Vinegar	Water and Sweetener (honey, sugar, or maple syrup)
PREPARATION TIME	Tea: 3–5 Minutes Infusion: 10–20 Minutes	30–45 Minutes	4–6 Weeks (shake jar daily to enhance extraction)	45 Minutes–1 Hour
STRENGTH	1–2 teaspoons of dried herbs or 2–3 teaspoons of fresh herbs per 1 cup (8 ounces) of water	1–2 tablespoons of dried herbs or 2–3 tablespoons of fresh herbs with 2 cups (16 ounces) of water	Fresh Herbs: 1 part herb to 2 parts alcohol (1:2) Dried Herbs: 1 part herb to 5 parts alcohol (1:5)	1 part herbal decoction/infusion to 1 part sweetener by volume
DOSAGE	1 cup, 1–3 times daily	1/2 to 1 cup, 1–3 times daily	20–40 drops (1–2 mL), diluted in water or tea, 1–3 times daily	1–2 teaspoons, 1–3 times daily
SHELF LIFE	Short (1 Day)	Short (1–2 Days)	Long (1–5 Years)	Medium (2–3 Months)
COMMON USE	Digestive Aid, Sleep Aid & Relaxation, Immune Support, Symptom Relief (colds)	Digestive Aid, Stress & Anxiety Relief, Immune Support, Symptom Relief (colds)	Digestive Aid, Stress & Anxiety Relief, Immune Support, Symptom Relief (colds)	Digestive Aid, Stress & Anxiety Relief, Immune Support, Symptom Relief (colds)
TASTE	Refreshing, Warm, & Soothing	Earthy, Warm, & Grounding	Potent, Concentrated, & Strong	Sweet, Smooth, & Herbaceous

HERBAL PREPARATIONS FOR EXTERNAL USE

	SALVE & BALM	POULTICE	ESSENTIAL OILS
VITAL PARTS	Infused Oils & Beeswax or Candelilla Wax	Herbs: fresh or dried, crushed or ground	Concentrated plant compounds from leaves, flowers, bark, or roots
SOLVENT	Oil (olive oil, coconut oil, almond oil)	Water to moisten the herbs and release their properties	Carrier Oil (e.g., coconut, jojoba) or used neat with caution
PREPARATION TIME	2–4 weeks (solar method) or 1–3 hours (heat method)	10–15 Minutes	Pre-extracted (distillation or cold-press extraction, professionally produced)
STRENGTH	8 parts herbal infused oil to 1 part beeswax by weight	Fresh Herbs: Use as-is, crushed or ground Dried Herbs: Add just enough water to create a thick paste	Typically used at a 1-3% dilution in carrier oil (1-3 drops essential oil per teaspoon of carrier)
DOSAGE	Apply a small amount topically to the affected area, 2–3 times daily, or as needed	Apply directly to the affected area for 15–30 minutes, 1–3 times daily	Apply topically diluted to the skin or use 3–5 drops in a diffuser or inhalation method
SHELF-LIFE	6–12 Months	Fresh for Each Use	3–10+ years when stored properly in dark, airtight bottles
COMMON USE	Skin Soothing, Wound Healing, Pain Relief, Respiratory Support	Detoxification, Wound Healing, Inflammation Relief, Skin Irritations, Pain Relief, Moisturizer	Aromatherapy, Stress Relief, Respiratory Support, Pain Relief, Relaxation, Mood Uplift
TOUCH	Nourishing, Soothing, & Silky	Warm or Cool, Comforting, & Herbal	Highly Concentrated, Potent, Aromatic (e.g., Floral, Citrus, Woody)

Chapter Four

PROFILES OF ESSENTIAL HERBS

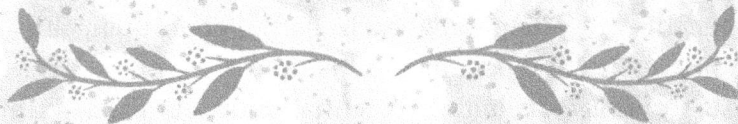

"Herbs are the medicine
of the future."
— Dr. Andrew Weil, Physician of Integrative
Medicine

Unlock the Healing Wisdom of 100 Essential Herbs

Step into the world of herbal mastery with this carefully curated guide of 100 essential herbs —a resource designed to empower, educate, and inspire. Blending ancient herbal traditions with modern scientific insights, each profile offers a comprehensive and practical exploration of nature's most powerful botanical allies.

This chapter is a guide to the plants that nature has so graciously provided—an invitation to reconnect with the earth and take charge of your health with the gifts of the natural world. You will learn to identify each herb through its distinct botanical characteristics, uncover its therapeutic properties, and explore its traditional and contemporary applications as a natural remedy. Whether used to promote vitality, restore balance, or support overall wellness, these herbs provide time-honored solutions for various health concerns.

To ensure effective and responsible use, each profile includes:
- High-quality images showcasing the most potent medicinal parts for accurate identification and optimal use.
- Astrological and zodiac correspondences to help you understand the cosmic influences behind each herb's healing properties.
- Step-by-step preparation methods, guiding you through making teas, tinctures, salves, poultices, decoctions, and more to maximize their benefits.
- Precise dosage recommendations, ensuring safe and effective use for adults, children, and those with specific health needs.
- Medicinal benefits, detailing how each herb supports health, from immunity and digestion to stress relief and pain management.
- Safety and precautions, including potential interactions, contraindications, and best practices for responsible use.

With this knowledge, you can confidently incorporate herbal remedies into your wellness routine while ensuring safe and effective results—one root, leaf, and flower at a time.

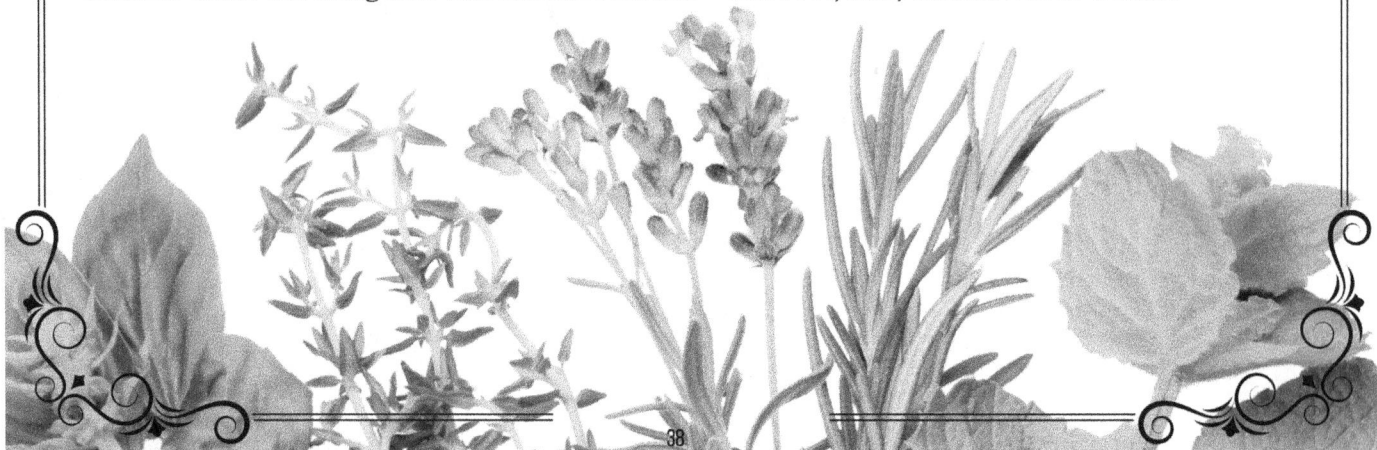

HOW TO NAVIGATE THE HERBAL PROFILES

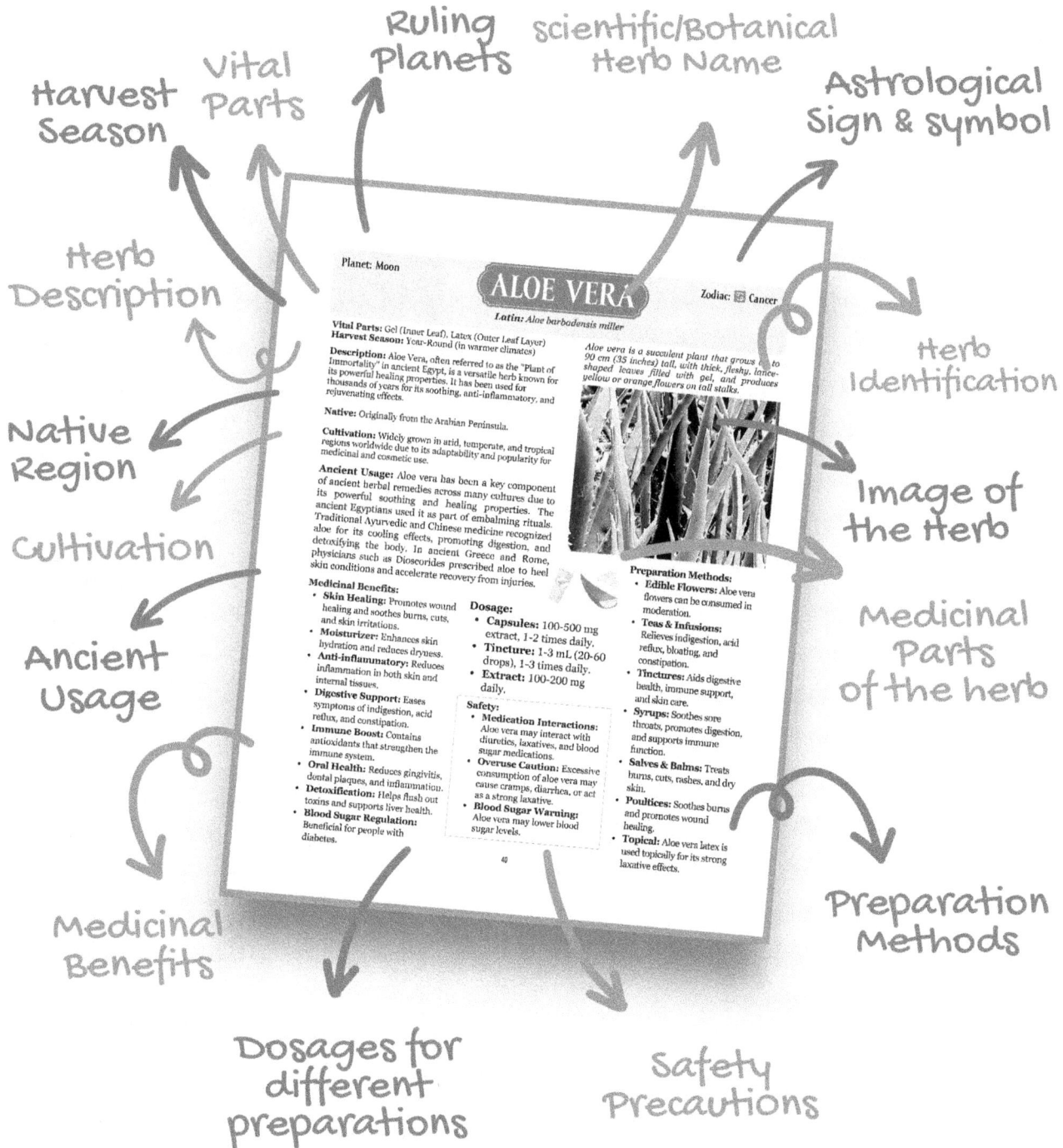

Harvest Season

Vital Parts

Ruling Planets

Scientific/Botanical Herb Name

Astrological Sign & Symbol

Herb Description

Herb Identification

Native Region

Image of the Herb

Cultivation

Medicinal Parts of the herb

Ancient Usage

Medicinal Benefits

Preparation Methods

Dosages for different preparations

Safety Precautions

Planet: Moon

ALOE VERA
Latin: Aloe barbadensis miller

Zodiac: ♋ Cancer

Vital Parts: Gel (Inner Leaf), Latex (Outer Leaf Layer)
Harvest Season: Year-Round (in warmer climates)

Description: Aloe Vera, often referred to as the "Plant of Immortality" in ancient Egypt, is a versatile herb known for its powerful healing properties. It has been used for thousands of years for its soothing, anti-inflammatory, and rejuvenating effects.

Native: Originally from the Arabian Peninsula.

Cultivation: Widely grown in arid, temperate, and tropical regions worldwide due to its adaptability and popularity for medicinal and cosmetic use.

Ancient Usage: Aloe vera has been a key component of ancient herbal remedies across many cultures due to its powerful soothing and healing properties. The ancient Egyptians used it as part of embalming rituals. Traditional Ayurvedic and Chinese medicine recognized aloe for its cooling effects, promoting digestion, and detoxifying the body. In ancient Greece and Rome, physicians such as Dioscorides prescribed aloe to heal skin conditions and accelerate recovery from injuries.

Aloe vera is a succulent plant that grows up to 90 cm (35 inches) tall, with thick, fleshy, lance-shaped leaves filled with gel, and produces yellow or orange flowers on tall stalks.

Medicinal Benefits:
- **Skin Healing:** Promotes wound healing and soothes burns, cuts, and skin irritations.
- **Moisturizer:** Enhances skin hydration and reduces dryness.
- **Anti-inflammatory:** Reduces inflammation in both skin and internal tissues.
- **Digestive Support:** Eases symptoms of indigestion, acid reflux, and constipation.
- **Immune Boost:** Contains antioxidants that strengthen the immune system.
- **Oral Health:** Reduces gingivitis, dental plaques, and inflammation.
- **Detoxification:** Helps flush out toxins and supports liver health.
- **Blood Sugar Regulation:** Beneficial for people with diabetes.

Dosage:
- **Capsules:** 100-500 mg extract, 1-2 times daily.
- **Tincture:** 1-3 mL (20-60 drops), 1-3 times daily.
- **Extract:** 100-200 mg daily.

Safety:
- **Medication Interactions:** Aloe vera may interact with diuretics, laxatives, and blood sugar medications.
- **Overuse Caution:** Excessive consumption of aloe vera may cause cramps, diarrhea, or act as a strong laxative.
- **Blood Sugar Warning:** Aloe vera may lower blood sugar levels.

Preparation Methods:
- **Edible Flowers:** Aloe vera flowers can be consumed in moderation.
- **Teas & Infusions:** Relieves indigestion, acid reflux, bloating, and constipation.
- **Tinctures:** Aids digestive health, immune support, and skin care.
- **Syrups:** Soothes sore throats, promotes digestion, and supports immune function.
- **Salves & Balms:** Treats burns, cuts, rashes, and dry skin.
- **Poultices:** Soothes burns and promotes wound healing.
- **Topical:** Aloe vera latex is used topically for its strong laxative effects.

40

ALOE VERA

Latin: Aloe barbadensis miller

Vital Parts: Gel (Inner Leaf), Latex (Outer Leaf Layer)
Harvest Season: Year-Round (in warmer climates)

Description: Aloe Vera, often referred to as the "Plant of Immortality" in ancient Egypt, is a versatile herb known for its powerful healing properties. It has been used for thousands of years for its soothing, anti-inflammatory, and rejuvenating effects.

Native: Originally from the Arabian Peninsula.

Cultivation: Widely grown in arid, temperate, and tropical regions worldwide due to its adaptability and popularity for medicinal and cosmetic use.

Ancient Usage: Aloe vera has been a key component of ancient herbal remedies across many cultures due to its powerful soothing and healing properties. The ancient Egyptians used it as part of embalming rituals. Traditional Ayurvedic and Chinese medicine recognized aloe for its cooling effects, promoting digestion, and detoxifying the body. In ancient Greece and Rome, physicians such as Dioscorides prescribed aloe to heel skin conditions and accelerate recovery from injuries.

Aloe vera is a succulent plant that grows up to 90 cm (35 inches) tall, with thick, fleshy, lance-shaped leaves filled with gel, and produces yellow or orange flowers on tall stalks.

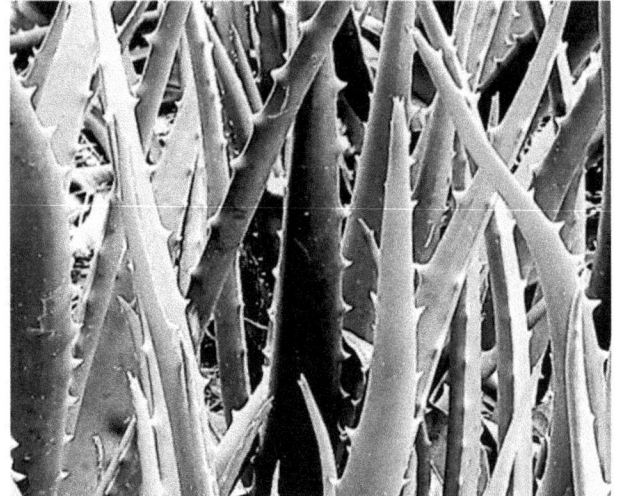

Medicinal Benefits:
- **Skin Healing:** Promotes wound healing and soothes burns, cuts, and skin irritations.
- **Moisturizer:** Enhances skin hydration and reduces dryness.
- **Anti-inflammatory:** Reduces inflammation in both skin and internal tissues.
- **Digestive Support:** Eases symptoms of indigestion, acid reflux, and constipation.
- **Immune Boost:** Contains antioxidants that strengthen the immune system.
- **Oral Health:** Reduces gingivitis, dental plaques, and inflammation.
- **Detoxification:** Helps flush out toxins and supports liver health.
- **Blood Sugar Regulation:** Beneficial for people with diabetes.

Dosage:
- **Capsules:** 100-500 mg extract, 1-2 times daily.
- **Tincture:** 1-3 mL (20-60 drops), 1-3 times daily.
- **Extract:** 100-200 mg daily.

Safety:
- **Medication Interactions:** Aloe vera may interact with diuretics, laxatives, and blood sugar medications.
- **Overuse Caution:** Excessive consumption of aloe vera may cause cramps, diarrhea, or act as a strong laxative.
- **Blood Sugar Warning:** Aloe vera may lower blood sugar levels.

Preparation Methods:
- **Edible Flowers:** Aloe vera flowers can be consumed in moderation.
- **Teas & Infusions:** Relieves indigestion, acid reflux, bloating, and constipation.
- **Tinctures:** Aids digestive health, immune support, and skin care.
- **Syrups:** Soothes sore throats, promotes digestion, and supports immune function.
- **Salves & Balms:** Treats burns, cuts, rashes, and dry skin.
- **Poultices:** Soothes burns and promotes wound healing.
- **Topical:** Aloe vera latex is used topically for its strong laxative effects.

ANGELICA

Latin: Angelica archangelica

Vital Parts: Roots, Stems, Leaves, Seeds
Harvest Season: Late Summer to Early Autumn

Description: Angelica, revered in traditional European herbal medicine, is a powerful herb known for its digestive, calming, and immune-boosting properties.

Native: Indigenous to northern and central Europe, particularly the Nordic regions and parts of Siberia.

Cultivation: Angelica thrives in cool, moist climates and is often cultivated in temperate regions worldwide. It prefers rich, well-drained soil and partial shade but can tolerate sunny environments with adequate moisture.

Ancient Usage: Angelica has been used in ancient herbal medicine for its powerful restorative and protective properties. In traditional European practices, it was believed to ward off evil spirits and plague, often used as a protective herb in rituals. The roots and stems were valued for improving digestion, relieving respiratory conditions, and promoting circulation. In traditional Chinese medicine, angelica was used to support women's reproductive health, balance hormones, and improve blood flow.

Angelica is a biennial herbaceous plant that can grow up to 2.5 meters (8 feet) tall. It features large, hollow stems with a purple hue and broad, deeply lobed leaves. The plant's greenish-white, umbrella-shaped flower clusters (umbels) appear during its second year of growth.

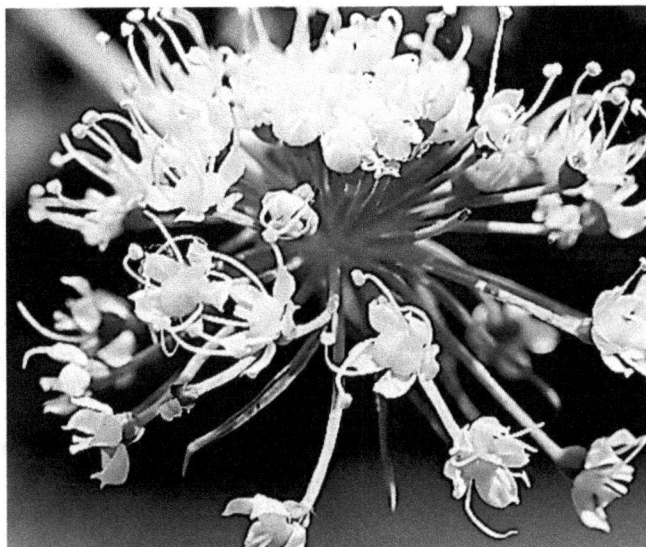

Medicinal Benefits:
- **Digestive Aid:** Relieves indigestion and bloating.
- **Respiratory Support:** Eases symptoms of colds, coughs, and bronchitis.
- **Circulation Booster:** Improves blood flow and may help with circulation-related issues.
- **Menstrual Support:** Regulates menstrual cycles and alleviates cramps.
- **Anti-inflammatory:** Reduces inflammation, joint pain, and arthritis.
- **Appetite Stimulant:** Encourages appetite.
- **Calming Agent:** Provides sedative effects and promotes relaxation.
- **Immune Support:** Contains antibacterial and antifungal properties.

Dosage:
- **Capsules:** 500-1,000 mg, 1-2 times daily.
- **Tea:** 1-2 grams dried root in 1 cup of water.
- **Tincture:** 1-2 mL (20-40 drops).

Safety:
- **Internal Use:** Excessive consumption may cause digestive upset or photosensitivity.
- **Allergy Risk:** Avoid if allergic to plants in the Apiaceae family (e.g., celery, carrot, parsley).

Preparation Methods:
- **Edible Flowers:** Angelica flowers are edible and often used as a garnish or candied for desserts.
- **Teas & Infusions:** Supports digestion, reduces bloating, and alleviates mild respiratory issues.
- **Decoctions:** Aids menstrual cramps, respiratory congestion, and digestive discomfort.
- **Tinctures:** Aids in digestion, reduces stress, and supports overall vitality.
- **Syrups:** Soothes coughs and eases throat irritation.
- **Salves & Balms:** Relieves muscle tension, improves circulation, and soothes skin irritations.
- **Poultices:** Promotes wound healing.
- **Topical:** Angelica essential oil can be applied to promote circulation and reduce inflammation.

Planet: Mercury

ANISE

Zodiac: ♍ Virgo

Latin: Pimpinella anisum

Vital Parts: Seeds, Leaves, Flowers
Harvest Season: Late Summer to Early Autumn

Description: Anise is an aromatic herb prized for its sweet, licorice-like flavor and medicinal properties. It has been used for centuries to aid digestion, reduce inflammation, and promote respiratory health.

Native: Originally from the eastern Mediterranean and Southwest Asia.

Cultivation: Anise is cultivated in warm, sunny regions with well-drained soil. It thrives in temperate climates and is widely grown across Europe, the Middle East, and parts of North America.

Ancient Usage: Anise has been prized in ancient herbal medicine for its aromatic and digestive-supporting properties. In ancient Egypt and Greece, it was used to relieve indigestion, bloating, and colic, often consumed as a tea or chewed after meals. Roman physicians, including Pliny the Elder, recommended anise to freshen breath, promote restful sleep, and alleviate respiratory ailments. In traditional Ayurvedic medicine, anise was used to stimulate appetite, support lung health, and reduce mucus buildup. Medieval European healers utilized anise in remedies for coughs, menstrual discomfort, and calming stress.

Anise is an annual herbaceous plant that typically grows to a height of 0.5 to 1 meter (1.5 to 3 feet). It has slender, ridged stems and feathery, bright green leaves that vary in shape. Anise produces small, white, star-shaped flowers arranged in delicate, flat-topped clusters known as umbels that give way to small, oval seeds.

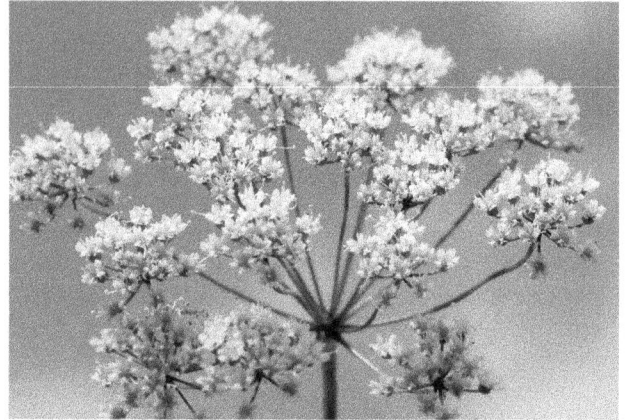

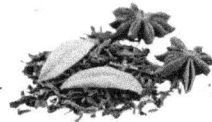

Medicinal Benefits:
- **Digestive Aid:** Relieves indigestion, gas, and bloating.
- **Respiratory Health:** Alleviates coughs and congestion.
- **Hormonal Balance:** Supports menstrual health and reduces menopausal symptoms.
- **Anti-inflammatory:** Reduces inflammation and supports immune health.
- **Antimicrobial:** Has antibacterial and antifungal properties to support overall health.
- **Sleep and Relaxation:** Helps promote restful sleep and reduce anxiety.

Dosage:
- **Capsules:** 500-1,000 mg, 1-2 times daily.
- **Tea:** 1-2 grams dried root in 1 cup water.
- **Tincture:** 1-2 mL (20-40 drops).

Safety:
- **Allergic Reactions:** Individuals allergic to anise or related plants (e.g., fennel, dill) should use caution.
- **Drug Interactions:** Use cautiously if taking hormonal or blood-thinning medications.

Preparation Methods:
- **Teas & Infusions:** Aids digestion, reduces bloating, and alleviates congestion.
- **Decoctions:** Aids colic, coughs, and menstrual discomfort.
- **Tinctures:** Supports digestion, relieves gas, and aids with anxiety.
- **Syrups:** Soothes coughs, eases sore throats, and supports respiratory health.
- **Salves & Balms:** Relieves muscle aches and joint discomfort.
- **Poultices:** Soothes minor skin irritations.
- **Topical:** Anise essential oil is potent and should always be diluted.

Planet: Saturn

ANRICA

Latin: Arnica montana

Vital Parts: Flowers
Harvest Season: Late Spring to Early Summer

Description: Arina is a lesser-known herb traditionally used in herbal medicine for its calming and restorative properties. It is valued for promoting relaxation, improving sleep quality, and supporting nervous system health.

Native: Originating from Central and Eastern Europe, particularly in mountainous and temperate forest regions.

Cultivation: Arina thrives in cool, temperate climates with moist, well-drained soil. It is primarily cultivated in Eastern European countries and regions with similar growing conditions.

Ancient Usage: Arnica has been used in ancient herbal medicine for its powerful anti-inflammatory and pain-relieving properties. Indigenous peoples of North America and European healers applied arnica poultices to bruises, sprains, and wounds to reduce swelling and promote healing. In traditional alpine medicine, it was known as a remedy for sore muscles and joint pain caused by overexertion or injury. Medieval herbalists recommended arnica to stimulate blood flow and speed recovery from trauma, such as contusions and fractures.

Arnica is a perennial herbaceous plant that typically grows to a height of 1 to 2 feet. It features erect, hairy stems and bright green, oval-shaped basal leaves that form a rosette near the ground. The plant's yellow-orange, daisy-like flowers bloom at the top of each stem.

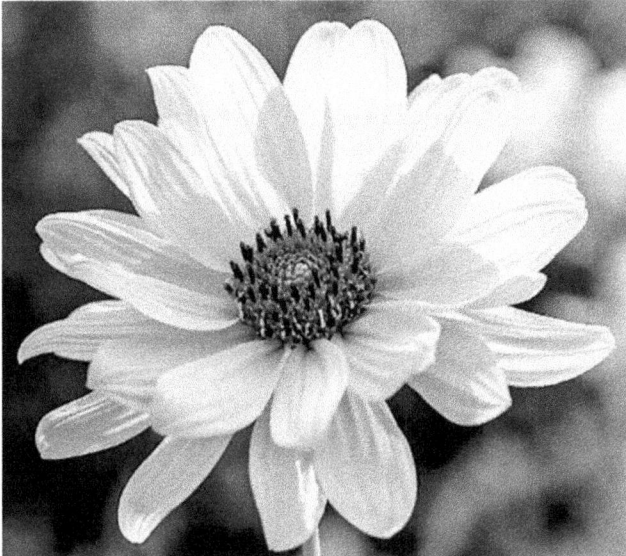

Medicinal Benefits:

- **Pain Relief:** Aids muscle aches, joint pain, and arthritis discomfort.
- **Anti-inflammatory:** Reduces swelling and inflammation from injuries and chronic conditions.
- **Bruise Healing:** Speeds up the healing process for bruises and soft tissue damage.
- **Post-injury Recovery:** Helps minimize pain, swelling, and bruising after surgeries or injuries.
- **Improved Circulation:** Promotes faster healing of wounds and injuries.
- **Topical Wound Care:** Reduces pain and inflammation in minor cuts, sprains, and strains.

Dosage:
- **Capsules:** 500-1,000 mg, 1-2 times daily.
- **Tea:** 1-2 grams dried root per cup of water.
- **Tincture:** 1-2 mL (20-40 drops).

Safety:
- **Moderation:** Excessive consumption could cause nausea.
- **Topical Use:** Dilute anise oil when applying to the skin to prevent irritation or reactions.
- **Allergies:** Avoid anise if you have allergies to plants in the carrot family (Apiaceae), such as fennel or celery.
- **Medication Interactions:** May interact with hormone-sensitive medications or anticoagulants.

Preparation Methods:
- **Teas & Infusions:** Aids digestion, reduces bloating, and soothes respiratory congestion.
- **Decoctions:** Addresses colic, coughs, and menstrual discomfort.
- **Tinctures:** Supports digestive health, relieves gas, and promotes relaxation.
- **Syrups:** Soothes coughs and eases throat irritation.
- **Salves & Balms:** Alleviates muscle aches and minor joint discomfort.
- **Poultices:** Soothes minor skin irritations and insect bites.

ARTICHOKE LEAF

Latin: Cynara scolymus

Vital Parts: Leaves
Harvest Season: Late Spring to Early Autumn

Description: Artichoke leaf is a well-known herbal remedy valued for its ability to support digestive health, promote liver function, and lower cholesterol levels.

Native: Originally from the Mediterranean region, particularly in areas with mild, coastal climates.

Cultivation: Artichoke thrives in warm, temperate regions with well-drained, nutrient-rich soil. It is widely cultivated in Mediterranean countries.

Ancient Usage: Artichoke leaf has a rich history, revered by ancient cultures for both its medicinal and culinary properties. The ancient Greeks referred to it as the "food of the gods," while the Romans called it Cynara, inspired by a myth about a woman turned into an artichoke by Zeus. Romans also believed artichokes had aphrodisiac qualities and often included them in extravagant feasts to boost vitality. Additionally, artichoke leaf was valued for its ability to stimulate bile production, making it a popular remedy for digestive issues and even hangovers.

Artichoke is a perennial herbaceous plant that can grow up to 1.5 meters (5 feet) tall. It has thick, sturdy stems and large, deeply lobed, silver-green leaves that can reach up to 80 centimeters (31 inches) in length. The plant produces globe-shaped flower buds surrounded by thick, fleshy bracts.

Medicinal Benefits:
- **Digestive Support:** Helps relieve bloating, nausea, and indigestion.
- **Liver Health:** Supports liver function and detoxification.
- **Cholesterol Reduction:** Lowers LDL ("bad") cholesterol and improves overall lipid profiles.
- **Antioxidant:** Provides protection against cellular damage from oxidative stress.
- **Blood Sugar Control:** May help regulate blood sugar levels, supporting metabolic health.
- **Anti-inflammatory:** Reduces inflammation in both the digestive and circulatory systems.

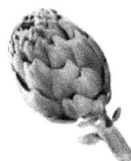

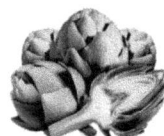

Dosage:
- **Capsules:** 500-1,000 mg, 1-2 times daily.
- **Tea:** 1-2 grams dried leaf per cup of water.
- **Tincture:** 1-2 mL (20-40 drops).

Safety:
- **Allergies:** Avoid if allergic to plants in the Asteraceae family (e.g., daisies, marigolds).
- **Gallstones:** Avoid artichoke leaf if you have gallstones or bile duct obstruction.
- **Medication Interactions:** May interact with cholesterol-lowering medications and diuretics.

Preparation Methods:
- **Edible Flowers:** Artichoke flowers include the fleshy base (the heart) and bracts.
- **Teas & Infusions:** Supports liver health, aids digestion, and helps regulate cholesterol levels.
- **Decoctions:** Artichoke leaves are simmered to make a stronger decoction for digestive complaints, bile production, and detoxification.
- **Tinctures:** Assists with liver detox, improves digestion, and supports heart health.
- **Syrups:** Soothes digestive discomfort and supports overall gut health.
- **Poultices:** Reduces inflammation and promotes localized healing of minor skin irritations.
- **Topical:** Primarily used internally for its anti-inflammatory benefits.

ASHWAGANDHA

Latin: Withania somnifera

Vital Parts: Roots, Leaves, Berries
Harvest Season: Late Autumn to Early Winter

Description: Ashwagandha is a renowned adaptogenic herb celebrated for its ability to reduce stress, improve energy levels, and enhance overall well-being. It contains bioactive compounds that have anti-inflammatory, antioxidant, and immune-boosting properties.

Native: Originally from the Indian subcontinent, particularly in drier regions of India, Pakistan, and Sri Lanka.

Cultivation: Ashwagandha thrives in warm, arid climates with well-drained, sandy or loamy soil. It is widely cultivated in India, the Middle East, and parts of Africa.

Ancient Usage: Ashwagandha has been revered for centuries in Ayurvedic medicine as a powerful adaptogen and rejuvenating herb. It was often referred to as "Rasayana," meaning a plant that promotes longevity, strength, and vitality. Ancient practitioners used ashwagandha to enhance energy, reduce stress, and support overall health, particularly for improving stamina and fertility. Additionally, it was valued for its calming effects on the nervous system, making it a popular remedy for anxiety, insomnia, and immune support.

Medicinal Benefits:
- **Stress Reduction:** Lowers cortisol levels, reducing anxiety.
- **Improved Sleep:** Promotes relaxation and sleep quality.
- **Energy and Endurance:** Boosts strength and stamina.
- **Cognitive Support:** Enhances memory, focus, and brain function.
- **Immune Modulation:** Strengthens the immune system and reduces inflammation.
- **Hormonal Balance:** Helps regulate thyroid and adrenal function.
- **Anti-inflammatory:** Reduces chronic inflammation and supports joint health.
- **Reproductive Health:** Improves fertility and boosts vitality.

Ashwagandha is a perennial shrub that typically grows to a height of 1.5 to 5 feet. It has woody stems and oval, green, velvety leaves that are arranged alternately along the branches. The plant produces small, pale green or yellow flowers, which eventually develop into small, round, orange-red berries encased in a papery husk.

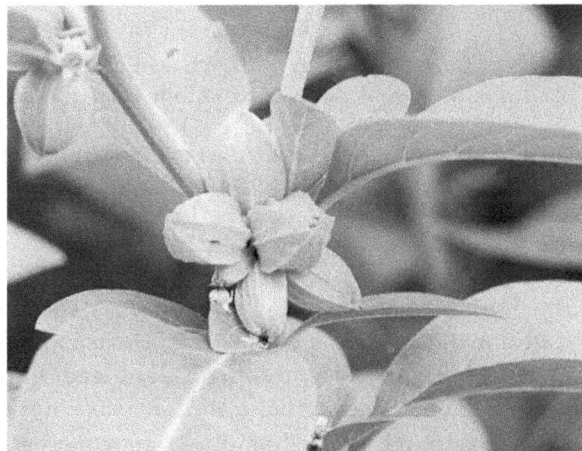

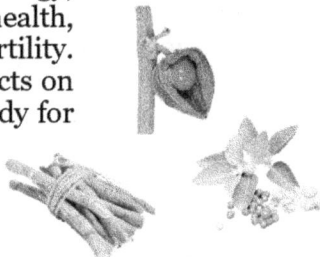

Dosage:
- **Powder:** 1-5 grams daily (approximately 1/4 to 1 teaspoon).
- **Standardized Extract:** 300-600 mg (with 5% withanolides).
- **Tincture:** 2-4 mL (40-80 drops).

Safety:
- **Internal Use:** Prolonged use may cause stomach upset.
- **Allergic Reactions:** Individuals sensitive to nightshades (e.g., potatoes) should use caution.
- **Drug Interactions:** Use cautiously if taking medications for thyroid function, sedatives, or blood pressure.

Preparation Methods:
- **Edible Flowers:** Ashwagandha flowers are edible.
- **Teas & Infusions:** Reduces stress, supports energy levels, and enhances well-being.
- **Decoctions:** Improves resilience to stress, boosts immunity, and supports sleep.
- **Tinctures:** Reduces stress, balances hormones, and provides cognitive support.
- **Syrups:** Supports sleep and anxiety and improves stamina.
- **Salves & Balms:** Soothes muscle tension, joint pain, and localized inflammation.
- **Poultices:** Reduces pain and swelling.

ASTRAGALUS

Latin: *Astragalus memranaceus*

Vital Parts: Root
Harvest Season: Late Summer to Early Autumn

Description: Astragalus is a powerful adaptogenic herb known for its immune-boosting, anti-inflammatory, and antioxidant properties. It is valued for enhancing energy, supporting the body's resistance to stress.

Native: Originally from northern and eastern regions of China, as well as parts of Mongolia and Korea.

Cultivation: Astragalus thrives in temperate climates with well-drained, sandy or loamy soil. It is primarily cultivated in China, where it has been a staple in traditional Chinese medicine for centuries.

Ancient Usage: Astragalus has been a cornerstone of traditional Chinese medicine for thousands of years, known as "Huang Qi," meaning "yellow leader," due to its prominence among herbal tonics. It was revered for its ability to strengthen the immune system, increase energy, and promote longevity. Ancient practitioners used astragalus to enhance the body's resistance to illness, particularly for respiratory infections and fatigue. Additionally, it was valued for its role in improving circulation, supporting kidney function, and accelerating wound healing.

Astragalus is a perennial herb that can grow up to 60 to 120 centimeters (2 to 4 feet) tall. It features upright, branched stems and pinnately compound leaves with multiple pairs of small, oval leaflets. The plant produces clusters of pale yellow or cream-colored, pea-shaped flowers that develop into small, elongated seed pods,

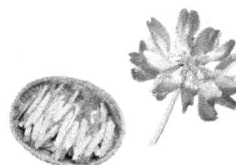

Medicinal Benefits:
- **Immune Support:** Boosts white blood cell production to fight infections.
- **Anti-inflammatory:** Reduces inflammation in chronic conditions like arthritis.
- **Antioxidant:** Protects cells from stress and disease.
- **Energy Boost:** Improves energy and reduces fatigue in chronic conditions.
- **Heart Health:** Enhances circulation, lowers blood pressure, and reduces cholesterol.
- **Kidney Support:** Improves kidney function and reduces protein loss in urine.

Dosage:
- **Dried Root:** 9-15 grams per day.
- **Capsules/Tablets:** 500-1,000 mg per dose.
- **Tincture:** 2-4 mL (40-80 drops) in water or juice.

Safety:
- **Autoimmune Disorders:** May worsen lupus, arthritis, or multiple sclerosis.
- **Medication Interactions:** May interact with immunosuppressive drugs, anticoagulants, and blood pressure medications.
- **Allergies:** Use caution if you are allergic to plants in the legume family (Fabaceae).

Preparation Methods:
- **Teas & Infusions:** Boosts immunity and supports energy levels.
- **Decoctions:** Supports immunity, stamina, and recovery from illness.
- **Tinctures:** Supports immune health, combats fatigue, and promotes resilience to stress.
- **Syrups:** Enhances immunity, soothes respiratory irritation, and supports vitality.
- **Salves & Balms:** Promotes wound healing and reduces inflammation.
- **Poultices:** Applied to wounds or minor skin irritations to promote healing and reduce swelling.

Planet: Saturn

BAY LEAF

Zodiac: ♑ Capricorn

Latin: Laurus nobilis

Vital Parts: Leaves
Harvest Season: Year-round - Peak Late Summer

Description: Bay leaf is an aromatic herb known for its ability to support digestive health, reduce inflammation, and provide antioxidant benefits. It is valued for its ability to relieve indigestion, promote respiratory health, and support heart function.

Native: Originally from the Mediterranean region, particularly around areas such as Turkey, Greece, and Italy.

Cultivation: Bay leaf thrives in warm, subtropical, and Mediterranean climates with well-drained soil. It is cultivated in many regions, including southern Europe, North Africa, and parts of North America.

Ancient Usage: Bay leaf has been highly valued since ancient times, particularly in Greek and Roman cultures, where it symbolized victory, wisdom, and protection. Known as "laurel," it was used to create wreaths for heroes, scholars, and athletes. Medicinally, bay leaves were used to support digestion, relieve indigestion, and soothe respiratory ailments. Additionally, they were believed to ward off evil spirits and were often burned in purification rituals to promote protection and mental clarity.

Bay leaf is an evergreen shrub or small tree that can grow up to 30 to 50 feet tall. It has smooth, dark green, leathery, glossy, elliptical leaves. The plant produces small, pale yellow flowers that appear in clusters and develop into dark purple or black berry-like fruits.

Medicinal Benefits:
- **Digestive Aid:** Relieves bloating, gas, and indigestion.
- **Anti-Inflammatory:** Reduces inflammation, arthritis, joint pain, and muscle soreness.
- **Respiratory Health:** Supports congestion and respiratory health.
- **Antimicrobial Properties:** Inhibits bacterial and fungal growth.
- **Heart Health:** Supports cholesterol and circulation.
- **Stress Relief:** Provides calming and anti-anxiety effects.
- **Blood Sugar Regulation:** Provides diabetes support.
- **Detoxification:** Supports liver function.

Dosage:
- **Tea:** 1-2 whole dried bay leaves per 250 mL (1 cup) of water.
- **Capsules:** 500-1,000 mg, 1-2 times daily.

Safety:
- **Moderation:** Excessive use may cause stomach upset.
- **Allergies:** Avoid if you have allergies to bay leaf or related plants (Lauraceae family).
- **Medication Interactions:** May interact with diabetes medications, and sedatives.
- **Blood Sugar Levels:** May lower blood sugar, those with diabetes should use caution.

Preparation Methods:
- **Teas & Infusions:** Aids digestion, reduces bloating, and supports respiratory health.
- **Decoctions:** Relieves cold symptoms, promotes circulation, and eases joint discomfort.
- **Tinctures:** Supports digestion, reduces inflammation, and relieves minor muscle pain.
- **Syrups:** Soothes sore throats and eases coughs.
- **Salves & Balms:** Relieves muscle aches, joint pain, and skin irritations.
- **Poultices:** Crushed bay leaves can soothe insect bites and relieve localized pain.
- **Topical:** Treats fungal infections, improves circulation, and soothes muscle tension.

BILBERRY

Latin: *Vaccinium myrtillus*

Vital Parts: Berries and Leaves
Harvest Season: Late Summer

Description: Bilberry is a nutrient-rich berry known for its powerful antioxidant, anti-inflammatory, and vision-supporting properties.

Native: Originally from northern and central Europe, with a natural range extending into parts of North America and Asia.

Cultivation: Bilberry thrives in cool, temperate climates with acidic, well-drained soil. It is commonly found growing in wild, forested areas and heathlands.

Ancient Usage: Bilberry, often referred to as the "vision herb," has been valued in traditional European herbal medicine for centuries. Medieval herbalists used it to improve night vision and strengthen eyesight, with British pilots during World War II reportedly consuming bilberry jam to enhance their night-flying abilities. The berries were also prized for their ability to promote circulation, treat varicose veins, and reduce inflammation In folklore, it was believed to protect against illnesses and was often gathered during seasonal rituals for vitality.

Bilberry is a low-growing deciduous shrub that typically reaches a height of 30 to 60 centimeters (1 to 2 feet). It has thin, green, angular stems and small, oval-shaped leaves with finely serrated edges. The plant produces small, bell-shaped pink or pale red flowers, which develop into dark blue or purple berries with a slightly tart flavor.

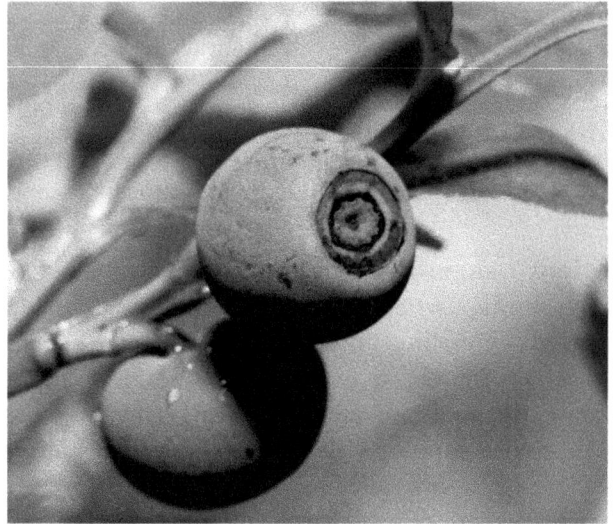

Medicinal Benefits:
- **Eye Health:** Enhances vision and reduces eye strain; aids macular degeneration and cataracts.
- **Circulation Support:** Improves blood flow, supports heart health, and reduces varicose veins.
- **Antioxidant Properties:** Protects cells from oxidative stress.
- **Blood Sugar Regulation:** Stabilizes blood sugar, making it beneficial for individuals with diabetes.
- **Anti-Inflammatory:** Reduces inflammation, benefiting those with arthritis or IBS.
- **Digestive Aid:** Relieves diarrhea by soothing the gut lining.

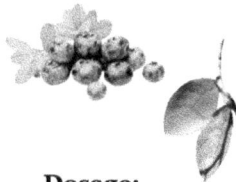

Dosage:
- **Standardized Extract:** 80-160 mg (25% anthocyanins) per dose.
- **Dried Bilberries/Powder:** 20-60 grams daily.
- **Tea:** 1-2 teaspoons of dried fruit or leaves per cup (250 mL) of water.
- **Tincture:** 2-4 mL (40-80 drops) in water or juice.

Safety:
- **Internal Use:** Excessive consumption may cause mild gastrointestinal discomfort.
- **Allergic Reactions:** Individuals allergic to berries or related plants should use caution.
- **Blood Thinning:** Use with caution if taking blood-thinning medications.

Preparation Methods:
- **Teas & Infusions:** Supports eye health, improves circulation, and aids in digestion.
- **Decoctions:** Soothes sore throats, alleviates diarrhea, and promotes urinary tract health.
- **Tinctures:** Supports vision, combats inflammation, and regulates blood sugar.
- **Syrups:** Soothes respiratory irritation, strengthens immunity, and supports cardiovascular health.
- **Salves & Balms:** Promotes wound healing and improves skin health.
- **Poultices:** Soothes irritated skin, reduces swelling, and promotes healing of wounds.

Planet: Mars

BLACK COHOSH

Zodiac: ♏ Scorpio

Latin: *Actaea racemosa*

Vital Parts: Roots, Rhizomes
Harvest Season: Late Summer to Early Autumn

Description: Black cohosh is an herb known for its ability to support women's health, particularly in alleviating symptoms of menopause, such as hot flashes, mood swings, and sleep disturbances.

Native: Originally from eastern North America, particularly in forested regions of the United States and Canada.

Cultivation: Black cohosh thrives in cool, temperate climates with moist, well-drained, and shaded soil. It is commonly cultivated and harvested in forested areas and herbal gardens.

Ancient Usage: Black cohosh, often called "black snakeroot," has been revered by Native American tribes for its powerful support of women's health. It was used to ease menstrual cramps, promote smooth childbirth, and alleviate menopausal symptoms such as hot flashes and mood swings. Native healers also relied on it to treat snakebites, respiratory conditions, and inflammation. In folklore, the plant was believed to possess protective qualities and was used in rituals to promote emotional balance and resilience.

Black cohosh is a tall, perennial herbaceous plant that can grow up to 1.5 to 2.5 meters (5 to 8 feet) in height. It features slender, branching stems and large, compound leaves with serrated, oval leaflets. The plant produces long, spiky small, white, fragrant flowers.

Medicinal Benefits:
- **Menopausal Support:** Alleviates hot flashes, night sweats, and mood swings.
- **Hormonal Balance:** Supports menstrual health, reduces cramps, and eases PMS.
- **Anti-Inflammatory:** Provides relief for joint pain and arthritis.
- **Nervous System Support:** Calms the nervous system, reduces anxiety, and promotes relaxation.
- **Muscle Relaxation:** Eases tension and spasms, particularly in the uterus.
- **Bone Health:** Reduces the risk of osteoporosis, especially in women.

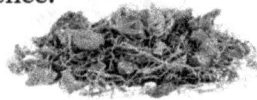

Dosage:
- **Standardized Extract:** 20-80 mg daily.
- **Tincture:** 2-4 mL (40-80 drops) in water or juice.
- **Tea:** 1-2 grams in 1 cup (250 mL) of water daily.

Safety:
- **Internal Use:** Prolonged use may cause headaches.
- **Drug Interactions:** May interact with hormone replacement therapy (HRT), birth control pills, or medications affecting the liver.

Preparation Methods:
- **Teas & Infusions:** Supports hormonal balance, eases menstrual cramps, and alleviates menopausal symptoms.
- **Decoctions:** Addresses more intense symptoms of PMS.
- Tinctures: Relieves hormonal imbalances.
- **Syrups:** Soothes throat irritation and support hormonal health.
- **Salves & Balms:** Black cohosh-infused oil can be incorporated into salves to relieve muscle aches, joint pain, and inflammation.
- **Poultices:** Can be made into a poultice and applied to sore muscles, inflamed joints, or minor skin irritations.

49

BLACK WALNUT

Latin: *Juglans nigra*

Vital Parts: Hulls, Bark, Leaves
Harvest Season: Late Summer to Early Autumn

Description: Black walnut is valued for its potent medicinal properties, particularly for promoting digestive health, supporting the body's natural detoxification processes, and combating parasitic infections.

Native: Originally from eastern North America, black walnut trees are commonly found in the United States and parts of southern Canada, thriving in forests and rich floodplains.

Cultivation: Black walnut trees prefer full sun and deep, fertile, well-drained soil. They are drought-tolerant once established and are often cultivated for both their medicinal properties and valuable hardwood.

Ancient Usage: Black walnut has been revered for centuries for its cleansing and protective properties. Native American tribes used the hulls to expel intestinal parasites, promote digestion, and support skin health by treating conditions like eczema and fungal infections. In European folklore, black walnut was believed to offer protection against negative energies and was often used in purification rituals. Traditional herbalists valued its properties to cleanse the blood and promote lymphatic drainage. The tree's strong, durable wood was also prized for building sacred objects, while the nut's rich, earthy flavor made it a valuable food source.

Black walnut is a large deciduous tree with a straight, dark-barked trunk and a broad, rounded canopy. Its compound leaves are lance-shaped, serrated leaflets. The tree produces small, greenish flowers—followed by round, green husks encasing hard-shelled, dark-brown nuts.

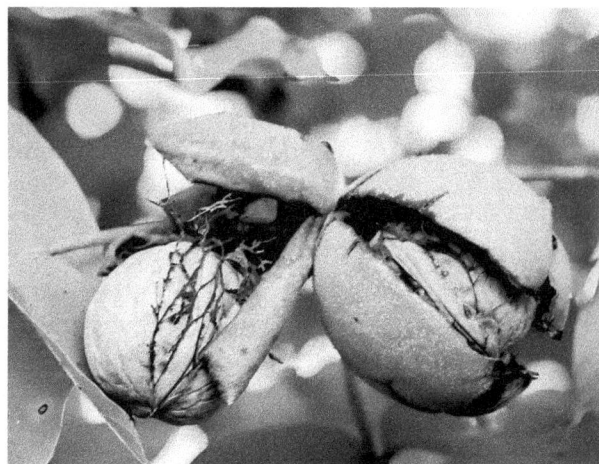

Medicinal Benefits:

- **Antimicrobial Properties:** Effective against bacteria, fungi, and parasites, making it useful for infections, ringworm, and candida.
- **Digestive Health:** Aids in treating intestinal worms, parasites, and digestive issues.
- **Detoxification:** Supports liver and kidney health by promoting natural detoxification.
- **Anti-Inflammatory:** Reduces inflammation and minor injuries.
- **Skin Health:** Treats acne, eczema, warts, and other skin conditions.
- **Immune Support:** Helps combat infections and illnesses.
- **Cardiovascular Health:** Supports heart health by reducing oxidative stress.

Dosage:
- **Standardized Extract:** 20-80 mg daily.
- **Tincture:** 2-4 mL (40-80 drops) in water or juice.
- **Tea:** 1-2 grams of dried black cohosh root boiled in 1 cup (250 mL) of water.

Safety:
- **Internal Use:** Excessive use may cause gastrointestinal discomfort.
- **Allergic Reactions:** Individuals allergic to nuts should avoid black walnut.
- **Drug Interactions:** May interact with blood-thinning or liver medications.

Preparation Methods:
- **Teas & Infusions:** Aids in digestion, detoxification, and immune health.
- **Decoctions:** Addresses parasites, fungal infections, and skin issues.
- **Tinctures:** Promotes gut health and combats infections.
- **Syrups:** Supports digestive health and addresses infections.
- **Salves & Balms:** Treat skin conditions like eczema, fungal infections, and minor wounds.
- **Poultices:** Draws out toxins, reduces inflammation, and treats fungal infections.
- **Topical:** Black walnut hull extract can be applied as a topical antiseptic or antifungal treatment for athlete's foot or ringworm.

BLESSED THISTLE

Latin: Cnicus benedictus

Vital Parts: Leaves, Stems, Flowers
Harvest Season: Late Spring to Early Summer

Description: Blessed thistle is known for its digestive and liver-supporting properties and is used to stimulate appetite and aid digestion and detoxification.

Native: Blessed thistle is native to the Mediterranean region, particularly in dry, rocky areas of southern Europe and western Asia.

Cultivation: Blessed thistle thrives in sunny locations with well-drained, moderately fertile soil. It is often cultivated in herbal gardens and can also grow wild in arid environments.

Ancient Usage: Blessed thistle, also known as the "holy herb," was highly valued during the Middle Ages for its protective and healing properties. It was believed to ward off the plague and evil spirits, earning its name for its association with divine protection and healing. European herbalists used blessed thistle to support digestion, stimulate appetite, and promote liver detoxification. It was also a common remedy for nursing mothers to increase milk production and for treating fevers and respiratory ailments. Monks often cultivated it in monastery gardens, believing it to be a gift from God for promoting health and vitality.

Blessed thistle is a spiny, annual herb that grows up to 3 feet tall with branched, hairy stems. Its deeply lobed, serrated leaves feature sharp thorns along the edges, giving it a distinct, protective appearance. The plant produces bright yellow, thistle-like flowers surrounded by spiny bracts, creating a striking contrast against its green foliage.

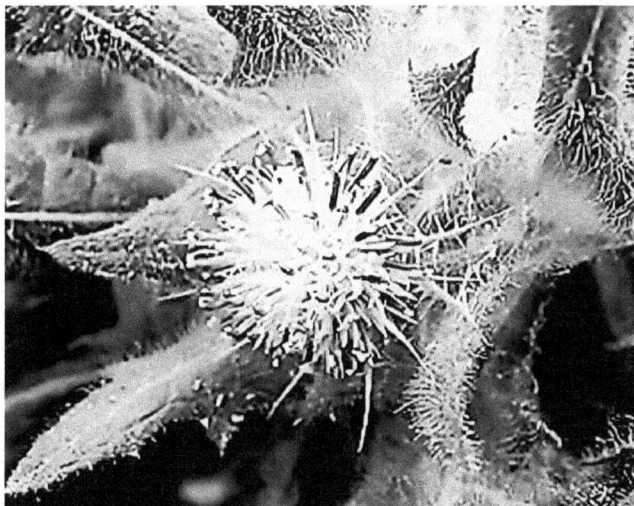

Medicinal Benefits:
- **Digestive Health:** Aids in digestion and relieves bloating, gas, and indigestion.
- **Liver Support:** Supports liver function and promotes overall detoxification.
- **Appetite Stimulant:** Supports low appetite from illness or low energy.
- **Women's Health:** Supports lactation and helps regulate menstrual cycles.
- **Immune Boosting:** Contains antimicrobials that combat infection
- **Wound Healing:** Soothes wounds and skin irritations.

Dosage:
- **Standardized Extract:** 300-500 mg daily.
- **Tincture:** 2-4 mL (40-80 drops) in water or juice, up to 3 times daily.
- **Tea:** 1-2 tsp dried herb per cup of water.

Safety:
- **Internal Use:** Excessive use may cause stomach upset.
- **Allergy Risk:** Individuals sensitive to plants in the Asteraceae family (e.g., ragweed, daisies) should use cautiously.
- **Drug Interactions:** May interact with liver and stomach medications.

Preparation Methods:
- **Teas & Infusions:** Supports digestion, stimulates appetite, and promotes liver health.
- **Decoctions:** Addresses digestive discomfort, improves bile production, and supports detoxification.
- **Tinctures:** Aids in digestive health, supports liver function, and helps regulate PMS.
- **Syrups:** Soothes cough, eases throat irritation, and supports immune health.
- **Salves & Balms:** Soothes minor skin irritations, wounds, and rashes.
- **Poultices:** Promotes wound healing and soothes insect bites.
- **Topical:** Treats localized inflammation and minor skin conditions.

Planet: Uranus

BLUE VERVAIN

Zodiac: ♒ Aquarius

Latin: Verbena hastata

Vital Parts: Flowers, Leaves, Stems
Harvest Season: Summer to Early Fall

Description: Blue vervain is an herb known for its calming and restorative effects, often used to alleviate stress, anxiety, and insomnia. It also supports women's health by relieving menstrual cramps.

Native: Blue vervain is native to North America, commonly found in meadows, wetlands, and along streams and ditches.

Cultivation: Blue vervain thrives in moist, well-drained soil with full sun to partial shade. It is often cultivated in herbal gardens and grows wild in wetlands and grasslands.

Ancient Usage: Blue vervain, sometimes referred to as the "herb of enchantment," has been revered for its calming and protective properties. In ancient Europe, it was considered sacred and used in rituals to ward off evil spirits, attract love, and promote peace. The Romans believed it held divine power, using it in religious ceremonies and medicinal applications to treat fevers and wounds. Native American tribes used blue vervain to relieve anxiety, insomnia, and respiratory conditions. It was associated with emotional balance, protection, and recovery in physical and spiritual health.

Blue vervain is a tall, slender herb that can grow up to 5 feet in height, with square-shaped, branching stems. Its opposite, lance-shaped leaves are serrated and dark green, adding to its elegant, upright form. The plant produces spikes of small, violet-blue flowers that bloom from bottom to top.

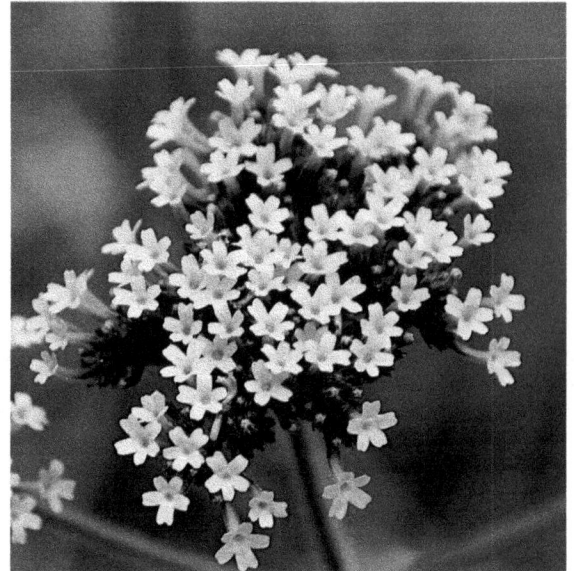

Medicinal Benefits:
- **Stress Relief:** Calms the nervous system and reduces stress and anxiety.
- **Sleep Aid:** Promotes restful sleep and helps alleviate insomnia.
- **Hormonal Balance:** Supports menstrual health, reduces cramps, and eases PMS.
- **Digestive Aid:** Relieves bloating, gas, and indigestion.
- **Anti-Inflammatory:** Reduces inflammation, making it useful for arthritis and muscle pain.
- **Immune Support:** Helps fight colds, flu, and respiratory infections.
- **Detoxification:** Acts as a gentle liver tonic, promoting liver health.

Dosage:
- **Standardized Extract:** 200-400 mg daily.
- **Tincture:** 2-4 mL (40-80 drops).
- **Tea:** 1-2 tsp dried herb per cup of water.

Safety:
- **Internal Use:** Excessive use may cause mild gastrointestinal discomfort or nausea.
- **Drug Interactions:** May interact with sedatives, antidepressants, and medications affecting liver function.

Preparation Methods:
- **Edible Flowers:** Blue vervain flowers are edible.
- **Teas & Infusions:** Calms the nervous system, relieves stress, and supports digestion.
- **Decoctions:** Addresses cramps, anxiety, and respiratory health.
- **Tinctures:** Reduces stress, balances hormones, and alleviates tension.
- **Syrups:** Soothes coughs, promotes relaxation, and supports respiratory health.
- **Salves & Balms:** Treats skin irritations and reduces muscle tension.
- **Poultices:** Reduces swelling, calms inflamed skin, and promotes wound healing.
- **Topical:** Reduces inflammation and eases muscle tension.

BORAGE

Latin: Borago officinalis

Vital Parts: Leaves, Flowers, Seeds
Harvest Season: Late Spring to Early Summer

Description: Borage is an herb known for its anti-inflammatory and adrenal-supporting properties, often used to promote healthy skin, balance hormones, and reduce stress.

Native: Borage is native to the Mediterranean region, particularly in dry, rocky areas of southern Europe and North Africa.

Cultivation: Borage thrives in fertile, well-drained soil with full sun. It is often cultivated in herb and gardens and grows easily in many temperate climates.

Ancient Usage: Borage has been used since ancient times and was often referred to as the "herb of gladness" or "courage herb." The ancient Romans believed that borage gave warriors courage before battle and served it in wine to inspire bravery. In medieval Europe, it was commonly used to lift spirits and ward off sadness, making it a popular remedy for melancholy. Ancient Greek herbalists, including Dioscorides, praised borage for its ability to strengthen the heart and relieve symptoms of exhaustion. It was associated with protection and in folklore and planted to promote emotional resilience.

Medicinal Benefits:
- **Hormonal Balance:** Alleviates symptoms of PMS and menopause.
- **Skin Health:** Soothes skin conditions like eczema, dermatitis, and acne.
- **Respiratory Support:** Helps relieve coughs, colds, and bronchitis.
- **Anti-Inflammatory:** Reduces inflammation in joints and tissues, aiding in arthritis.
- **Digestive Health:** Calms stomach upset and promotes digestion.
- **Heart Health:** Improves circulation and reduces inflammation.
- **Mood Support:** Helps reduce stress and anxiety.
- **Diuretic Properties:** Helps eliminate excess fluid.

Borage is a hardy, annual herb that grows up to 2 to 3 feet tall, with hollow, branched stems covered in coarse, bristly hairs. Its large, oval leaves have a rough, fuzzy texture, giving the plant a distinct feel. Borage features star-shaped, vibrant blue flowers with black stamens that bloom in clusters.

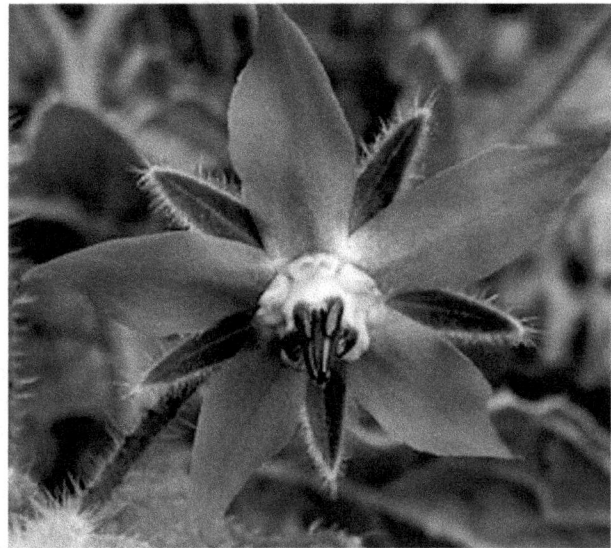

Dosage:
- **Standardized Extract:** 300-600 mg daily.
- **Tincture:** 2-4 mL (40-80 drops).
- **Tea:** 1-2 tsp dried leaves or flowers per cup of water.

Safety:
- **Internal Use:** Long-term or excessive use of leaves may pose risks to liver health.
- **Children:** Safe for older children in small amounts for respiratory or digestive issues.
- **Drug Interactions:** May interact with liver medications.

Preparation Methods:
- **Edible Flowers:** Borage flowers are edible and often used in foods.
- **Teas & Infusions:** Supports adrenal health, reduces stress, and promotes relaxation.
- **Decoctions:** Relieves respiratory conditions and promotes urinary health.
- **Tinctures:** Reduces stress, balances hormones, and supports skin health.
- **Syrups:** Soothes sore throats, supports respiratory health, and calms nerves.
- **Salves & Balms:** Treats dry skin, reduces inflammation, and supports wound healing.
- **Poultices:** Soothes minor burns, insect bites, and inflamed areas.
- **Topical:** Used topically to support eczema and psoriasis.

BURDOCK

Latin: *Arctium lappa*

Vital Parts: Roots, Leaves, Seeds
Harvest Season: Late Summer to Early Autumn

Description: Burdock is an herb known for its powerful detoxifying and blood-purifying properties, often used to support liver and kidney health. It helps remove toxins from the body, promoting healthy skin and alleviates acne, eczema, and psoriasis.

Native: Burdock is native to Europe and Asia but has naturalized in North America, thriving in fields, along roadsides, and in disturbed soils.

Cultivation: Burdock thrives in fertile, well-drained soil with full sun to partial shade. It is commonly cultivated in herbal gardens and grows wild in various open environments.

Ancient Usage: Burdock has been used for centuries in traditional herbal medicine and was often referred to as a "blood purifier." In ancient China, it was valued for its ability to detoxify the body and support healthy skin, often used to treat conditions like boils and rashes. In medieval Europe, burdock was a popular remedy for gout, arthritis, and other inflammatory conditions. Native American tribes used burdock root to aid digestion, support kidney function, and relieve pain. Burdock was believed to protect against negative influences, and its burs inspired the invention of Velcro.

Burdock is a biennial herb that can grow up to 6 feet tall, with branching stems and large, heart-shaped, grayish-green leaves. The plant's broad leaves are soft and velvety underneath, while the stem leaves become smaller and more pointed. It produces thistle-like, purple flower heads surrounded by hooked bracts that develop into burrs, which cling to clothing and animal fur.

Medicinal Benefits:
- **Detoxification:** Promotes liver and kidney function.
- **Skin Health:** Treats acne, eczema, psoriasis, and other skin conditions.
- **Digestive Health:** Soothes indigestion and aids gut health.
- **Anti-Inflammatory:** Reduces inflammation in joints, skin, and tissues.
- **Immune Support:** Strengthens immunity and combats infections.
- **Blood Sugar Regulation:** Beneficial for those with diabetes or metabolic syndrome.
- **Lymphatic Support:** Aids in the body's natural detoxification processes.
- **Heart Health:** Improves circulation and helps regulate cholesterol levels.

Dosage:
- **Standardized Extract:** 200-500 mg daily.
- **Tea:** 1-2 tsp per cup of water.
- **Tincture:** 2-4 mL (40-80 drops).

Safety:
- **Children:** Safe for older children in small amounts for skin or digestive issues.
- **Allergy Risk:** Those allergic to the Asteraceae family (e.g., daisies) should use cautiously.
- **Drug Interactions:** May interact with diuretics, anticoagulants, and blood sugar medications.

Preparation Methods:
- **Teas & Infusions:** Supports digestion and promotes detoxification.
- **Decoctions:** Supports liver health, kidney function, and inflammation.
- **Tinctures:** Aids in detoxification, supports immune health, and helps manage acne or eczema.
- **Syrups:** Supports respiratory health and soothes sore throats.
- **Salves & Balms:** Treats dry skin, reduces inflammation, and promotes healing.
- **Poultices:** Reduces swelling, soothes insect bites, and supports the healing of wounds.
- **Topical:** Relieves skin irritation and rashes.

CALENDULA

Latin: Tagetes erecta

Vital Parts: Flowers, Petals
Harvest Season: Early Summer to Late Autumn

Description: Calendula is an herb known for its skin-healing and anti-inflammatory properties, often used to soothe wounds, burns, and rashes.

Native: Calendula is native to southern Europe and parts of the Mediterranean region, thriving in warm, temperate climates.

Cultivation: Calendula thrives in well-drained, fertile soil with full sun to partial shade. It is often grown in herb and flower gardens for its medicinal and ornamental qualities.

Ancient Usage: Calendula, often known as "marigold" or the "herb of the sun," has been revered for its skin-healing and protective properties since ancient times. The Romans and Greeks used calendula flowers to treat wounds, burns, and skin irritations, believing it could promote rapid healing. In medieval Europe, calendula was used in medicine and spiritual practices, often included in rituals to ward off evil and bring good fortune. Its vibrant flowers symbolized warmth, vitality, and renewal.

Calendula is a hardy, flowering herb that grows up to 1 to 2 feet tall, with slightly hairy, branching stems. Its oblong, light green leaves have a soft, sticky texture. The plant is known for its vibrant, daisy-like flowers in shades of orange and yellow, blooming in clusters.

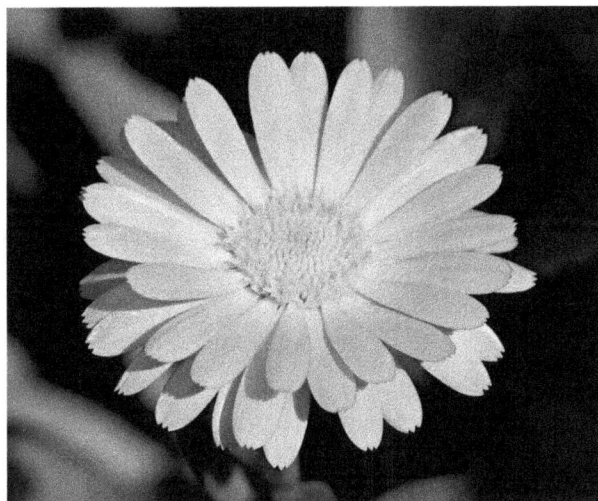

Medicinal Benefits:

- **Skin Health:** Promotes healing, reduces inflammation, and prevents infection.
- **Anti-Inflammatory:** Effective for eczema, dermatitis, and hemorrhoids.
- **Digestive Health:** Alleviates inflammation in the stomach and intestines.
- **Immune Support:** Helps to combat infections.
- **Menstrual Health:** Regulates cycles by promoting blood flow and reducing uterine inflammation.
- **Oral Health:** Reduces gum inflammation and mouth sores.
- **Detoxification:** Aids in the removal of waste and toxins.

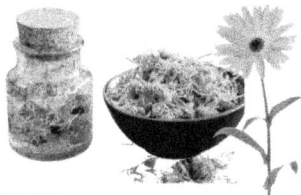

Dosage:
- **Standardized Extract:** 300-600 mg daily.
- **Tincture:** 2-4 mL (40-80 drops), up to 3 times daily.
- **Tea:** 1-2 tsp per cup of water, 2-3 times daily.
- **Capsules:** 500-1,000 mg of dried herb, 1-2 times daily.

Safety:
- **Children:** Safe for children for wounds or rashes.
- **Allergy Risk:** Those allergic to the Asteraceae family (e.g., daisies) should use cautiously.

Preparation Methods:
- **Edible Flowers:** Calendula flowers are edible.
- **Teas & Infusions:** Supports digestion and soothes inflammation.
- **Decoctions:** Supports liver detoxification and reduces inflammation.
- **Tinctures:** Aids in immune support and wound healing.
- **Syrups:** Soothes sore throats and supports respiratory health.
- **Salves & Balms:** Treats wounds, burns, and rashes.
- **Poultices:** Reduces swelling, promotes healing, and soothes insect bites or minor wounds.
- **Topical:** Treats acne, eczema, and other skin irritations.

CARAWAY

Latin: Carum carvi

Vital Parts: Seeds
Harvest Season: Late Summer to Early Autumn

Description: Caraway is an herb known for its digestive-supporting properties, often used to relieve bloating, gas, and indigestion.

Native: Caraway is native to Europe, North Africa, and western Asia, thriving in meadows and open, temperate regions.

Cultivation: Caraway grows best in well-drained, fertile soil with full sun. It is commonly cultivated in herb gardens and grows wild in meadows and grasslands.

Ancient Usage: Caraway, often called the "seed of protection," has been valued since ancient times for its digestive-supporting properties. The Egyptians used caraway seeds to relieve indigestion and bloating, and they were found in burial sites as a symbol of protection in the afterlife. In medieval Europe, caraway was believed to prevent theft and wandering spirits, often used to ward off negative influences. Folklore suggested that caraway seeds could guard against evil and promote fidelity.

Caraway is a biennial herb that reaches up to 2 feet in height, with smooth, slender stems and finely divided, feathery leaves. Its small, white or pale pink flowers form delicate, umbrella-shaped clusters (umbels). The plant produces crescent-shaped, aromatic seeds.

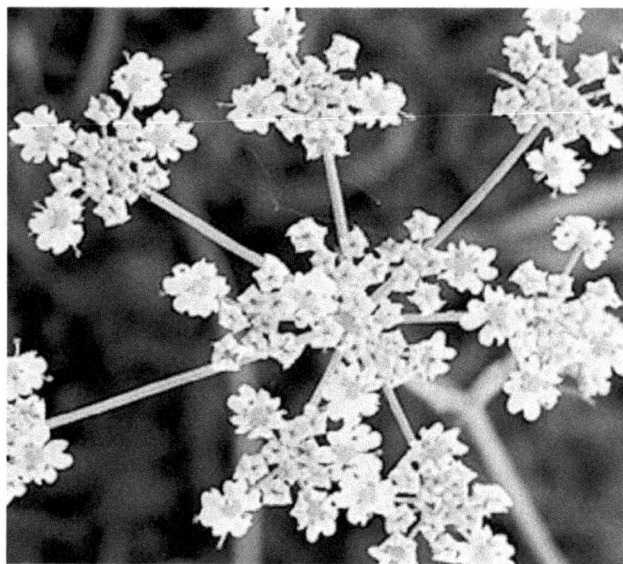

Medicinal Benefits:

- **Digestive Health:** Alleviates symptoms of IBS and colic.
- **Antimicrobial Properties:** Combats harmful bacteria, fungi, and yeast.
- **Respiratory Health:** Soothes coughs and clears congestion when used in teas or inhalations.
- **Appetite Stimulation:** Encourages healthy appetite and improves digestion.
- **Menstrual Health:** Reduces menstrual cramps and regulates cycles due to its antispasmodic properties.
- **Skin Health:** Soothes skin irritations and minor wounds.
- **Anti-Inflammatory:** Aids arthritis and muscle soreness.

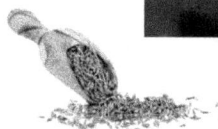

Dosage:
- **Standardized Extract:** 200-400 mg daily.
- **Tincture:** 2-4 mL (40-80 drops), up to 3 times daily.
- **Tea:** 1-2 tsp of crushed seeds per cup of water, 2-3 times daily for digestion.
- **Capsules:** 500-1,000 mg of dried seeds, 1-2 times daily.

Safety:
- **Internal Use:** Overuse may cause digestive upset.
- **Children:** Safe in small amounts.
- **Allergy Risk:** Those sensitive to plants in the Apiaceae family (e.g., parsley, celery) should use cautiously.

Preparation Methods:
- **Edible Flowers:** Caraway flowers are edible.
- **Teas & Infusions:** Reduces bloating and aids in relaxation.
- **Decoctions:** Addresses respiratory congestion.
- **Tinctures:** Supports digestion, reduces menstrual cramps, and promotes appetite.
- **Syrups:** Soothes sore throats and calms coughs.
- **Salves & Balms:** Relieves muscle soreness, joint pain, and minor skin irritations.
- **Poultices:** Soothes muscle tension and inflammation.
- **Topical:** Relieves acne, eczema, and minor irritations.

Planet: Jupiter

CARDAMOM

Zodiac: ⚹ Sagittarius

Latin: Elettaria cardamomum

Vital Parts: Seeds, Pods
Harvest Season: Late Summer to Early Winter

Description: Cardamom is an aromatic herb known for its digestive and respiratory-supporting properties. It is often used to relieve indigestion while promoting healthy lung function and soothing coughs.

Native: Cardamom is native to the tropical forests of southern India and Sri Lanka.

Cultivation: Cardamom thrives in warm, humid climates with well-drained, fertile soil and partial shade. It is cultivated on farms and in herb gardens in tropical regions.

Ancient Usage: Cardamom, often referred to as the "queen of spices," has been prized for its aromatic and medicinal qualities since ancient times. In Ayurvedic and traditional Chinese medicine, it was used to improve digestion, relieve gas, and soothe stomach discomfort. The ancient Egyptians chewed cardamom seeds to freshen breath and used it in perfumes and sacred rituals. Hippocrates valued cardamom for its warming properties, using it to alleviate respiratory issues and promote circulation.

Medicinal Benefits:
- **Digestive Health:** Relieves bloating, gas, indigestion, and nausea.
- **Respiratory Support:** Alleviates colds, bronchitis, and asthma.
- **Anti-Inflammatory:** Reduces inflammation, IBS, and arthritis.
- **Detoxification:** Promotes liver and kidney function by eliminating toxins.
- **Immune Support:** Combats infections.
- **Oral Health:** Prevents gum infections and tooth decay.
- **Heart Health:** Improves circulation and regulates blood pressure.
- **Mood Enhancement:** Reduces stress, anxiety, and mental fatigue.

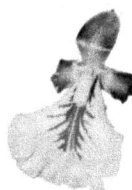

Cardamom is a tropical, perennial herb that grows up to 10 feet tall, with thick, reed-like stems and long, lance-shaped green leaves. It features small, yellow flowers with purple-veined lips that bloom near the base of the plant. The plant produces small, green pods containing aromatic seeds, which are valued for their spicy-sweet flavor.

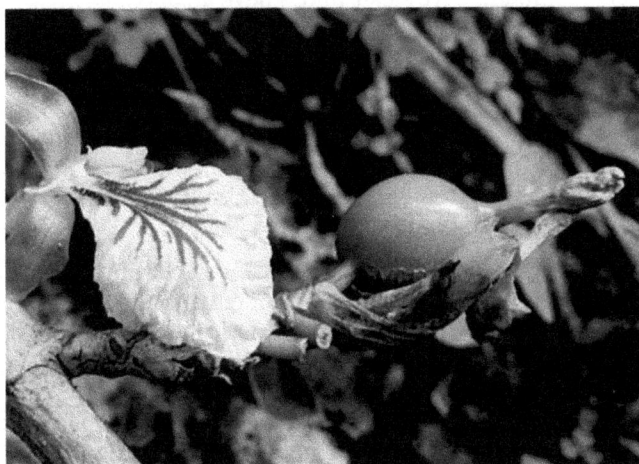

Dosage:
- **Standardized Extract:** 300-600 mg daily.
- **Tincture:** 2-4 mL (40-80 drops), up to 3 times daily.
- **Tea:** 1-2 crushed cardamom pods per cup of water, 2-3 times daily.
- **Capsules:** 500-1,000 mg of dried seed powder, 1-2 times daily.

Safety:
- **Children:** Safe for children in small amounts for digestive and respiratory support.
- **Drug Interactions:** May interact with anticoagulants and digestion medications.

Preparation Methods:
- **Edible Flowers:** Cardamom flowers are aromatic and edible.
- **Teas & Infusions:** Aids digestion and reduces bloating.
- **Decoctions:** Relieves congestion, promotes circulation, and soothes digestive discomfort.
- **Tinctures:** Supports digestion, inflammation, and nausea.
- **Syrups:** Soothes sore throats, eases coughs, and supports respiratory health.
- **Salves & Balms:** Improves circulation and relieves muscle tension.
- **Poultices:** Soothes skin irritations, reduces swelling, and provides relief for tension.
- **Topical:** Relieves muscle aches and improves circulation.

57

CATNIP

Latin: *Nepeta cataria*

Vital Parts: Leaves, Flowers, Stems
Harvest Season: Late Spring to Early Autumn

Description: Catnip is an herb known for its calming and sedative effects, often used to promote relaxation, improve sleep, and relieve anxiety.

Native: Catnip is native to Europe and parts of Asia but has naturalized in North America.

Cultivation: Catnip grows best in well-drained soil with full sun to partial shade. It is commonly cultivated in herb gardens and can also be found growing wild in fields and along roadsides.

Ancient Usage: Catnip, often called "catmint," has been valued for its calming and medicinal properties since ancient times. Native American tribes used catnip to treat colds, coughs, and fever, often brewing it as a tea to promote sweating and relieve respiratory ailments. In medieval Europe, catnip was used to ease anxiety, improve sleep, and alleviate digestive discomfort. It was also believed to ward off evil spirits and promote relaxation, with herbalists using it to soothe children's colic and teething pain.

Medicinal Benefits:
- **Stress and Anxiety Relief:** Reduces restlessness and irritability.
- **Sleep Aid:** Promotes relaxation and improves sleep quality.
- **Digestive Health:** Relieves bloating, gas, and stomach cramps.
- **Menstrual Health:** Alleviates menstrual cramps and promotes relaxation of uterine muscles.
- **Respiratory Support:** Helps ease coughs, colds, and bronchitis.
- **Pain Relief:** Aids headaches, muscle tension, and minor aches.
- **Immune Support:** Helps the body combat infections.

Catnip is a perennial herb that grows up to 3 feet tall, with square, branching stems and heart-shaped, gray-green leaves covered in fine hairs. The leaves have serrated edges and emit a minty fragrance when crushed. It produces small clusters of white to pale lavender flowers with purple spots.

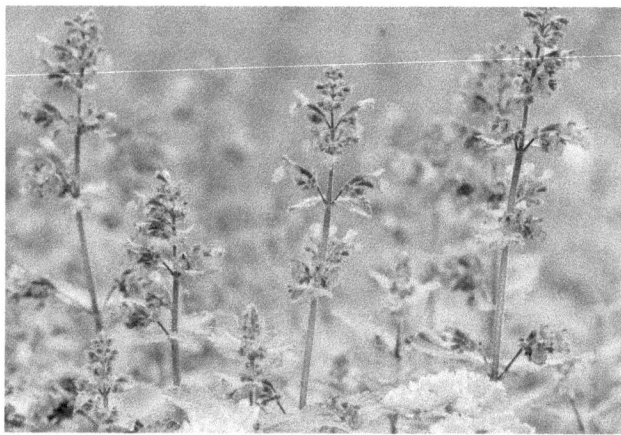

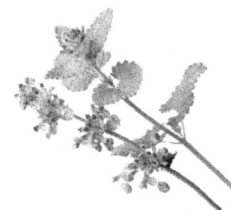

Dosage:
- **Standardized Extract:** 200-400 mg daily.
- **Tincture:** 2-4 mL (40-80 drops), up to 3 times daily.
- **Tea:** 1-2 tsp of dried leaves per cup of water, 2-3 times daily.
- **Capsules:** 500-1,000 mg of dried herb, 1-2 times daily.

Safety:
- **Internal Use:** Excessive use may cause nausea or dizziness.
- **Children:** Safe for children in small amounts, particularly for digestive upset, colic, or mild restlessness.
- **Allergy Risk:** Those sensitive to mint-family plants (Lamiaceae) should use cautiously.

Preparation Methods:
- **Edible Flowers:** Catnip flowers are edible and can be used in salads or herbal dishes.
- **Teas & Infusions:** Helps with relaxation, digestion, and reducing stress.
- **Decoctions:** Used for its calming and digestive properties.
- **Tinctures:** Supports stress relief, digestion, and mild pain management.
- **Syrups:** Soothes coughs, promotes restful sleep, and supports respiratory health.
- **Salves & Balms:** Reduces inflammation .
- **Poultices:** Catnip leaves can reduce swelling and alleviate discomfort from insect bites.
- **Topical:** Reduces minor skin irritations and swelling.

CAYENNE

Latin: Capsicum annuum

Vital Parts: Fruits (Peppers)
Harvest Season: Late Summer to Early Autumn

Description: Cayenne is known for its powerful circulation-boosting and pain-relieving properties. It is often used to stimulate digestion, improve metabolism, and reduce inflammation.

Native: Cayenne is native to Central and South America, thriving in tropical and subtropical climates.

Cultivation: Cayenne thrives in warm climates with well-drained, fertile soil and full sun. It is commonly grown in herb and vegetable gardens.

Ancient Usage: Cayenne, often referred to as "red pepper" or the "spice of life," has been used for centuries for its powerful medicinal and culinary properties. It was highly valued by the Aztecs and Mayans who used it to stimulate circulation, reduce pain, and boost energy. Traditional healers used cayenne to treat colds, sore throats, and digestive issues. In European herbal medicine, it was used to improve blood flow, alleviate joint pain, and support heart health. Cayenne's reputation as a "fire herb" made it a popular ingredient in protective rituals and remedies to enhance vitality and strength.

Cayenne is a bushy, perennial pepper plant that can grow up to 3 feet tall, with smooth, green stems and narrow, lance-shaped leaves. It produces small, white flowers that develop into long, tapered red peppers. The peppers have a glossy surface, known for their intense heat and vibrant color.

Medicinal Benefits:
- **Stress and Anxiety Relief:** Promotes relaxation and reduces anxiety.
- **Sleep Aid:** Helps alleviate insomnia and supports sleep.
- **Digestive Support:** Relieves stomach cramps, gas, and bloating.
- **Menstrual Pain Relief:** Reduces menstrual cramps and discomfort through.
- **Cold and Flu Relief:** Reduces fever and alleviates coughs.
- **Anti-Inflammatory Properties:** Reduces swelling, inflammation, and skin irritations.
- **Headache and Migraine Relief:** Relieves tension headaches when consumed as tea or infusion.

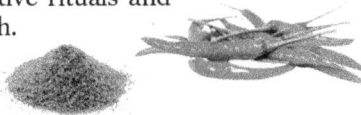

Dosage:
- **Standardized Extract:** 200-400 mg of capsaicin extract daily.
- **Tincture:** 2-4 mL (40-80 drops), up to 3 times daily.
- **Tea:** 1/4 to 1/2 tsp of cayenne powder per cup of water, taken once daily.
- **Capsules:** 500-1,000 mg of powder, 1-2 times daily.

Safety:
- **Internal Use:** Excessive consumption may cause stomach irritation or heartburn.
- **Topical Use:** Avoid direct contact with eyes, open wounds, or mucous membranes.

Preparation Methods:
- **Teas & Infusion:** Stimulates circulation, supports digestion, and relieves congestion.
- **Decoctions:** Used for its warming effects, pain relief, and respiratory support.
- **Tinctures:** Enhances circulation, relieves joint pain, and supports heart health.
- **Syrups:** Soothes sore throats, clears congestion, and boosts immunity.
- **Salves & Balms:** Alleviates muscle pain, reduces joint inflammation, and promotes blood flow.
- **Poultices:** Stimulates circulation, reduces pain, and warms the affected area (use caution to avoid irritation).
- **Topical:** Cayenne-infused oil or creams can be applied to reduce muscle pain and stimulate circulation.

CHICKWEED

Latin: Stellaria media

Vital Parts: Leaves, Stems, Flowers
Harvest Season: Spring to Early Summer

Description: Chickweed is known for its soothing and anti-inflammatory properties, often used to promote skin healing and relieve itching and irritation.

Native: Chickweed is native to Europe and Asia but has naturalized in many regions of North America.

Cultivation: Chickweed thrives in cool, moist environments with partial shade and well-drained soil. It grows wild in gardens, meadows, and disturbed areas.

Ancient Usage: Chickweed, often referred to as the "star herb," has been used in traditional herbal medicine for its soothing and anti-inflammatory properties. Ancient European herbalists applied chickweed to wounds, rashes, and irritated skin to promote healing and reduce itching. It was also consumed as a nutritious wild green, valued for its high vitamin and mineral content. In folklore, chickweed was believed to symbolize hope and resilience, renewal, and vitality.

Medicinal Benefits:
- **Skin Healing:** Soothes rashes, eczema, psoriasis, and bug bites.
- **Anti-Inflammatory:** Aids joint pain, injuries, and irritated skin.
- **Digestive Aid:** Eases bloating, indigestion, and mild constipation while promoting healthy digestion.
- **Respiratory Support:** Acts as an expectorant to loosen mucus and relieve coughs, colds, and bronchitis symptoms.
- **Nutrient Boost:** High in vitamins A, C, and D, as well as minerals like magnesium and iron.
- **Weight Management:** Supports metabolism and detoxification.
- **Immune Support:** Helps the body combat infections and recover from illnesses.

Chickweed is a low-growing, annual herb with creeping stems that can spread several feet across. Its small, oval, opposite leaves are bright green and smooth, with pointed tips. The plant produces tiny, star-shaped white flowers with deeply notched petals, blooming throughout the year.

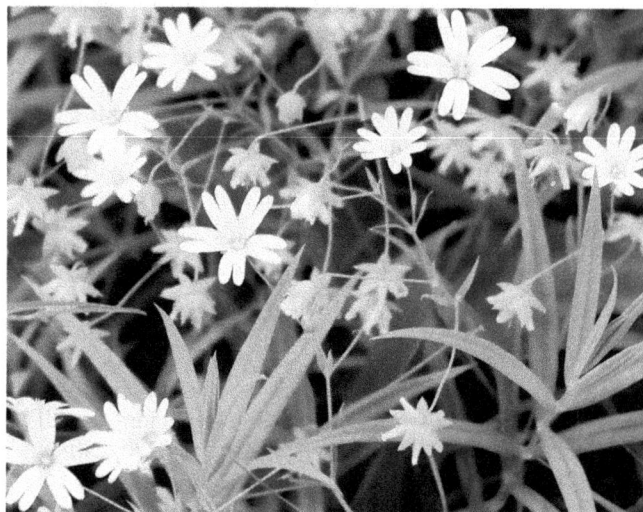

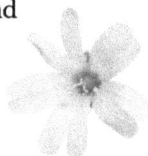

Dosage:
- **Standardized Extract:** 200-400 mg daily.
- **Tincture:** 2-4 mL (40-80 drops), up to 3 times daily.
- **Tea:** 1-2 tsp of dried herb per cup of water, 2-3 times daily.
- **Capsules:** 500-1,000 mg of dried herb, 1-2 times daily.

Safety:
- **Internal Use:** Excessive intake may cause digestive discomfort.
- **Allergy Risk:** Individuals sensitive to plants in the Caryophyllaceae family should test before use.
- **Drug Interactions:** May interact with diuretics or medications affecting water balance.

Preparation Methods:
- **Edible Flowers:** Chickweed flowers are edible and can be added to foods.
- **Teas & Infusions:** Soothes inflammation, supports digestion, and promotes urinary health.
- **Decoctions:** Supports respiratory congestion, detoxification, and inflammation.
- **Tinctures:** Supports lymphatic drainage, soothes skin conditions, and reduces inflammation.
- **Syrups:** Calms coughs, soothes sore throats, and supports respiratory health.
- **Salves & Balms:** Treats eczema, minor wounds, rashes, and skin conditions.
- **Poultices:** Reduces swelling, soothes irritated skin, and relieves discomfort from insect bites and minor wounds.
- **Topical:** Calms itchy, inflamed skin and treats minor wounds.

Planet: Moon

CHAMOMILE

Zodiac: ♋ Cancer

Latin: Matricaria chamomilla

Vital Parts: Flowers
Harvest Season: Late Spring to Early Autumn

Description: Chamomile is known for its calming and anti-inflammatory properties, often used to promote relaxation, improve sleep, and soothe digestive discomfort.

Native: Chamomile is native to Europe and western Asia and is now widely cultivated around the world.

Cultivation: Chamomile thrives in well-drained, moderately fertile soil with full sun. It is commonly grown in herb gardens for medicinal purposes.

Ancient Usage: Chamomile, often called the "herb of tranquility," has been cherished for its calming and healing properties since ancient times. The Egyptians associated it with the sun god Ra and used it to treat fevers and skin ailments. The Greeks and Romans valued chamomile for its ability to soothe digestive discomfort, promote restful sleep, and reduce inflammation. In medieval Europe, it was used in medicine and rituals to promote relaxation and peace, often scattered on floors during gatherings to create a calming atmosphere.

Chamomile is a low-growing, herbaceous plant that reaches about 1 to 2 feet in height, with slender, branched stems and finely divided, feathery leaves. It produces small, daisy-like flowers with white petals and a yellow, conical center.

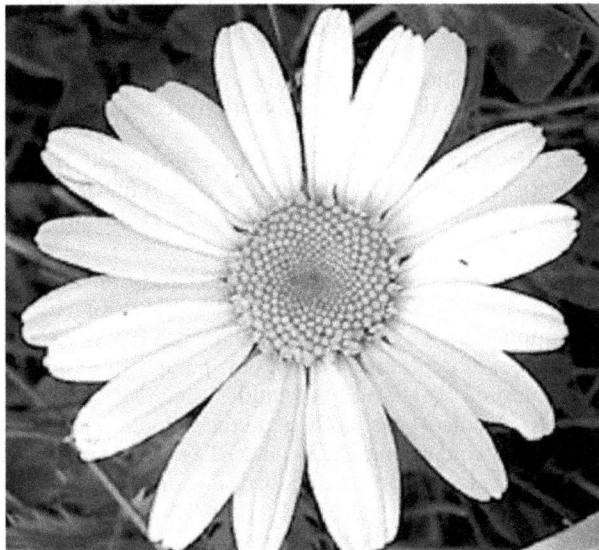

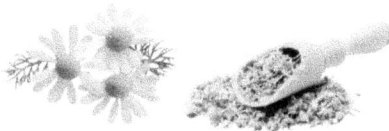

Medicinal Benefits:
- **Stress and Anxiety Relief:** Reduces stress, anxiety, and mild depression.
- **Sleep Aid:** Improves sleep quality by calming the nervous system.
- **Digestive Health:** Soothes indigestion, bloating, and nausea.
- **Anti-Inflammatory:** Reduces inflammation and aids IBS.
- **Immune Support:** Helps the body combat colds, flu, and infections.
- **Skin Health:** Treats minor wounds, burns, eczema, and rashes.
- **Menstrual Health:** Alleviates cramps and balances hormones.

Dosage:
- **Standardized Extract:** 300-600 mg daily.
- **Tincture:** 2-4 mL (40-80 drops), up to 3 times daily.
- **Tea:** 1-2 tsp of dried flowers per cup of water, 2-3 times daily.
- **Capsules:** 500-1,000 mg of dried herb, 1-2 times daily.

Safety:
- **Internal Use:** Excessive use may cause mild digestive upset.
- **Children:** Safe for children for colic, digestive upset, and stress.
- **Allergy Risk:** Those allergic to plants in the Asteraceae family (e.g., ragweed, daisies) should use cautiously.
- **Drug Interactions:** May interact with blood-thinning medications and sedatives.

Preparation Methods:
- **Edible Flowers:** Chamomile flowers are edible.
- **Teas & Infusions:** Reduces stress, supports digestion, and promotes restful sleep.
- **Decoctions:** Soothes inflammation and promotes relaxation.
- **Tinctures:** Aids in stress relief, digestion, pain, and inflammation.
- **Syrups:** Soothes sore throats, calms coughs, and supports respiratory health.
- **Salves & Balms:** Treats skin irritations, rashes, burns, and wounds.
- **Poultices:** Reduces swelling, eases muscle tension, and promotes healing.
- **Topical:** Reduces inflammation, calms irritated skin, and soothes rashes.

CHICORY

Latin: *Cichorium intybus*

Vital Parts: Roots, Leaves, Flowers
Harvest Season: Late Spring to Early Autumn

Description: Chicory is known for its liver-supporting and digestive-enhancing properties, often used to stimulate bile production and improve digestion.

Native: Chicory is native to Europe and western Asia and has become naturalized in North America.

Cultivation: Chicory thrives in well-drained, moderately fertile soil with full sun. It grows wild in fields and along roadsides and is also cultivated for its roots and leaves.

Ancient Usage: Chicory, often called the "blue herb," has been used since ancient times for its liver-supporting and digestive-enhancing properties. The ancient Egyptians used it to purify the blood and promote liver and gallbladder health. The Romans valued chicory as both a medicinal plant and a wild green, consuming it to aid digestion and improve vitality. In European folklore, chicory was believed to have magical protective properties, with legends claiming that carrying its flowers could unlock doors and bring protection from harm.

Chicory is a hardy, perennial herb that can grow up to 4 feet tall, with tough, branching stems and lance-shaped, toothed basal leaves. The plant is known for its striking, sky-blue flowers, which are arranged along the stems and open in the morning.

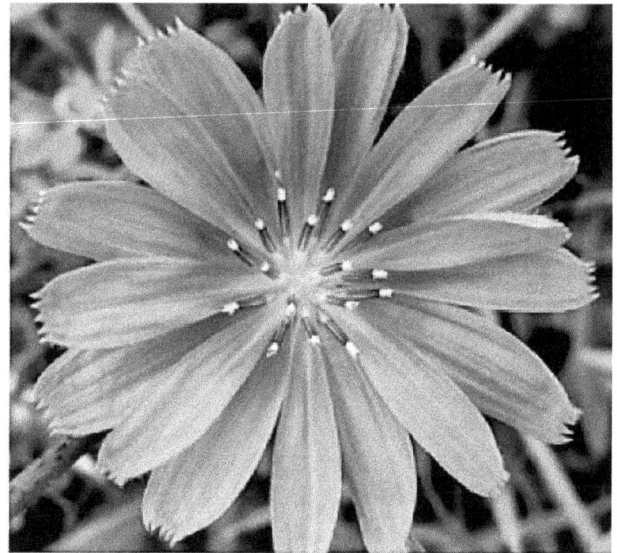

Medicinal Benefits:
- **Digestive Health:** Improves digestion and relieves constipation by promoting healthy gut flora.
- **Liver Support:** Aids in detoxification and supports liver function.
- **Kidney Health:** Helps flush toxins and reduce water retention.
- **Blood Sugar Regulation:** Helps stabilize blood sugar levels by slowing the absorption of carbohydrates.
- **Anti-Inflammatory:** Reduces inflammation in the digestive tract, joints, and other tissues, aiding IBS.
- **Immune Support:** Boosts the immune system by fostering a healthy gut microbiome.
- **Heart Health:** Helps lower cholesterol levels and improve circulation.

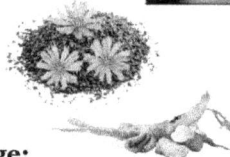

Dosage:
- **Standardized Extract:** 300-600 mg daily.
- **Tincture:** 2-4 mL (40-80 drops), up to 3 times daily.
- **Tea:** 1-2 tsp of dried root per cup of water, 2-3 times daily.
- **Capsules:** 500-1,000 mg of dried root, 1-2 times daily.

Safety:
- **Internal Use:** Excessive consumption may cause bloating.
- **Children:** Safe for older children for digestive support.
- **Allergy Risk:** Individuals allergic to plants in the Asteraceae family (e.g., ragweed, daisies) should use cautiously.
- **Drug Interactions:** May interact with blood sugar medications or diuretics.

Preparation Methods:
- **Edible Flowers:** Chicory flowers are edible and can be used fresh.
- **Teas & Infusions:** Supports digestion and promotes liver health.
- **Decoctions:** Improves liver function, reduces joint inflammation, and supports detoxification.
- **Tinctures:** Aids in digestion, promotes liver health, and supports heart function.
- **Syrups:** Soothes coughs, supports digestion, and promotes respiratory health.
- **Salves & Balms:** Alleviates skin irritations and swelling.
- **Poultices:** Reduces inflammation, soothes irritated skin, and eases joint pain.
- **Topical:** Soothes inflamed skin and promotes healing.

CINNAMON

Zodiac: ♌ Leo

Latin: Cinnamomum verum

Vital Parts: Bark, Leaves
Harvest Season: Year-round in tropical climates

Description: Cinnamon is known for its antioxidant, antimicrobial, and blood sugar-regulating properties. It is often used to support inflammation.

Native: Cinnamon is native to South and Southeast Asia, particularly Sri Lanka and southern India.

Cultivation: Cinnamon thrives in warm, tropical climates with well-drained, fertile soil. It is cultivated for its inner bark, which is harvested, dried, and used in herbal medicine.

Ancient Usage: Cinnamon, often referred to as the "spice of kings," has been treasured for its warming and healing properties for thousands of years. The ancient Egyptians used it in embalming rituals and as a key ingredient in sacred incense. In ancient China and India, cinnamon was a prized remedy for improving digestion, boosting circulation, and relieving respiratory ailments.

Cinnamon is an evergreen tree that can grow up to 50 feet tall, with smooth, reddish-brown bark and glossy, elongated green leaves. The leaves are thick and leathery, with pointed tips and prominent veins. The tree produces small, pale-yellow flowers forming clusters, followed by dark purple berries, though the inner bark is the primary part harvested for its aromatic spice.

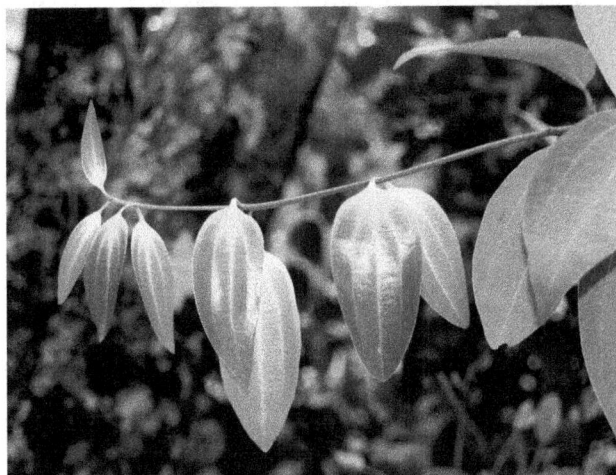

Medicinal Benefits:
- **Blood Sugar Regulation:** Helps improve insulin sensitivity.
- **Digestive Health:** Soothes indigestion, bloating, and gas.
- **Anti-Inflammatory:** Reduces inflammation in joints and muscles.
- **Immune Support:** Combats bacterial, viral, and fungal infections.
- **Heart Health:** Improves circulation and reduces cholesterol levels.
- **Respiratory Health:** Soothes coughs, clears congestion, and alleviates colds.
- **Antioxidant Properties:** Neutralizes free radicals, protecting cells from stress.

Dosage:
- **Standardized Extract:** 300-600 mg daily.
- **Tincture:** 2-4 mL (40-80 drops), up to 3 times daily.
- **Tea:** 1-2 tsp or a cinnamon stick per cup of water, 2-3 times daily.
- **Capsules:** 500-1,000 mg of powder, 1-2 times daily.

Safety:
- **Internal Use:** Excessive use may cause liver toxicity.
- **Children:** Safe for children in small amounts for digestive and respiratory support.
- **Allergy Risk:** Individuals sensitive to cinnamon should use cautiously.
- **Drug Interactions:** May interact with blood-thinning medications, diabetes drugs, and liver medications.

Preparation Methods:
- **Teas & Infusions:** Supports digestion, balances blood sugar levels, and reduces inflammation.
- **Decoctions:** Relieves respiratory congestion, improves circulation, and supports immune health.
- **Tinctures:** Aids in regulating blood sugar, enhances digestion, and promotes overall vitality.
- **Syrups:** Soothes coughs, supports respiratory health, and eases throat irritation.
- **Salves & Balms:** Provides warmth to sore muscles and alleviates aches.
- **Poultices:** Reduces inflammation, soothes irritated skin, and promotes healing of minor wounds.
- **Topical:** Cinnamon essential oil, when diluted, can be applied topically to improve circulation, relieve muscle pain, and reduce inflammation.

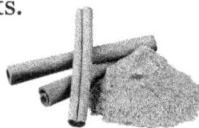

CLEAVERS

Latin: *Galium aparine*

Vital Parts: Leaves, Stems, Flowers

Harvest Season: Spring to Early Summer

Description: Cleavers is known for its gentle diuretic and lymphatic-cleansing properties, often used to support detoxification and reduce swelling.

Native: Cleavers is native to Europe, Asia, and North America, commonly found in woodlands and hedgerows.

Cultivation: Cleavers thrives in moist, shaded areas with well-drained soil. It grows wild in forests, gardens, and along fences.

Ancient Usage: Cleavers, sometimes called "goosegrass," has been used in traditional medicine for its gentle detoxifying and lymphatic-cleansing properties. Ancient herbalists in Europe and Asia used cleavers to promote kidney health and support skin healing. In folklore, cleavers were believed to aid in spiritual purification and were associated with clearing physical and emotional blockages.

Cleavers is a sprawling, annual herb with slender, square stems that can grow several feet long. Its narrow, lance-shaped leaves grow in whorls of six to eight around the stem, covered with tiny, hook-like hairs that can cling to surfaces. Small, white, star-shaped flowers bloom at leaf junctions, followed by tiny, bristly seeds that stick to fur and clothing.

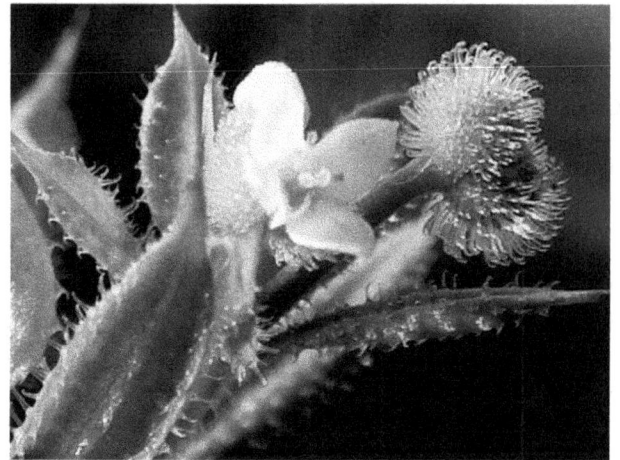

Medicinal Benefits:

- **Lymphatic Support:** Helps reduce swelling and supports immune health.
- **Diuretic Properties:** Promotes kidney health by increasing urine flow.
- **Skin Health:** Clears acne, eczema, and skin irritations.
- **Anti-Inflammatory:** Soothes irritated tissues and joints.
- **Digestive Aid:** Eases mild stomach discomfort and supports digestion.
- **Detoxification:** Acts as a gentle cleanser for the liver and kidneys.
- **Immune Support:** Aids in recovery from illnesses.

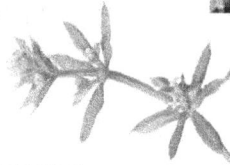

Dosage:
- **Standardized Extract:** 200-400 mg daily.
- **Tincture:** 2-4 mL (40-80 drops), 2-3 times daily.
- **Tea:** 1-2 tsp of dried herb per cup of water, 2-3 times daily.
- **Capsules:** 500-1,000 mg of dried herb, 1-2 times daily.

Safety:
- **Internal Use:** Excessive consumption may cause mild digestive upset.
- **Allergy Risk:** Those with sensitivities to the Rubiaceae family should use cautiously.
- **Drug Interactions:** May enhance the effects of diuretics.

Preparation Methods:

- **Teas & Infusions:** Aids detoxification and promotes urinary health.
- **Decoctions:** Soothes skin conditions and inflammation.
- **Tinctures:** Aids in detoxifying the lymphatic system.
- **Syrups:** Soothes sore throats, and supports immunity.
- **Salves & Balms:** Treats skin irritations, reduces swelling, and promotes healing.
- **Poultices:** Reduces inflammation, eases skin irritation, and soothes wounds.
- **Topical:** Reduces swelling, calms irritated skin, and supports lymphatic health.

CLOVE

Latin: *Syzygium aromaticum*

Vital Parts: Flower Buds
Harvest Season: Late Summer to Early Winter

Description: Clove is known for its powerful antimicrobial, analgesic, and digestive-supporting properties. It is often used to relieve toothaches, freshen breath, and improve digestion.

Native: Clove is native to the Maluku Islands (Spice Islands) in Indonesia.

Cultivation: Clove thrives in tropical climates with well-drained, fertile soil. The dried flower buds are used in herbal medicine, typically prepared as essential oils, teas, or powders.

Ancient Usage: Clove, often referred to as the "spice of warmth," has been valued for its powerful antiseptic and pain-relieving properties since ancient times. The ancient Chinese and Indian civilizations used clove to treat toothaches, freshen breath, and support digestion. In medieval Europe, clove was ward off illness and reduce fevers. Folklore held that clove could protect against negative energy, and it was often carried for physical and spiritual protection.

Clove is an evergreen tree that grows up to 40 feet tall, with smooth, gray bark and large, glossy, oval-shaped leaves. The tree produces clusters of small, red-pink flower buds, which are harvested before blooming and dried to become the familiar clove spice.

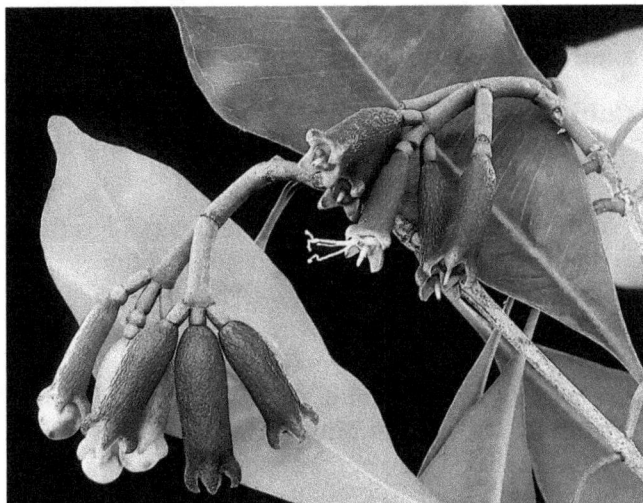

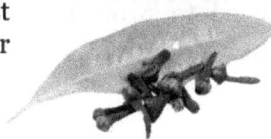

Medicinal Benefits:
- **Digestive Aid:** Stimulates digestion, reduces bloating, and alleviates nausea.
- **Pain Relief:** Acts as a natural analgesic, particularly for toothaches and gum pain.
- **Anti-Inflammatory:** Reduces inflammation and joint pain.
- **Antimicrobial Properties:** Fights bacterial, viral, and fungal infections.
- **Immune Support:** High in antioxidants.
- **Respiratory Health:** Eases coughs, colds, and congestion when used in teas or inhalations.
- **Circulatory Health:** Promotes healthy blood flow and helps regulate blood sugar levels.

Dosage:
- **Standardized Extract:** 200-500 mg daily.
- **Tincture:** 2-4 mL (40-80 drops), 2-3 times daily.
- **Tea:** 1-2 tsp of clove buds per cup of water, 2-3 times daily.
- **Capsules:** 500-1,000 mg of ground cloves, 1-2 times daily.

Safety:
- **Internal Use:** Excessive consumption may cause stomach irritation.
- **Topical Use:** Always dilute clove oil before topical application.
- **Allergy Risk:** Those with sensitivities to the Myrtaceae family should use cautiously.
- **Drug Interactions:** May interact with blood-thinning medications.

Preparation Methods:
- **Edible Flowers:** Clove buds are commonly used as a spice.
- **Teas & Infusions:** Supports digestion, nausea, and soothes sore throats.
- **Decoctions:** Relieves respiratory congestion and supports oral health.
- **Tinctures:** Aids in digestion, supports circulation, and provides relief from tooth pain.
- **Syrups:** Soothes coughs, calms sore throats, and promotes respiratory health.
- **Salves & Balms:** Relieves muscle aches, improves circulation, and soothes wounds.
- **Poultices:** Reduces pain, eases swelling, and promotes healing of wounds.
- **Topical:** Relieves pain, reduces inflammation, and soothes toothaches.

COLTSFOOT

Latin: *Tussilago farfara*

Vital Parts: Leaves, Flowers
Harvest Season: Early Spring to Late Summer

Description: Coltsfoot is known for its ability to soothe respiratory conditions, often used to relieve coughs, bronchitis, and sore throats.

Native: Coltsfoot is native to Europe and Asia but has naturalized in parts of North America.

Cultivation: Coltsfoot thrives in moist, nutrient-rich soil with full to partial sun. It grows in meadows, along streams, and in disturbed areas.

Ancient Usage: Coltsfoot, sometimes called the "cough herb," has been used for centuries to soothe respiratory ailments. The Greeks and Romans, including Dioscorides, recommended coltsfoot to relieve coughs, asthma, and bronchitis by loosening mucus and calming irritation. During the Middle Ages, it was widely used in Europe as a remedy for lung conditions and fevers. Coltsfoot was often burned as incense to purify the air and was believed to protect against respiratory infections.

Medicinal Benefits:
- **Respiratory Health:** Soothes coughs, bronchitis, and asthma.
- **Anti-Inflammatory:** Alleviates inflammation in the respiratory tract.
- **Digestive Aid:** Eases mild gastrointestinal discomfort, including indigestion and bloating.
- **Skin Healing:** Treats minor wounds, burns, and skin irritations.
- **Immune Support:** Strengthens the immune system during recovery from colds and flu.
- **Sore Throat Relief:** Coats irritated mucous membranes.

Coltsfoot is a low-growing, perennial herb with stout, unbranched stems that produce bright yellow, dandelion-like flowers early in spring. Its large, heart-shaped leaves appear after the flowers have bloomed and have a soft, downy underside.

Dosage:
- **Standardized Extract:** 200-400 mg daily.
- **Tincture:** 2-4 mL (40-80 drops), 2-3 times daily.
- **Tea:** 1-2 tsp per cup of water, 2-3 times daily.
- **Capsules:** 500-1,000 mg, 1-2 times daily.

Safety:
- **Internal Use:** Avoid long-term use, as coltsfoot contains PAs, which can harm the liver.
- **Allergy Risk:** Individuals with sensitivities to plants in the daisy family (Asteraceae) should use cautiously.
- **Drug Interactions:** May interact with medications affecting the liver.

Preparation Methods:
- **Edible Flowers:** Coltsfoot flowers are edible and can be used as a garnish.
- **Teas & Infusions:** Soothes coughs, relieves respiratory discomfort, and supports lung health.
- **Decoctions:** Addresses bronchial congestion, reduces inflammation, and promotes respiratory healing.
- **Tinctures:** Aids in alleviating coughs and mucus, supporting respiratory health.
- **Syrups:** Calms sore throats, soothes dry coughs, and supports lung function.
- **Salves & Balms:** Relieves skin irritations, reduces inflammation, and promotes healing of wounds and rashes.
- **Poultices:** Reduces swelling, soothes irritation, and promotes wound healing.
- **Topical:** Soothes skin irritations and minor wounds.

COMFREY

Latin: *Symphytum officinale*

Vital Parts: Leaves, Roots
Harvest Season: Late Spring to Early Autumn

Description: Comfrey is known for its ability to promote wound healing and support bone and tissue repair. It contains allantoin, which helps stimulate cell regeneration. Comfrey is commonly used externally to treat bruises, sprains, and inflamed joints.

Native: Comfrey is native to Europe and parts of Asia.

Cultivation: Comfrey thrives in moist, fertile soil with full sun to partial shade. It is cultivated in herbal gardens for its healing properties.

Ancient Usage: Comfrey, known as "knitbone" in ancient times, has been revered for its ability to promote the healing of bones, wounds, and tissues. Ancient Greek physicians such as Dioscorides and Galen used comfrey to treat fractures, sprains, and ulcers. In medieval Europe, comfrey poultices and salves were commonly applied to accelerate the healing of injuries. Folklore associated comfrey with physical restoration, and it was planted near homes to protect and promote health.

Comfrey is a hardy, perennial herb that can grow up to 4 feet tall, with thick, hairy stems and large, lance-shaped, rough-textured leaves. Its bell-shaped flowers, which range from purple to pink or white, bloom in clusters on curved stalks.

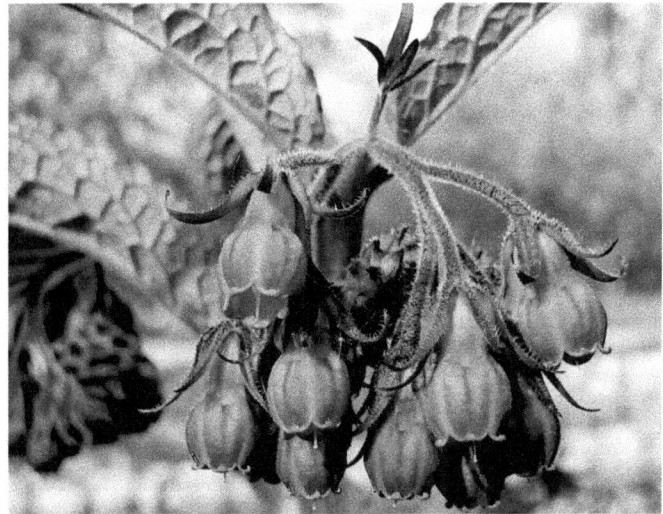

Medicinal Benefits:
- **Wound Healing:** Accelerates healing of cuts, scrapes, burns, and bruises.
- **Pain Relief:** Alleviates joint pain, muscle aches, and sprains.
- **Bone and Tissue Repair:** Supports healing of fractures, sprains, and tendon injuries.
- **Skin Health:** Treats minor skin irritations, rashes, and ulcers.
- **Anti-Inflammatory:** Reduces swelling and inflammation in joints and muscles, aiding arthritis.
- **Scar Reduction:** Helps minimize scarring when used on healing wounds.

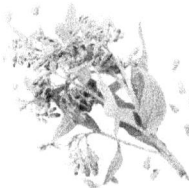

Dosage:
- **Standardized Extract:** Not recommended internally due to potential liver toxicity.
- **Tincture:** 2-4 mL (40-80 drops), used topically for wound healing.

Safety:
- **Internal Use:** Comfrey should not be taken internally due to its pyrrolizidine alkaloids.
- **Topical Use:** Safe when applied to unbroken skin.
- **Drug Interactions:** May interact with anticoagulants or medications for liver health.

Preparation Methods:
- **Edible Flowers:** Comfrey flowers can be used sparingly in salads or as a decorative garnish.
- **Teas & Infusions:** Supports digestion, soothes inflammation, and promotes respiratory health.
- **Decoctions:** Addresses joint pain, promotes wound healing, and supports skin repair.
- **Tinctures:** Reduces inflammation, soothes pain, and aids tissue repair.
- **Salves & Balms:** Treats bruises, sprains, minor wounds, and joint pain, promoting faster healing.
- **Poultices:** Reduces swelling, soothes sprains, and promotes tissue repair.
- **Topical:** Best used externally due to its pyrrolizidine alkaloids, which may be harmful if ingested.

CORIANDER

Latin: *Coriandrum sativum*

Vital Parts: Leaves, Seeds
Harvest Season: Spring to Early Autumn

Description: Coriander is known for its digestive-supporting and anti-inflammatory properties. It is often used to relieve bloating, gas, and indigestion, while also promoting detoxification.

Native: Coriander is native to the Mediterranean region and southwestern Asia.

Cultivation: Coriander thrives in well-drained, fertile soil with full sun. It is cultivated worldwide for both its seeds and leaves (cilantro).

Ancient Usage: Coriander, often called "the spice of happiness," has been used in traditional medicine for its digestive and detoxifying properties. Ancient Egyptians included coriander seeds in tombs as a symbol of eternal life. The Greeks and Romans used coriander as a remedy for indigestion. In Ayurvedic and Chinese medicine, it was believed to cool the body and promote detoxification of the liver.

Coriander is an annual herb that grows up to 2 feet tall, with slender, branching stems and bright green, finely divided, lacy leaves. The plant produces small, white or pale pink flowers that form umbrella-shaped clusters (umbels). After flowering, it develops round seeds known as coriander, a spice, while the leaves - cilantro, are a popular culinary herb.

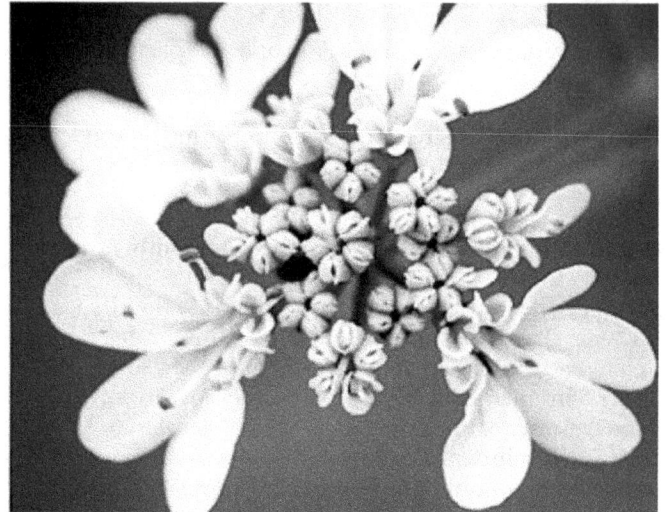

Medicinal Benefits:
- **Digestive Health:** Stimulates digestion, reduces bloating, and alleviates indigestion.
- **Anti-Inflammatory:** Reduces inflammation, benefiting arthritis and sore muscles.
- **Antimicrobial Properties:** Combats bacteria and fungi, supporting gut and skin health.
- **Detoxification:** Promotes detoxification of heavy metals from the body.
- **Heart Health:** Helps lower cholesterol and regulate blood pressure.
- **Blood Sugar Regulation:** Supports healthy blood sugar levels and is beneficial for diabetes.
- **Immune Support:** Contains antimicrobials and antioxidants.

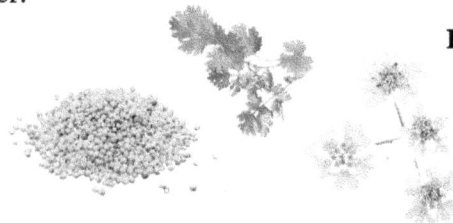

Dosage:
- **Standardized Extract:** 200-400 mg daily.
- **Tincture:** 2-4 mL (40-80 drops), up to 3 times daily.
- **Tea:** 1-2 tsp of crushed seeds per cup of water, 2-3 times daily.
- **Capsules:** 500-1,000 mg of dried seeds, 1-2 times daily.

Safety:
- **Children:** Safe in food in small amounts.
- **Allergy Risk:** Individuals allergic to plants in the Apiaceae family (e.g., fennel, parsley) should exercise caution.

Preparation Methods:
- **Edible Flowers:** Coriander flowers are edible.
- **Teas & Infusions:** Aids digestion and reduces inflammation.
- **Decoctions:** Supports detoxification and bloating.
- **Tinctures:** Aids digestion, regulates blood sugar, and reduces inflammation.
- **Syrups:** Soothes sore throats and supports respiratory health.
- **Salves & Balms:** Relieves muscle soreness, reduces inflammation, and supports skin health.
- **Poultices:** Soothes skin irritations, swelling, and wound healing.
- **Topical:** Relieves muscle tension, inflamed skin, and promotes relaxation.

Planet: Neptune

COWSLIP

Zodiac: ♓ Pisces

Latin: Primula veris

Vital Parts: Flowers, Leaves, Roots
Harvest Season: Spring to Early Summer

Description: Cowslip is valued for its sedative and anti-inflammatory properties. Traditionally used to relieve symptoms of anxiety, insomnia, and restlessness.

Native: Cowslip is native to Europe and parts of western Asia, thriving in meadows, grasslands, and open woodlands.

Cultivation: Cowslip prefers well-drained, slightly alkaline soils and thrives in partial sun to full sun. It grows best in temperate climates with adequate moisture. Cultivated primarily for its flowers.

Ancient Usage: Cowslip, sometimes called the "fairy flower," has been valued since medieval times for its ability to promote relaxation and relieve respiratory conditions. European herbalists used cowslip to treat coughs, colds, and insomnia, often preparing it as a soothing tea. In folklore, cowslip was associated with fairies and magic, believed to bring good fortune and protection to those who planted it near their homes.

Cowslip is a low-growing, perennial herb that reaches about 6 to 12 inches in height, with a rosette of wrinkled, oval leaves that have toothed edges. It produces clusters of fragrant, bell-shaped yellow flowers with orange centers, hanging from thin stalks.

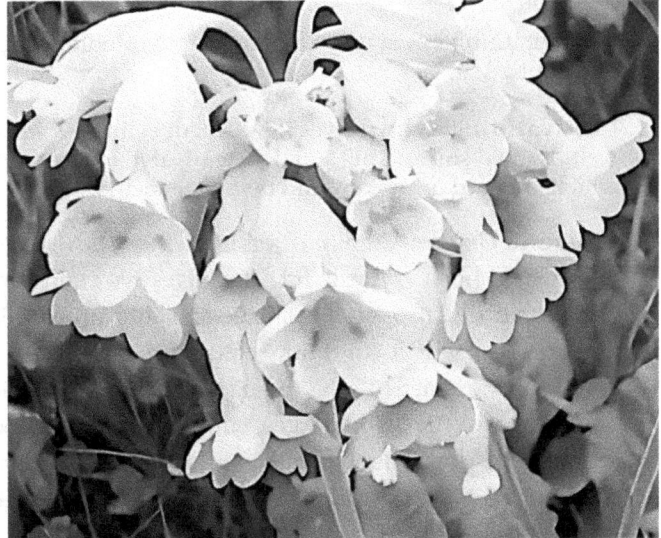

Medicinal Benefits:
- **Respiratory Health:** Soothes coughs, bronchitis, and other respiratory issues.
- **Nervous System Support:** Eases anxiety, restlessness, and insomnia.
- **Anti-Inflammatory:** Relieves joint pain, arthritis, and headaches.
- **Skin Health:** Soothes minor wounds, burns, and skin irritations.
- **Digestive Aid:** Alleviates bloating, gas, and indigestion.
- **Immune Support:** The flowers contain vitamin C and other antioxidants.

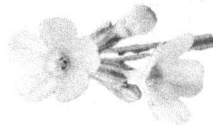

Dosage:
- **Standardized Extract:** 200-400 mg daily.
- **Tincture:** 2-4 mL (40-80 drops), up to 3 times daily.
- **Tea:** 1-2 tsp of crushed seeds per cup of water, 2-3 times daily.
- **Capsules:** 500-1,000 mg of dried seeds, 1-2 times daily.

Safety:
- **Internal Use:** Excessive consumption may cause stomach upset.
- **Allergy Risk:** Individuals sensitive to primrose may experience allergic reactions.
- **Sustainability:** Overharvesting has made wild cowslip less common. Cultivate sources responsibly.

Preparation Methods:
- **Edible Flowers:** Cowslip flowers are edible.
- **Teas & Infusions:** Relieves stress, promotes relaxation, and supports respiratory health.
- **Decoctions:** Addresses respiratory issues, soothes coughs, and reduces inflammation.
- **Tinctures:** Calms the nervous system, relieves headaches, and supports respiratory health.
- **Syrups:** Soothes coughs and eases throat irritation.
- **Salves & Balms:** Treats skin irritations, reduces inflammation, and promotes healing of wounds.
- **Poultices:** Reduces swelling, bruises, and inflammation.
- **Topical:** Calms skin irritations and minor wounds.

CUMIN

Latin: Cuminum cyminum

Vital Parts: Seeds
Harvest Season: Late Summer to Early Autumn

Description: Cumin is known for its digestive properties, helping to relieve bloating and indigestion.

Native: Cumin is native to the eastern Mediterranean and South Asia.

Cultivation: Cumin thrives in warm, dry climates with well-drained soil and full sun. It is cultivated for its seeds, which are used in cooking and herbal medicine.

Ancient Usage: Cumin, often known as the "spice of life," has been prized for its digestive and anti-inflammatory properties since ancient times. The Egyptians used it in both culinary and medicinal applications, particularly to aid digestion and boost immunity. In the Middle Ages, cumin was considered a symbol of love and loyalty, often carried during weddings to ensure fidelity. In traditional Ayurvedic and Middle Eastern medicine, cumin was used to support respiratory health and improve metabolism.

Medicinal Benefits:
- **Digestive Health:** Stimulates enzyme production and alleviates bloating,, gas, and indigestion.
- **Anti-Inflammatory:** Relieves arthritis and muscle pain.
- **Antimicrobial Properties:** Helps combat bacterial and fungal infections.
- **Antioxidant Support:** Neutralizes free radicals and protects cells from stress.
- **Blood Sugar Regulation:** Improves insulin sensitivity and helps regulate blood sugar levels.
- **Immune Boosting:** Contains antimicrobial and antioxidant properties.
- **Respiratory Health:** Helps clear congestion and soothes coughs.

Cumin is an annual herb that grows up to 1 to 2 feet tall, with slender, branching stems and finely divided, feathery leaves. The plant produces small, white or pale pink flowers arranged in delicate, umbrella-shaped clusters (umbels), and its seeds are narrow, elongated, and aromatic.

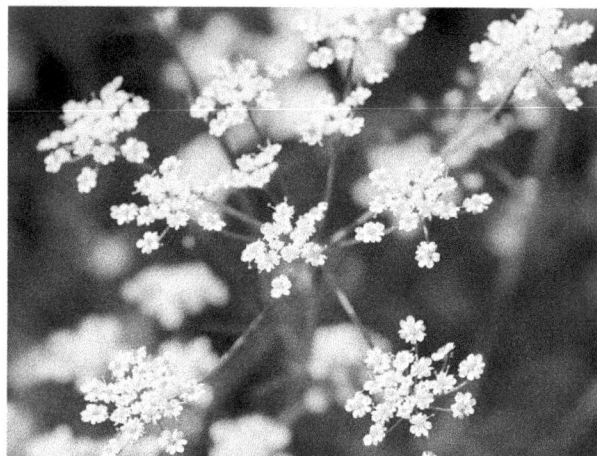

Dosage:
- **Standardized Extract:** 200-400 mg daily.
- **Tincture:** 2-4 mL (40-80 drops), up to 3 times daily.
- **Tea:** 1-2 tsp crushed seeds per cup of water, 2-3 times daily.
- **Capsules:** 500-1,000 mg of ground cumin, 1-2 times daily.

Safety:
- **Internal Use:** Excessive consumption may cause digestive upset.
- **Topical Use:** Cumin essential oil should be diluted before applying to the skin to avoid irritation.
- **Children:** Safe in food amounts.
- **Allergy Risk:** Individuals allergic to plants in the Apiaceae family (e.g., fennel, parsley) should use cautiously.

Preparation Methods:
- **Teas & Infusions:** Reduces bloating and enhances metabolism.
- **Decoctions:** Supports respiratory health, detoxification, and digestion.
- **Tinctures:** Promotes digestion, reduces inflammation, and enhances immunity.
- **Syrups:** Soothes sore throats, clears congestion, and supports respiratory health.
- **Salves & Balms:** Relieves muscle aches and joint pain.
- **Poultices:** Soothes inflamed skin, reduces swelling, and reduces abdominal discomfort.
- **Topical:** Alleviates muscle tension and bloating.

DANDELION

Latin: Taraxacum officinale

Vital Parts: Leaves, Roots, Flowers
Harvest Season: Spring to Early Autumn

Description: Dandelion is a well-known diuretic and detoxifier, traditionally used to support liver health, digestion, and kidney function. It is rich in vitamins and minerals and reduces inflammation.

Native: Dandelion is native to Europe and Asia but has naturalized worldwide.

Cultivation: Dandelions grow in a variety of soil types but prefer well-drained soil and full sun. Often considered a weed, dandelion is prized for its leaves, roots, and flowers.

Ancient Usage: Dandelion, sometimes called the "herb of the sun," has been used for centuries for its detoxifying and diuretic properties. Ancient Chinese and Arabic healers used dandelion to support liver health, reduce inflammation, and promote digestion. In medieval Europe, dandelion was valued for its ability to cleanse the blood and treat skin ailments. Folklore associated dandelions with wishes and renewal, with the seeds symbolizing the dispersal of hope and prosperity.

Dandelion is a hardy, perennial herb with a deep taproot and a rosette of toothed, lance-shaped green leaves. Its bright yellow flowers bloom on hollow stems and later transform into white, fluffy seed heads that disperse in the wind. The entire plant, including the roots, leaves, and flowers, is known for its detoxifying properties and nutritional value.

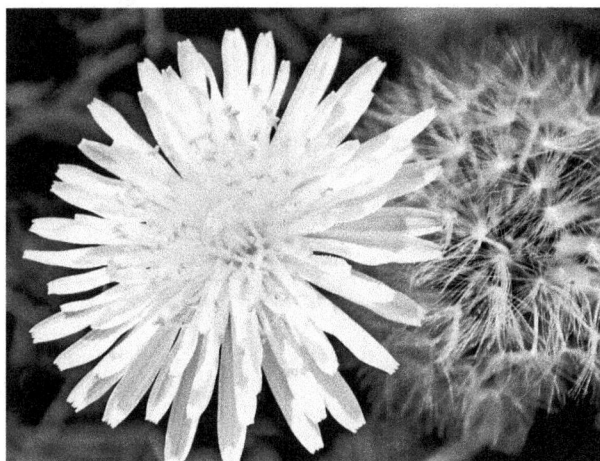

Medicinal Benefits:
- **Liver Support:** Stimulates bile production, aids detoxification, and supports digestion.
- **Digestive Aid:** Eases bloating, indigestion, and constipation.
- **Kidney Health:** Acts as a natural diuretic, encouraging urination and reducing water retention.
- **Anti-Inflammatory:** Supports arthritis and joint pain.
- **Blood Sugar Regulation:** Improves insulin sensitivity, which is beneficial for diabetes.
- **Skin Health:** Treats acne, eczema, and other skin conditions.
- **Heart Health:** Lowers cholesterol and blood pressure.
- **Immune Support:** Strengthens the immune system and combats stress.

Dosage:
- **Standardized Extract:** 300-600 mg daily.
- **Tincture:** 2-4 mL (40-80 drops), 2-3 times daily.
- **Tea:** 1-2 tsp of leaves or root per cup of water 2-3 times daily.
- **Capsules:** 500-1,000 mg of dried herb, 1-2 times daily.

Safety:
- **Internal Use:** Excessive use may cause mild stomach discomfort.
- **Drug Interactions:** May interact with diuretics, blood sugar-lowering medications, or anticoagulants.

Preparation Methods:
- **Edible Flowers:** Dandelion flowers are edible and can be added to dishes.
- **Teas & Infusions:** Supports digestion and liver detoxification and acts as a natural diuretic.
- **Decoctions:** Improves liver function, supports kidney health, and aids in detoxification.
- **Tinctures:** Supports digestion, reduces inflammation, and promotes vitality.
- **Syrups:** Soothes coughs and supports respiratory health.
- **Salves & Balms:** Relieves muscle aches, reduces joint inflammation, and soothes minor skin irritations.
- **Poultices:** Reduces swelling, soothes insect bites, and aids in wound healing.
- **Topical:** Soothes skin irritations and reduces inflammation.

DEVIL'S CLAW

Latin: *Harpagophytum procumbens*

Vital Parts: Roots (Tubers)
Harvest Season: Late Summer to Early Autumn

Description: Devil's Claw is valued for its anti-inflammatory and analgesic properties. It is commonly used to reduce pain and inflammation for arthritis, back pain, and muscle stiffness.

Native: Devil's Claw is native to the arid regions of southern Africa, particularly Namibia, Botswana, and South Africa.

Cultivation: Devil's Claw prefers sandy, well-drained soil and a warm, dry climate. Its tuberous roots are harvested for use in herbal medicine.

Ancient Usage: Devil's claw, often called the "root of relief," has been used for centuries in African traditional medicine to alleviate joint pain, inflammation, and digestive issues. Indigenous tribes valued it for its ability to treat arthritis and back pain. In European herbal medicine, it became popular in the 20th century as a natural remedy for chronic pain and rheumatic conditions. Folklore regarded the plant as a symbol of protection against harmful spirits, likely due to its claw-shaped seed pods.

Medicinal Benefits:

- **Anti-Inflammatory:**
  Supports arthritis, gout, and other joint disorders.
- **Pain Relief:** Provides natural analgesic effects for back pain, muscle aches, and headaches.
- **Digestive Health:**
  Stimulates appetite and eases bloating and indigestion.
- **Joint Mobility:** Supports flexibility and reduces stiffness, supporting osteoarthritis.
- **Wound Healing:** Promotes healing of skin wounds and reduces swelling.

Devil's claw is a low-growing, perennial herb with sprawling, vine-like stems and deeply lobed, grayish-green leaves. Its striking, claw-shaped seed pods give the plant its name, while the trumpet-shaped, pink to red-purple flowers bloom at the tips of the stems.

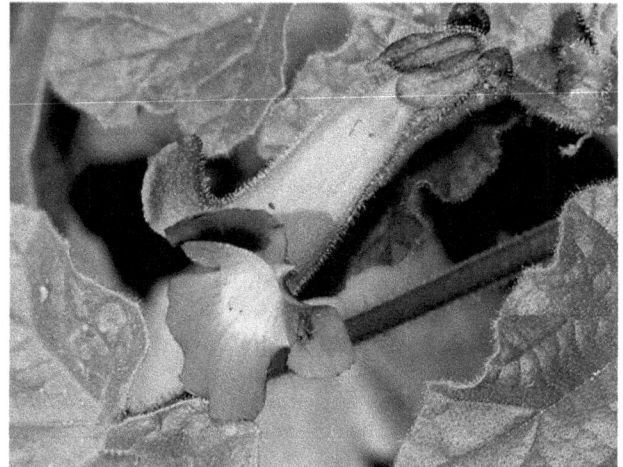

Dosage:
- **Standardized Extract:** 300-600 mg daily.
- **Tincture:** 2-4 mL (40-80 drops), up to 3 times daily.
- **Tea:** 1-2 tsp per cup of water, 2-3 times daily.
- **Capsules:** 500-1,000 mg of root powder, 1-2 times daily.

Safety:
- **Digestive Sensitivity:** May cause mild gastrointestinal discomfort.
- **Drug Interactions:** Use caution if taking anticoagulants or medications for heart conditions.

Preparation Methods:
- **Teas & Infusions:** Alleviates inflammation, supports joint health, and aids digestion.
- **Decoctions:** Addresses arthritis pain, reduces inflammation, and supports liver health.
- **Tinctures:** Devil's claw root is preserved in alcohol or glycerin to create a tincture that supports pain relief, enhances mobility, and aids in reducing inflammation.
- **Syrups:** Soothes inflammation-related discomfort.
- **Salves & Balms:** Relieves muscle pain, reduces joint swelling, and improves mobility.
- **Poultices:** Reduces inflammation, eases joint pain, and promotes healing.
- **Topical:** Relieves joint pain and inflammation.

ECHINACEA

Latin: Echinacea purpurea

Vital Parts: Roots, Leaves, Flowers
Harvest Season: Late Summer to Early Autumn

Description: Echinacea is renowned for its immune-boosting properties. It is commonly used to reduce the severity and duration of colds and flu.

Native: Echinacea is native to North America, particularly the prairies and woodlands of the central and eastern United States.

Cultivation: Echinacea thrives in well-drained, loamy soil and full sun. It is grown for its roots and aerial parts, which are prepared as teas, tinctures, and syrups.

Ancient Usage: Echinacea, sometimes referred to as the "immune herb," has been used by Native American tribes for its infection-fighting and wound-healing properties. Tribes such as the Lakota and Cheyenne used it to treat snakebites, fevers, and sore throats. European settlers adopted echinacea as a remedy for colds, flu, and skin infections. It became a staple in 19th-century American folk medicine as a general immune booster and protector against epidemics.

Medicinal Benefits:
- **Immune Support:** Reduces colds, flu, and other infections.
- **Anti-Inflammatory:** Aids sore throats, sinusitis, and skin irritations.
- **Wound Healing:** Promotes healing of cuts, scrapes, and burns.
- **Antimicrobial Properties:** Fights bacteria, viruses, and fungi.
- **Respiratory Health:** Relieves congestion, coughs, and bronchitis.
- **Lymphatic Support:** Promotes detoxification and reduces swelling in the lymph nodes.
- **Skin Health:** Treats acne and boils.

Echinacea is a hardy, perennial herb that can grow up to 4 feet tall, with rough, hairy stems and lance-shaped, dark green leaves. It produces large, daisy-like flowers with purple or pink petals surrounding a spiny, cone-shaped brownish-orange center.

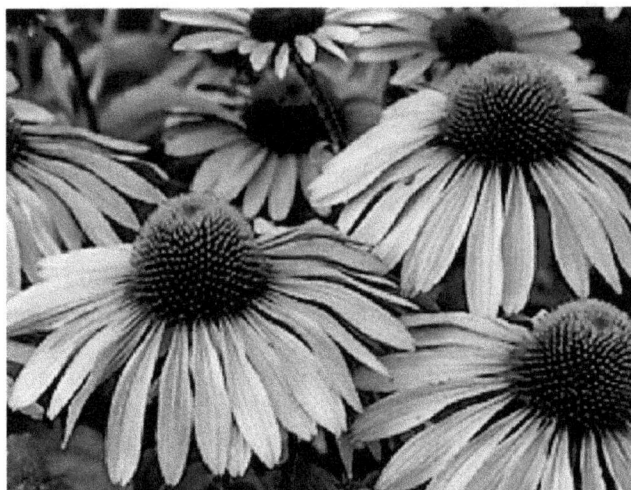

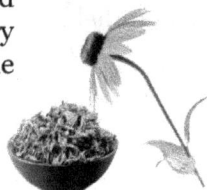

Dosage:
- **Standardized Extract:** 200-400 mg daily.
- **Tincture:** 2-4 mL (40-80 drops), 2-3 times daily.
- **Tea:** 1-2 tsp dried root or flowers per cup of water, 2-3 times daily.
- **Capsules:** 500-1,000 mg of dried herb, 1-2 times daily.

Safety:
- **Internal Use:** Prolonged use may cause mild stomach discomfort.
- **Allergic Reactions:** Individuals allergic to plants in the Asteraceae family (e.g., daisies, ragweed) should exercise caution.
- **Drug Interactions:** May interact with immunosuppressive medications.

Preparation Methods:
- **Edible Flowers:** Echinacea flowers are edible.
- **Teas & Infusions:** Boosts immunity and supports respiratory health.
- **Decoctions:** Enhances immune function, reduces cold symptoms, and supports overall wellness.
- **Tinctures:** Strengthens immunity and fights infections.
- **Syrups:** Soothes sore throats and calms coughs.
- **Salves & Balms:** Treats skin irritations and cuts.
- **Poultices:** Reduces swelling, soothes insect bites, and promotes healing of wounds.
- **Topical:** Promotes wound healing and reduces inflammation.

ELDER

Latin: *Sambucus nigra*

Vital Parts: Berries, Flowers
Harvest Season: Late Summer to Early Autumn

Description: Elder is best known for its antiviral and immune-supporting properties. It is commonly used to alleviate symptoms of colds, flu, and infections.

Native: Elder is native to Europe, North Africa, and parts of Asia but has naturalized in North America.

Cultivation: Elder prefers moist, well-drained soil and full to partial sun. Both the flowers and berries are used in herbal remedies, typically as syrups, tinctures, and teas to support immune health and reduce cold and flu symptoms.

Ancient Usage: Elder, often called the "medicine chest of the people," has been used in herbal medicine for its powerful immune-boosting and respiratory-supporting properties. Ancient Greek and Roman physicians, including Hippocrates, praised elder for treating colds, flu, and inflammation. In medieval Europe, elder was used to reduce fevers and relieve congestion. Folklore held that elder trees were sacred and offered protection, with a belief that harming an elder tree could bring misfortune.

Medicinal Benefits:
- **Immune Support:** Helps prevent colds and flu.
- **Respiratory Health:** Soothes congestion, sinusitis, bronchitis, and allergies.
- **Fever Reduction:** Promotes sweating to reduce fevers.
- **Anti-Inflammatory:** Beneficial for arthritis, sore throats, and skin irritations.
- **Digestive Aid:** Eases bloating, indigestion, and stomach upset.
- **Skin Health:** Soothes rashes, sunburn, and acne.
- **Detoxification:** Stimulates the kidneys.

Elder is a fast-growing, deciduous shrub or small tree that can reach up to 20 feet in height, with multiple stems and smooth, gray bark. Its compound leaves are composed of 5 to 11 lance-shaped, serrated leaflets. The plant produces clusters of small, creamy-white flowers, followed by dark purple or black berries

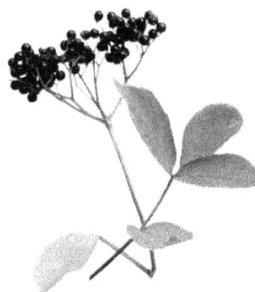

Dosage:
- **Standardized Extract:** 300-600 mg daily.
- **Tincture:** 2-4 mL (40-80 drops), 2-3 times daily.
- **Tea:** 1-2 tsp per cup of water, 2-3 times daily.
- **Syrup:** 1-2 tablespoons daily.
- **Capsules:** 500-1,000 mg of powder, 1-2 times daily.

Safety:
- **Internal Use:** Excessive consumption may cause gastrointestinal discomfort.
- **Allergic Reactions:** Individuals with sensitivities to plants in the Adoxaceae family should use cautiously.
- **Drug Interactions:** May interact with diuretics, blood sugar-lowering medications, or immunosuppressive drugs.

Preparation Methods:
- **Edible Flowers:** Elderflowers are edible and can be used raw.
- **Teas & Infusions:** Supports immunity, alleviates cold symptoms, and reduces fever.
- **Decoctions:** Boosts immunity, soothes respiratory discomfort, and reduces inflammation.
- **Tinctures:** Strengthens immunity, fights colds, and supports respiratory health.
- **Syrups:** Soothes sore throats, reduces cold duration, and boosts overall immunity.
- **Salves & Balms:** Treats minor skin irritations, promotes wound healing, and reduces inflammation.
- **Poultices:** Reduces swelling, soothes bruises, and promotes healing.
- **Topical:** Elder leaves and unripe berries should not be ingested due to their potential toxicity.

EPHEDRA

Latin: *Ephedra sinica*

Vital Parts: Stems
Harvest Season: Late Spring to Early Summer

Description: Ephedra is valued for its stimulant properties and ability to support respiratory and circulatory health. Traditionally, it has been used to alleviate asthma, allergies, and congestion. It is known to enhance energy and promote weight loss.

Native: Ephedra is native to arid and semi-arid regions of Asia, the Mediterranean, and parts of North and South America.

Cultivation: Ephedra thrives in dry, sandy, or rocky soils with excellent drainage and full sunlight. The stems are harvested and dried for use in herbal remedies.

Ancient Usage: Ephedra, often referred to as "ma huang" in traditional Chinese medicine, has a long history of use for respiratory health and energy enhancement. Ancient Chinese practitioners used it to treat asthma, bronchitis, and nasal congestion. In Ayurveda, it was valued for its ability to stimulate circulation. In Native American traditions, ephedra was used to alleviate colds, coughs, and fevers.

Ephedra is a low-growing, perennial shrub with a distinct, leafless appearance. It typically reaches heights of 1 to 4 feet and has slender, green, jointed stems that resemble twigs. The plant's leaves are small and scale-like, located at the nodes of the stems. Ephedra produces inconspicuous, yellowish-green flowers, followed by small, cone-like structures containing seeds.

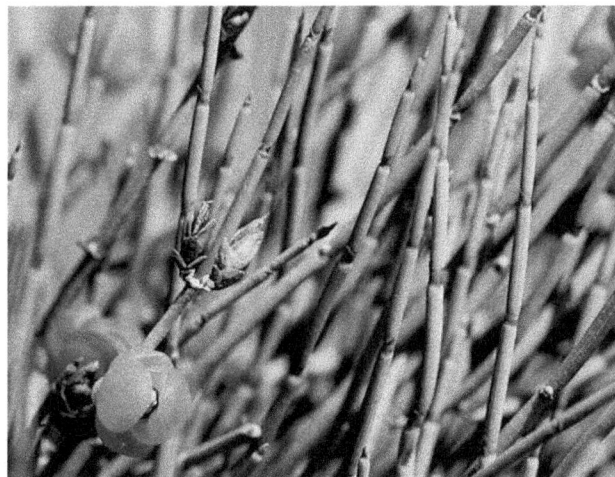

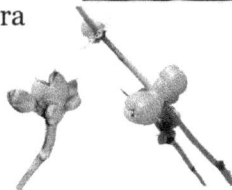

Medicinal Benefits:
- **Respiratory Health:** Relieves asthma, bronchitis, and congestion.
- **Energy Boost:** Improves energy and combats fatigue.
- **Weight Management:** Increases metabolism and supports weight loss efforts.
- **Circulatory Support:** Dilates blood vessels, helping with cold extremities.
- **Fever Reduction:** Promotes sweating to break fevers and detoxify the body.
- **Allergy Relief:** Eases symptoms of seasonal allergies and sinus congestion.

- **Tincture:** 0.5-1 mL (10-20 drops), up to 3 times daily.
- **Tea:** 1-2 grams per cup of water, up to 2 times daily.
- **Capsules:** 300-600 mg of powder, 1-2 times daily.

Safety:
- **Internal Use:** Ephedra contains potent alkaloids. Excessive use can cause rapid heart rate, high blood pressure, and anxiety.
- **Children:** Not recommended for children.
- **Drug Interactions:** May interact with stimulants, decongestants, and heart and blood pressure medications.

Preparation Methods:
- **Teas & Infusions:** Clears nasal congestion, eases breathing, and boosts energy.
- **Decoctions:** Supports severe respiratory issues, such as asthma or bronchitis.
- **Tinctures:** Supports respiratory health, enhances energy, and improves circulation.
- **Syrups:** Soothes coughs, clears congestion, and aids the respiratory system.
- **Salves & Balms:** Relieves muscle aches, joint pain, and inflammation.
- **Poultices:** Reduces swelling, soothes sore muscles, and relieves joint pain.

EUCALYPTUS

Latin: *Eucalyptus globulus*

Vital Parts: Leaves, Bark, Essential Oil
Harvest Season: Year-Round

Description: Eucalyptus is renowned for its antimicrobial and decongestant properties. It is used to relieve symptoms of respiratory infections, colds, and sinus congestion.

Native: Eucalyptus is native to Australia and surrounding islands, though it has been widely cultivated in subtropical and Mediterranean climates worldwide.

Cultivation: Eucalyptus prefers well-drained soil and full sunlight. The leaves are harvested for use in infusions, essential oils, and inhalation therapies.

Ancient Uses: Eucalyptus has been an essential part of traditional Aboriginal medicine in Australia for centuries. Aboriginal healers used eucalyptus leaves to treat wounds, reduce fevers, and relieve respiratory ailments. The leaves were crushed and inhaled to clear sinus congestion or used in steam baths for colds. Later, European settlers incorporated eucalyptus oil into remedies for coughs, sore throats, and infections. Its reputation earned it the nickname "fever tree."

Medicinal Benefits:
- **Respiratory Health:** Clears congestion, soothes coughs, and aids colds, bronchitis, asthma, and sinus infections.
- **Antimicrobial Properties:** Fights bacterial, viral, and fungal infections.
- **Pain Relief:** Eases muscle aches, joint pain, and headaches.
- **Immune Support:** Combats infections.
- **Skin Health:** Treats wounds, insect bites, and skin irritations.
- **Oral Health:** Freshens breath, reduces gum inflammation, and combats oral infections.
- **Mental Clarity:** Enhances focus, reduces mental fatigue, and promotes relaxation.

Eucalyptus is a fast-growing evergreen tree that can reach heights of over 200 feet in some species, with a straight trunk and smooth or peeling bark in shades of gray, brown, or cream. Its long, narrow, aromatic leaves are bluish-green and leathery in texture. The plant features clusters of small, white or cream-colored flowers with numerous stamens, followed by hard, woody fruit capsules known as gumnuts.

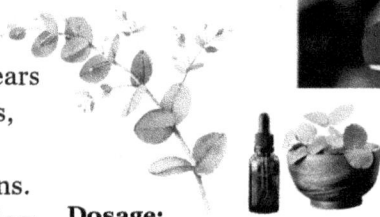

Dosage:
- **Essential Oil (Inhalation):** Add 5-10 drops to a bowl of hot water. Inhale steam for 5-10 minutes.
- **Tincture:** 2-4 mL (40-80 drops), up to 3 times daily.
- **Tea:** 1-2 tsp per cup of water, 2-3 times daily.
- **Capsules:** 300-500 mg powder daily.

Safety:
- **Internal Use:** Eucalyptus oil should never be ingested, as it is toxic.
- **Topical Use:** Undiluted oil may cause skin irritation.
- **Children:** Safe for older children for respiratory or topical support.
- **Drug Interactions:** May interact with diabetes and sedative medications.

Preparation Methods:
- **Teas & Infusions:** Relieves respiratory congestion, sore throats, and supports immunity.
- **Decoctions:** Clears sinuses, alleviates respiratory issues, and promotes relaxation.
- **Tinctures:** Supports respiratory health, reduces inflammation, and alleviates minor aches.
- **Syrups:** Soothes coughs and clears congestion.
- **Salves & Balms:** Relieves muscle aches, joint pain, and improves circulation.
- **Poultices:** Reduces swelling, soothes insect bites, and promotes wound healing.
- **Topical:** Essential oil is provides respiratory relief and muscle pain.

EVENING PRIMROSE

Latin: *Oenothera biennis*

Vital Parts: Seeds, Flowers, Leaves
Harvest Season: Late Summer to Early Autumn

Description: Evening primrose is known for its high content of gamma-linolenic acid (GLA), an essential fatty acid. It is commonly used to support hormonal balance, alleviate symptoms of PMS and menopause, and promote skin health.

Native: Evening primrose is native to North America but has spread to Europe and other temperate regions.

Cultivation: Evening primrose thrives in well-drained, sandy soil and full sun. Its seeds are harvested for oil, while the whole plant can be used in herbal medicine.

Ancient Usage: Evening primrose, sometimes called the "night bloom," has been used for centuries for its hormonal and skin-supporting properties. Native American tribes used the plant to promote wound healing, reduce inflammation, and ease menstrual pain. European herbalists adopted evening primrose in the 17th century, valuing its oil-rich seeds for relieving eczema, arthritis, and hormonal imbalances. Folklore associated the plant with renewal and feminine energy, symbolizing balance and healing for body and mind.

Evening primrose is a tall, biennial herb that grows up to 5 feet tall, with sturdy, reddish stems and lance-shaped leaves arranged alternately along the stem. It produces large, yellow, fragrant flowers that bloom in the evening and close by morning.

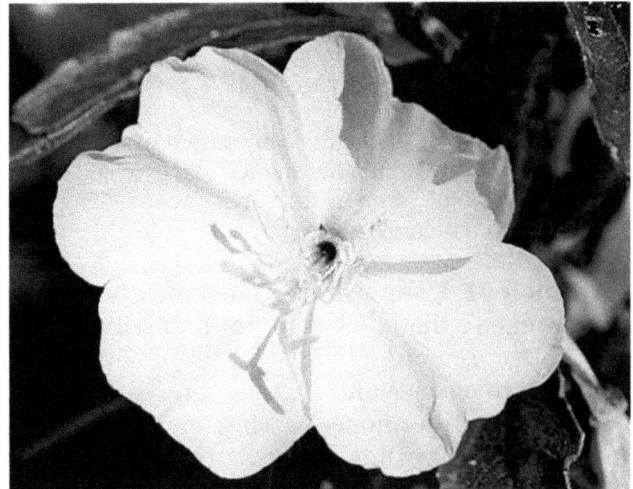

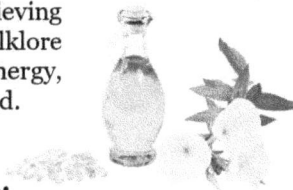

Medicinal Benefits:
- **Hormonal Balance:** Supports menopause and hormonal acne.
- **Skin Health:** Reduces inflammation and irritation for eczema, psoriasis, and dryness.
- **Anti-Inflammatory:** Eases joint pain and stiffness, supporting arthritis.
- **Hair & Scalp Health:** Encourages healthy hair growth and reduces dandruff.
- **Circulation Support:** Enhances blood flow and supports healthy blood pressure levels.
- **Wound Healing:** Promotes healing of minor wounds, scrapes, and cuts.

Dosage:
- **Standardized Extract:** 500-1,000 mg of oil daily.
- **Tincture:** 2-4 mL (40-80 drops), 2-3 times daily.
- **Capsules:** 500-1,000 mg of oil, 1-3 times daily.

Safety:
- **Internal Use:** High doses may cause headaches, nausea, or digestive upset.
- **Allergic Reactions:** People with allergies to plants in the Onagraceae family may experience skin sensitivity.
- **Drug Interactions:** May interact with blood thinners, antiplatelet medications, seizure medications, and drugs that affect hormones.

Preparation Methods:
- **Edible Flowers:** Evening primrose flowers are edible. They can be used raw in salads or as a garnish, adding a sweet flavor to dishes.
- **Teas & Infusions:** Supports hormonal balance, soothes menstrual discomfort, and promotes relaxation.
- **Decoctions:** Addresses skin conditions, supports digestion, and reduces inflammation.
- **Tinctures:** Aids in balancing hormones, soothing PMS symptoms, and promoting skin health.
- **Syrups:** Soothes coughs and supports respiratory health.
- **Salves & Balms:** Treats eczema, inflammation, and irritated skin.
- **Poultices:** Reduces swelling, soothes rashes, and promotes wound healing.
- **Topical:** Soothes dry skin, eczema, and inflammation.

FALSE UNICORN

Latin: *Chamaelirium luteum*

Vital Parts: Root and Rhizome
Harvest Season: Late Summer to Early Autumn

Description: False unicorn is valued for its hormone-regulating properties and is traditionally used to support reproductive health, particularly in women.

Native: False unicorn is native to the woodlands of eastern North America.

Cultivation: False unicorn prefers moist, rich, well-drained soil and partial shade. The root is used in herbal preparations, often as tinctures or capsules, to promote hormonal balance and reproductive health.

Ancient Usage: False unicorn, often called the "women's herb," has been traditionally used by Native American tribes for its ability to support reproductive health. It was particularly valued for balancing hormones, easing menstrual pain, and promoting fertility. Early European settlers learned of its use to treat conditions such as ovarian inflammation and infertility. In folklore, it was believed to enhance feminine vitality and offer protection for pregnancy.

False unicorn is a low-growing, perennial herb with a single, unbranched stem and long, narrow, lance-shaped leaves clustered near the base. The plant produces a tall flowering spike with small, star-shaped white or greenish flowers.

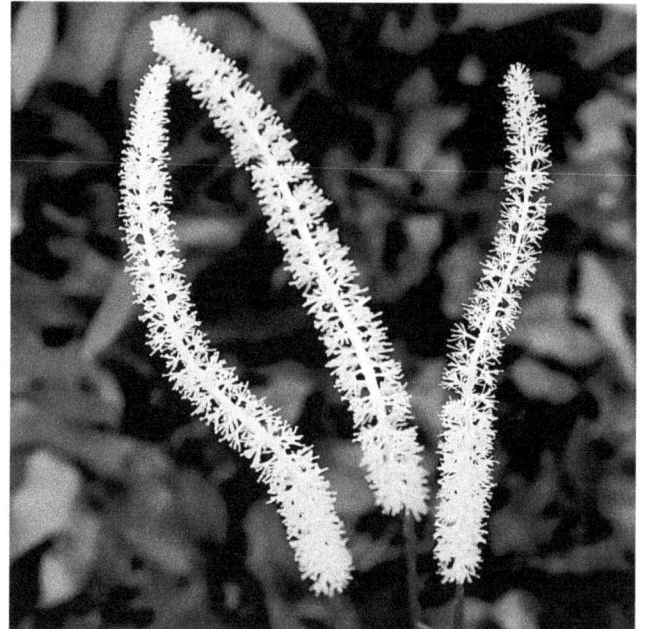

Medicinal Benefits:

- **Reproductive Health:** Balances hormones and supports menstrual issues.
- **Fertility Support:** Enhances uterine tone and function.
- **Ovarian Health:** Helps alleviate symptoms of ovarian cysts and polycystic ovary syndrome (PCOS).
- **Digestive Health:** Eases mild bloating, cramping, and nausea.
- **Urinary Health:** Reduces the risk of UTI and inflammation.
- **Endocrine Balance:** Believed to support overall hormonal balance.

Dosage:
- **Standardized Extract:** 200-400 mg daily.
- **Tincture:** 2-4 mL (40-80 drops), 2-3 times daily.
- **Capsules:** 500-1,000 mg of dried root, 1-2 times daily.
- **Tea:** 1-2 tsp of dried root per cup of water, 1-2 times daily.

Safety:
- **Internal Use:** Excessive use may lead to digestive discomfort.
- **Allergic Reactions:** Individuals sensitive to herbs in the Melanthiaceae family may experience reactions.
- **Drug Interactions:** May interact with hormonal medications.

Preparation Methods:
- **Teas & Infusions:** Supports reproductive health, balances hormones, and alleviates PMS.
- **Decoctions:** Supports kidney function and aids digestive health.
- **Tinctures:** Aids in balancing hormones, supporting uterine health, and menopausal issues.
- **Syrups:** Soothes coughs, supports vitality, and promotes fertility.
- **Salves & Balms:** Soothes skin irritations and promotes tissue repair.
- **Poultices:** Reduces swelling, and irritation.
- **Topical:** Addresses minor skin irritations and inflammation.

FENNEL

Latin: Foeniculum vulgare

Vital Parts: Bulb, Seeds, Leaves
Harvest Season: Late Summer to Early Autumn

Description: Fennel is widely used to aid digestion, reduce bloating and gas, and soothe colic. It has antimicrobial and anti-inflammatory properties and supports respiratory health by easing coughs and loosening mucus.

Native: Fennel is native to the Mediterranean region but is cultivated worldwide.

Cultivation: Fennel thrives in well-drained, fertile soil and full sun. Its seeds and leaves are used in herbal medicine.

Ancient Usage: Fennel, known as the "herb of vision," has been used since ancient times to support digestion, promote lactation, and improve respiratory health. The ancient Greeks and Romans believed fennel had protective properties, often using it to strengthen eyesight and purify the body. In medieval Europe, fennel was hung over doors to ward off evil spirits and protect homes. The seeds were also used to relieve bloating, gas, and colic, making fennel a staple in culinary and medicinal practices.

Fennel is a tall, aromatic, perennial herb that can grow up to 6 feet tall, with feathery, finely divided leaves and hollow, ribbed stems. It produces umbrella-shaped clusters (umbels) of small, yellow flowers.

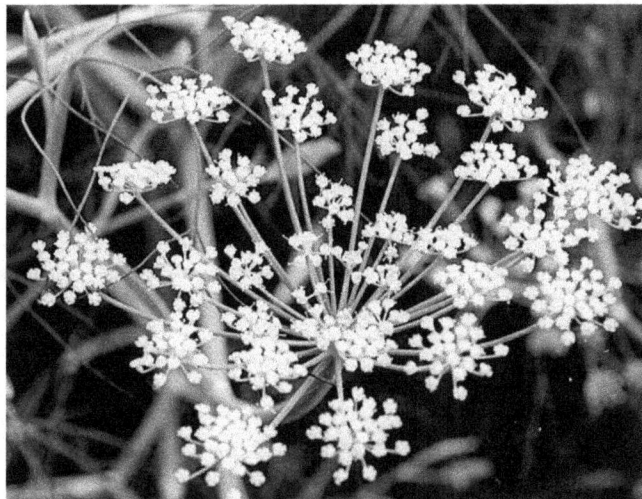

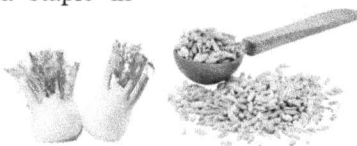

Medicinal Benefits:
- **Digestive Health:** Eases bloating and indigestion.
- **Colic Relief:** Alleviates colic and stomach cramps in infants and young children.
- **Respiratory Support:** Reduces mucus, coughs, colds, and bronchitis.
- **Hormonal Balance:** Regulates menstrual cycles and alleviates symptoms of PMS and menopause.
- **Lactation Support:** Promotes milk production in nursing mothers.
- **Anti-Inflammatory:** Supports the digestive and respiratory tracts.
- **Immune Support:** Contains antioxidants and antimicrobials
- **Appetite Stimulant:** Encourages healthy appetite and digestion.

Dosage:
- **Standardized Extract:** 300-600 mg daily.
- **Tincture:** 2-4 mL (40-80 drops), 2-3 times daily.
- **Tea:** 1-2 tsp of crushed seeds per cup of water, 2-3 times daily.
- **Capsules:** 500-1,000 mg of ground seeds, 1-2 times daily.

Safety:
- **Children:** Safe in small amounts for colic and digestive discomfort.
- **Allergy Risk:** Individuals allergic to the Apiaceae-family of plants (e.g., carrots, celery) should use cautiously.
- **Drug Interactions:** May interact with hormone and blood thinning medications.

Preparation Methods:
- **Edible Flowers:** Flowers are edible and used fresh.
- **Teas & Infusions:** Supports digestion and bloating.
- **Decoctions:** Addresses colic, soothes coughs, and promotes respiratory health.
- **Tinctures:** Aids in digestion, supports hormonal balance, and reduces inflammation.
- **Syrups:** Soothes sore throats, coughs, and digestive discomfort.
- **Salves & Balms:** Treats skin irritations, reduces inflammation, and improves circulation.
- **Poultices:** Reduces swelling, eases irritation, and promotes healing of minor wounds.
- **Topical:** Improves circulation and reduces bloating.

FENUGREEK

Latin: *Trigonella foenum-graecum*

Vital Parts: Seeds, Leaves
Harvest Season: Late Summer to Early Autumn

Description: Fenugreek is a herb known for its seeds, which are rich in protein, fiber, and minerals like iron and magnesium.

Native: Fenugreek is native to the Mediterranean region, Southern Europe, and parts of Asia. It is widely cultivated in many countries around the world due to its versatile uses.

Cultivation: Fenugreek thrives in well-drained soil with moderate moisture and plenty of sunlight. It is typically grown as an annual, and its seeds are harvested for various uses, including culinary and medicinal purposes. Fenugreek can be grown in a variety of soil types but prefers slightly alkaline conditions.

Ancient Usage: Fenugreek, often referred to as the "spice of strength," has been used in traditional Indian and Middle Eastern medicine to promote digestion, increase milk production in nursing mothers, and support hormonal balance. The ancient Egyptians used fenugreek seeds for embalming and as a remedy for respiratory ailments. In Ayurvedic medicine, it was valued for boosting energy, improving blood sugar control, and reducing inflammation.

Fenugreek is an annual herb that grows up to 2 feet tall, with erect, branching stems and trifoliate (three-part) leaves. It produces small, pale yellow flowers that develop into slender, curved pods containing hard, aromatic seeds.

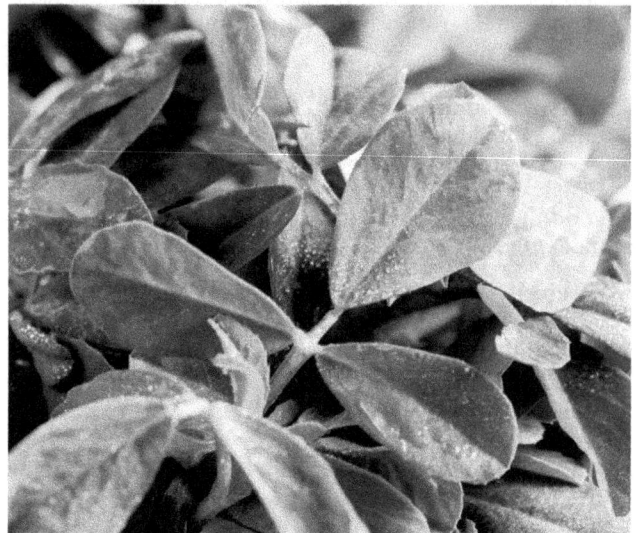

Medicinal Benefits:
- **Digestive Aid:** Relieves bloating, indigestion, and constipation.
- **Lactation Support:** Stimulates milk production in mothers.
- **Blood Sugar Regulation:** Improves insulin sensitivity, making it beneficial for diabetes.
- **Hormonal Balance:** Supports menstrual health and alleviates PMS.
- **Anti-Inflammatory:** Supports arthritis and muscle pain.
- **Heart Health:** Lowers cholesterol and triglycerides.
- **Appetite Stimulation:** Useful for recovery from illness.
- **Skin and Hair Health:** Reduces dandruff, and improves skin hydration and elasticity.

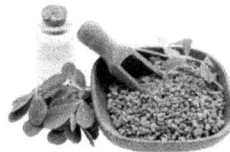

Dosage:
- **Standardized Extract:** 300-600 mg daily.
- **Tincture:** 2-4 mL (40-80 drops), 2-3 times daily.
- **Tea:** 1-2 tsp of seeds per cup of water, 2-3 times daily.
- **Capsules:** 500-1,000 mg of ground seeds, 1-2 times daily.

Safety:
- **Allergic Reactions:** Individuals allergic to legumes (pea family) should use caution.
- **Drug Interactions:** May enhance the effects of blood sugar-lowering and anticoagulant medications.

Preparation Methods:
- **Edible Flowers:** Fenugreek flowers are edible.
- **Teas & Infusions:** Supports digestion, balances blood sugar levels, and promotes lactation.
- **Decoctions:** Reduces inflammation and supports detoxification.
- **Tinctures:** Improves digestion and reduces inflammation.
- **Syrups:** Soothes sore throats, supports respiratory health, and alleviates digestive discomfort.
- **Salves & Balms:** Soothes skin irritations and supports healing.
- **Poultices:** Reduces joint pain and soothes irritated skin.
- **Topical:** Reduces swelling and eases muscle pain.

FIREBUSH

Latin: Hamelia patens

Vital Parts: Leaves, Flowers, Berries
Harvest Season: Year-Round in Tropical Climates

Description: Firebush is prized for its anti-inflammatory, antimicrobial, and wound-healing properties. Traditionally, it has been used to treat skin infections, inflammation, and digestive disorders.

Native: Firebush is native to tropical and subtropical regions of the Americas, including Florida and the Caribbean.

Cultivation: Firebush thrives in well-drained soil and full to partial sun. Its leaves and flowers are used in herbal remedies.

Ancient Usage: Firebush, sometimes known as "wildfire plant," has been used by indigenous cultures of Central and South America for its anti-inflammatory and wound-healing properties. Traditional healers also employed firebush to support immune health and reduce symptoms of respiratory infections. In folklore, the plant's vibrant red flowers symbolized strength and protection, with its fiery appearance believed to ward off negative energy.

Medicinal Benefits:
- **Anti-Inflammatory:** Aids arthritis, muscle pain, and skin irritations.
- **Wound Healing:** Speeds the healing of cuts, scrapes, and minor wounds.
- **Fever Reduction:** Reduces fevers and promotes sweating during illness.
- **Immune Support:** Defends against infections and illnesses.
- **Digestive Aid:** Relieves symptoms of diarrhea, stomach cramps, and indigestion.
- **Skin Health:** Treats rashes, insect bites, and other skin irritations.
- **Pain Relief:** Provides pain relief for minor injuries and headaches.

Firebush is a fast-growing, perennial shrub that can reach up to 10 feet tall, with slender, reddish-brown stems and elongated, lance-shaped green leaves. The plant is known for its vibrant, tubular orange to red flowers that attract hummingbirds and butterflies.

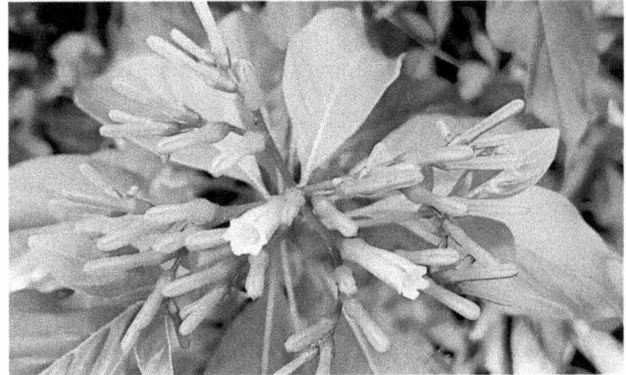

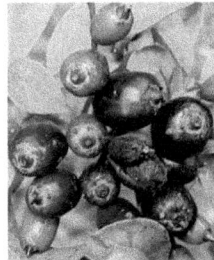

Dosage:
- **Standardized Extract:** 200-500 mg daily.
- **Tincture:** 2-4 mL (40-80 drops), 2-3 times daily.
- **Tea:** 1-2 tsp per cup of water, 2-3 times daily.

Safety:
- **Internal Use:** Overuse may cause mild stomach discomfort.
- **Children:** Safe for children in small for colic or digestive discomfort.
- **Allergy Risk:**
- Individuals who are allergic to plants in the Apiaceae family (e.g., carrots, celery, parsley) should use caution.
- **Drug Interactions:** May enhance hormone or blood-thinning medications.

Preparation Methods:
- **Edible Flowers:** Firebush flowers are edible and used raw.
- **Teas & Infusions:** Supports immune health, reduces inflammation, and alleviates digestive discomfort.
- **Decoctions:** Treats colds, soothes respiratory issues, and supports wound healing.
- **Tinctures:** Aids in reducing inflammation, supporting immune function, and promoting vitality.
- **Syrups:** Soothes coughs, calms sore throats, and supports respiratory health.
- **Salves & Balms:** Treats minor skin irritations, promotes wound healing, and reduces inflammation.
- **Poultices:** Applied directly to the skin to reduce swelling, soothe insect bites, and promote healing of wounds.

FRANKINCENSE

Latin: *Boswellia sacra*

Vital Parts: Resin

Harvest Season: Late Spring to Early Autumn

Description: Frankincense is renowned for its anti-inflammatory, immune-boosting, and stress-relieving properties.

Native: Frankincense is native to regions of the Arabian Peninsula, northeastern Africa, and parts of India.

Cultivation: Frankincense trees thrive in dry, rocky soil and arid climates. The resin is harvested and used in herbal medicine, often in the form of essential oils, tinctures, and incense to promote relaxation.

Ancient Usage: Frankincense, often called the "king of oils," has been revered for centuries for its spiritual and medicinal uses. Ancient Egyptians used it in sacred rituals, embalming practices, and to treat wounds and infections. In traditional Ayurvedic and Chinese medicine, frankincense was valued for reducing inflammation, improving circulation, and promoting respiratory health. Folklore associated it with purification and divine protection, often burned as incense to ward off negative energy and enhance meditation.

Frankincense is a slow-growing, drought-tolerant tree with multiple, twisting stems and papery, peeling bark. Its leaves are pinnate, with multiple small, oval leaflets clustered near the branch tips. The tree produces small, white to pale yellow flowers, but it is best known for its aromatic resin, harvested from cuts in the bark.

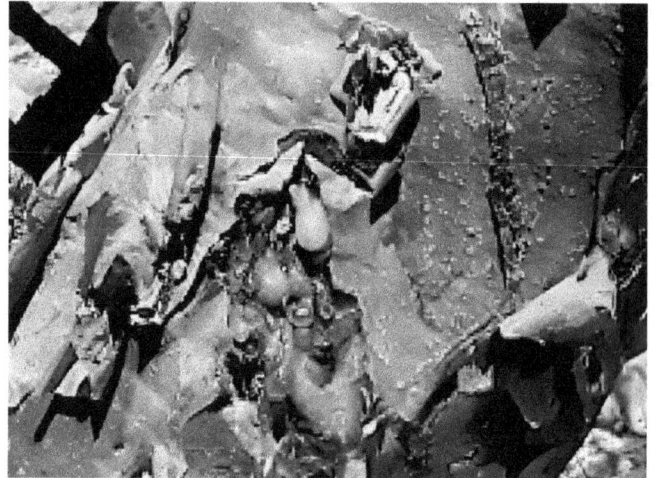

Medicinal Benefits:

- **Anti-Inflammatory:** Aids arthritis, asthma, and IBD.
- **Pain Relief:** Eases joint pain, muscle aches, and headaches.
- **Immune Support:** Helps the body fight bacterial, viral, and fungal infections.
- **Respiratory Health:** Aids bronchitis, asthma, and colds.
- **Digestive Health:** Reduces bloating, cramping, and inflammation.
- **Skin Health:** Treats wounds, scars, eczema, and acne.
- **Stress Relief:** Promotes relaxation and reduces anxiety for emotional balance and sleep.
- **Oral Health:** Reduces gum inflammation and bad breath.

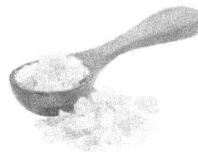

Dosage:

- **Standardized Extract:** 300-600 mg daily.
- **Tincture:** 2-4 mL (40-80 drops), 2-3 times daily.
- **Capsules:** 500-1,000 mg daily.
- **Tea:** 1-2 tsp per one cup of hot water, 1-2 times daily.

Safety:
- **Internal Use:** High doses may cause mild digestive upset.
- **Topical Use:** Undiluted essential oil may cause skin irritation.
- **Children:** Safe for older children for respiratory or skin issues.
- **Allergy Risk:** Those with sensitivities to resins should use cautiously.
- **Drug Interactions:** May interact with anticoagulants or medications for inflammation

Preparation Methods:

- **Teas & Infusions:** Supports digestion, promotes relaxation, and enhances respiratory health.
- **Decoctions:** Reduces inflammation, soothes respiratory discomfort, and supports immune health.
- **Tinctures:** Reduces inflammation and promotes joint health.
- **Syrups:** Soothes coughs and supports respiratory health.
- **Salves & Balms:** Reduces inflammation, soothes joint pain, and promotes skin rejuvenation.
- **Poultices:** Reduces swelling, promotes wound healing, and soothes irritated skin.
- **Topical Only:** Frankincense essential oil can be applied to the skin to promote healing but should not be ingested.

GARLIC

Latin: *Allium sativum*

Vital Parts: Bulbs, Cloves
Harvest Season: Late Summer to Autumn

Description: Garlic is valued for its potent antimicrobial, antioxidant, and cardiovascular-supporting properties.

Native: Garlic is native to Central Asia and northeastern Iran but has been cultivated worldwide.

Cultivation: Garlic grows best in well-drained, fertile soil with full sun. The bulbs are used in herbal medicine, often in the form of tinctures, capsules, or raw consumption.

Ancient Usage: Garlic, known as the "stinking rose," has been used for thousands of years for its powerful properties. Ancient Egyptians consumed it to enhance strength and endurance, particularly among laborers building the pyramids. In Greek and Roman medicine, garlic was used to treat infections and protect against disease. Folklore regarded garlic as a protector against evil spirits and vampires, with cloves often hung in homes for protection and healing.

Garlic is a hardy, perennial herb that grows up to 3 feet tall, with long, slender, green leaves and a bulb consisting of multiple cloves covered in papery skin. It produces small, white to pink flowers arranged in spherical clusters on tall, leafless stalks.

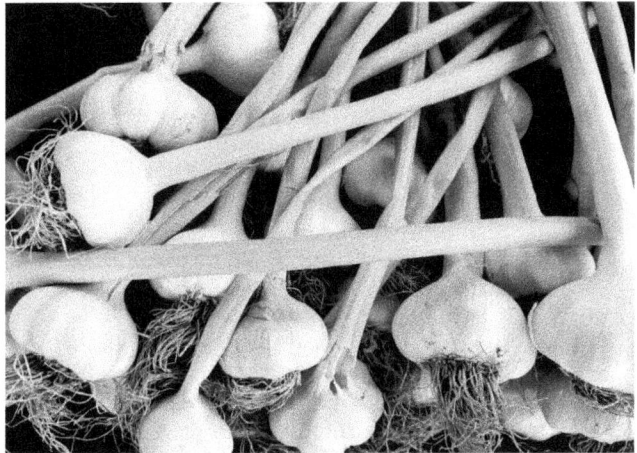

Medicinal Benefits:
- **Immune Support:** Fights colds, flu, and infections.
- **Antimicrobial Properties:** Exhibits antibacterial, antiviral, and antifungal effects.
- **Heart Health:** Lowers cholesterol levels, improves blood circulation, and reduces blood pressure.
- **Digestive Health:** Reduces bloating and combats harmful gut bacteria.
- **Anti-Inflammatory:** Reduces inflammation, benefiting arthritis.
- **Detoxification:** Aids in removing heavy metals and toxins from the body.
- **Blood Sugar Regulation:** Aids in diabetes and supports insulin resistance.
- **Antioxidant Properties:** Reduces the risk of chronic diseases.

Dosage:
- **Standardized Extract:** 300-600 mg of allicin daily.
- **Tincture:** 2-4 mL (40-80 drops), 2-3 times daily.
- **Capsules:** 500-1,000 mg of garlic powder, 1-2 times daily.
- **Raw:** 1-2 cloves daily.

Safety:
- **Internal Use:** Excessive use may cause stomach upset, heartburn, or bad breath.
- **Drug Interactions:** May enhance the effects of blood-thinning medications and lower blood pressure.

Preparation Methods:
- **Edible Flowers:** Garlic flowers, (scapes) are edible.
- **Teas & Infusions:** Supports immunity, improves circulation, and alleviates cold symptoms.
- **Decoctions:** Reduces inflammation, supports respiratory health, and addresses stomach discomfort.
- **Tinctures:** Promotes heart health, boosts immunity, and fights infections.
- **Syrups:** Soothes coughs, supports respiratory health, and boosts overall wellness.
- **Salves & Balms:** Treats fungal infections, reduces swelling, and soothes insect bites.
- **Poultices:** Reduces swelling, draws out infections, and promotes healing.

GENTIAN

Latin: Gentiana lutea

Vital Parts: Roots
Harvest Season: Late Summer to Early Autumn

Description: Gentian is renowned for its digestive-supporting properties. It is commonly used to stimulate appetite, improve digestion, and alleviate issues such as indigestion and bloating.

Native: Gentian is native to mountainous regions of Europe, Asia, and North and South America.

Cultivation: Gentian thrives in well-drained, slightly acidic soil and full to partial sun. It prefers cooler climates and is often found in alpine meadows. The roots are primarily used in herbal medicine.

Ancient Usage: Gentian, often referred to as the "bitter root," has been used since ancient times to support digestion and stimulate appetite. The plant was named after King Gentius of Illyria, who is said to have discovered its medicinal properties. Ancient Greek and Roman healers used gentian to treat fevers, digestive disorders, and wounds. In folklore, gentian was believed to strengthen both physical and spiritual endurance, symbolizing vitality and resilience.

Gentian is a perennial herb that can grow up to 4 feet tall, with erect, hollow stems and large, lance-shaped green leaves. The plant produces striking, trumpet-shaped flowers in shades of deep blue or purple. Its thick, bitter-tasting root has been traditionally used to stimulate digestion and appetite.

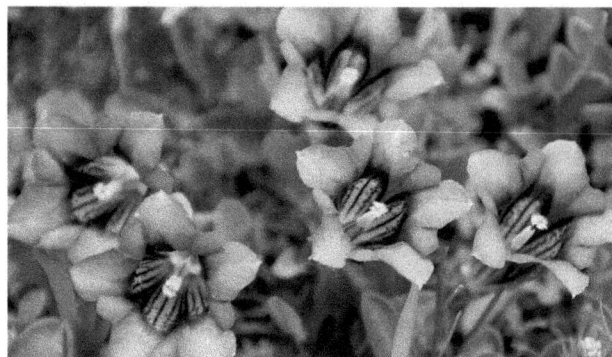

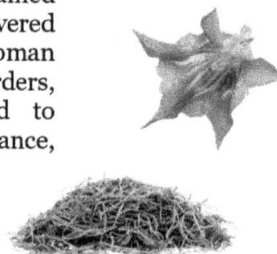

Medicinal Benefits:
- **Digestive Health:** Alleviates indigestion, bloating, and flatulence.
- **Appetite Stimulation:** Beneficial for those recovering from illness or low appetite.
- **Liver Health:** Supports liver function and detoxification.
- **Immune Support:** Promotes nutrient absorption and vitality.
- **Energy and Vitality:** Combats fatigue and improves energy.
- **Antimicrobial Properties:** Exhibits antibacterial and antifungal effects, aiding in the treatment of infections.
- **Fever Reduction:** Lowers fevers and promotes recovery during illnesses.

Dosage:
- **Standardized Extract:** 200-400 mg daily.
- **Tincture:** 2-4 mL (40-80 drops), 2-3 times daily.
- **Tea:** 1-2 tsp of dried root per cup of water, 2-3 times daily.
- **Capsules:** 500-1,000 mg of dried root, 1-2 times daily.

Safety:
- **Internal Use:** Excessive use may cause stomach irritation.
- **Drug Interactions:** May interact with medications for acid reflux or ulcers.
- **Allergy Risk:** Individuals with sensitivity to bitter herbs should use cautiously.

Preparation Methods:
- **Teas & Infusions:** Stimulates digestion, appetite, and aids liver health.
- **Decoctions:** Treats digestive complaints, supports detoxification, and boosts vitality.
- **Tinctures:** Supports digestion, appetite, and liver function.
- **Syrups:** Soothes digestive upset.
- **Salves & Balms:** Gentian root is rarely used in salves.
- **Poultices:** Reduces inflammation, soothes minor wounds, and supports healing.
- **Capsules & Powders:** Provides digestive support.

GINGER

Latin: *Zingiber officinale*

Vital Parts: Roots, Rhizomes
Harvest Season: Late Summer to Early Winter

Description: Ginger is well-known for its powerful digestive and anti-nausea properties. It is commonly used to alleviate nausea, motion sickness, and indigestion.

Native: Ginger is native to Southeast Asia and has been cultivated for thousands of years in tropical and subtropical regions worldwide.

Cultivation: Ginger thrives in warm, humid climates with well-drained, fertile soil and partial shade. The rhizomes (underground stems) are harvested for use in herbal medicine.

Ancient Usage: Ginger, sometimes called the "root of warmth," has been used for centuries to promote digestion, reduce nausea, and support circulation. Ancient Chinese and Indian healers valued ginger for its ability to balance the body's internal energy and relieve respiratory ailments. It was a key ingredient in Ayurvedic remedies to reduce inflammation and improve immunity.

Ginger is a tropical herb that grows up to 3 feet tall, with upright, reed-like stems and long, narrow, lance-shaped leaves. Its small, yellow-green flowers with purple accents grow on short spikes near the base of the plant.

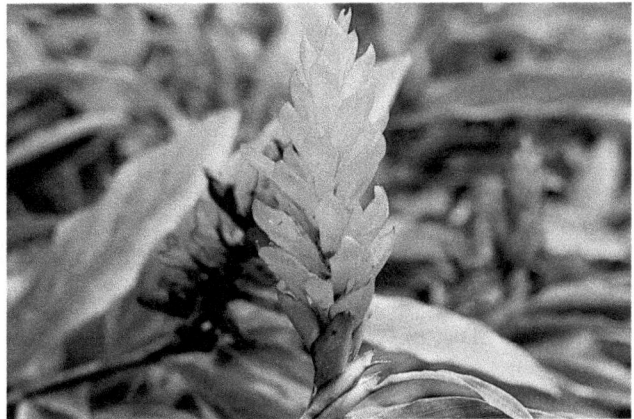

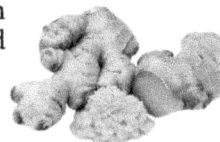

Medicinal Benefits:
- **Digestive Aid:** Relieves nausea, indigestion, and bloating.
- **Anti-Inflammatory:** Beneficial for arthritis, joint pain, and soreness.
- **Nausea Relief:** Eases morning and motion sickness.
- **Immune Support:** Aids colds, flu, and respiratory infections.
- **Pain Relief:** Alleviates cramps, headaches, and muscle pain.
- **Heart Health:** Improves circulation and reduces cholesterol.
- **Blood Sugar Regulation:** Beneficial for managing diabetes.
- **Antioxidant Properties:** Aids stress and anxiety.

Dosage:
- **Standardized Extract:** 300-600 mg daily.
- **Tincture:** 2-4 mL (40-80 drops), 2-3 times daily.
- **Tea:** 1-2 tsp per cup of water, 2-3 times daily.
- **Capsules:** 500-1,000 mg of dried ginger, 1-2 times daily.

Safety:
- **Topical Use:** Direct application may cause irritation.
- **Internal Use:** High doses may cause heartburn, diarrhea, or stomach upset.
- **Drug Interactions:** May enhance the effects of blood-thinning medications and lower blood sugar.

Preparation Methods:
- **Edible Flowers:** Ginger flowers are edible.
- **Teas & Infusions:** Relieves nausea, supports digestion, and boosts immunity.
- **Decoctions:** Alleviates colds, soothes sore throats, and reduces inflammation.
- **Tinctures:** Aids in digestion, supports circulation, and relieves joint pain.
- **Syrups:** Soothes coughs, calms sore throats, and promotes respiratory health.
- **Salves & Balms:** Relieves muscle pain, reduces inflammation, and improves circulation.
- **Poultices:** Reduces swelling, eases joint pain, and promotes healing of muscles.

GINKGO BILOBA

Latin: Ginkgo biloba

Vital Parts: Leaves, Seeds
Harvest Season: Late Summer to Early Autumn

Description: Ginkgo biloba is renowned for its ability to support cognitive function and improve circulation. It is often used to enhance memory, concentration, and mental clarity.

Native: Ginkgo biloba is native to China and is considered one of the oldest living tree species on Earth.

Cultivation: Ginkgo thrives in well-drained soil and full sun. It is highly adaptable and can tolerate urban environments. The leaves are harvested and used in herbal medicine.

Ancient Usage: Ginkgo biloba, often called the "living fossil," has been used for thousands of years in traditional Chinese medicine to enhance memory, improve circulation, and support brain health. Ancient healers believed it could strengthen the mind and promote longevity. Ginkgo was also used to treat asthma and bronchitis. Folklore associated the ginkgo tree with resilience and protection, with its leaves symbolizing endurance and vitality.

Ginkgo biloba is a large, deciduous tree that can reach over 100 feet in height, with a straight trunk and fan-shaped, bright green leaves that turn golden yellow in the fall. It produces small, inconspicuous flowers, with female trees developing fleshy, foul-smelling fruits containing seeds.

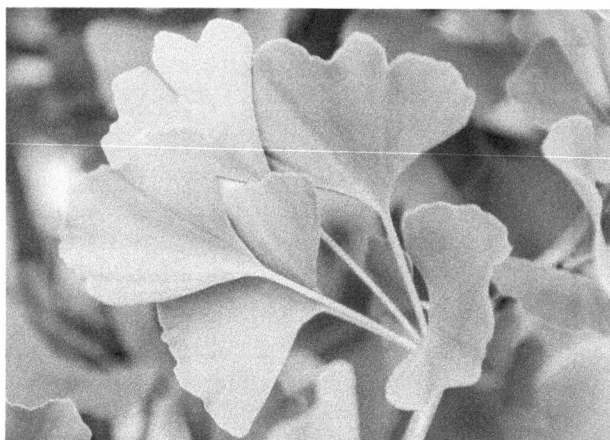

Medicinal Benefits:
- **Cognitive Support:** Improves memory, focus, and mental clarity. Aids in Alzheimer's disease and dementia.
- **Circulatory Health:** Aids in circulation and peripheral artery disease.
- **Antioxidant Properties:** Reduces the risk of chronic health conditions.
- **Mood Support:** Helps alleviate symptoms of anxiety, depression, and stress.
- **Eye Health:** Reduces the risk of age-related macular degeneration.
- **Anti-Inflammatory:** Reduces swelling in the brain and joints, and aids in arthritis and headaches.
- **Tinnitus Relief:** Helps reduce ringing in the ears caused by circulatory issues.

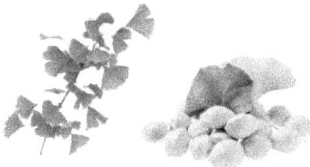

Dosage:
- **Standardized Extract:** 120-240 mg daily.
- **Tincture:** 2-4 mL (40-80 drops), 2-3 times daily.
- **Capsules:** 500-1,000 mg, 1-2 times daily.
- **Tea:** 1-2 tsp per cup of water, 1-2 times daily.

Safety:
- **Internal Use:** High doses may cause nausea, dizziness, or headaches.
- **Children:** Not recommended for young children.
- **Allergy Risk:** Those sensitive to ginkgo or related plants should test a small amount before use.

Preparation Methods:
- **Teas & Infusions:** Supports cognitive health, improves circulation, and reduces symptoms of anxiety.
- **Decoctions:** Enhances memory, supports blood flow, and reduces inflammation.
- **Tinctures:** Aids in improving brain function, reduces symptoms of dizziness, and promotes vascular health.
- **Syrups:** Supports respiratory health, promotes mental clarity, and boosts overall wellness.
- **Salves & Balms:** Reduces inflammation, soothes skin irritations, and improves circulation.
- **Poultices:** Reduces swelling, soothes irritation, and supports wound healing.
- **Topical:** Use caution with topical applications to avoid irritation.

GINSENG

Latin: *Panax ginseng*

Parts: Roots
Harvest Season: Autumn

Description: Ginseng is valued for its adaptogenic properties, helping the body manage stress and improve energy, stamina, and immune function. It is used to boost mental performance, physical endurance, and vitality.

Native: Panax ginseng is native to East Asia (China and Korea), while Panax quinquefolius (American ginseng) is native to North America.

Cultivation: Ginseng prefers cool, shaded environments with rich, well-drained soil. It is a slow-growing plant, with roots harvested after several years of growth.

Ancient Usage: Ginseng, known as the "root of life," has been revered in East Asian medicine for its adaptogenic and revitalizing properties. Ancient Chinese herbalists used it to increase energy, improve focus, and support the immune system. It was also valued for promoting longevity. In folklore, ginseng was believed to restore both physical and spiritual balance, often regarded as a symbol of health and vitality.

Medicinal Benefits:
- **Energy and Stamina:** Boosts physical and mental energy, reduces fatigue, and enhances endurance.
- **Cognitive Support:** Improves focus, memory, and mental clarity.
- **Immune Support:** Helps the body combat infections and illnesses.
- **Stress Relief:** Helps the body cope with physical, emotional, and environmental stressors.
- **Blood Sugar Regulation:** Beneficial for individuals with diabetes and metabolic syndrome.
- **Anti-Inflammatory:** Aids in arthritis and chronic pain.
- **Heart Health:** Improves circulation and regulates blood pressure.
- **Sexual Health:** Enhances libido and improves erectile dysfunction.

Ginseng is a slow-growing perennial herb with a single, unbranched stem and compound leaves made up of five serrated leaflets. The plant grows up to 60 cm (24 inches) tall and produces small, greenish-white flowers in umbels, which develop into bright red berries. Its thick, pale, gnarled root is highly valued for its medicinal uses.

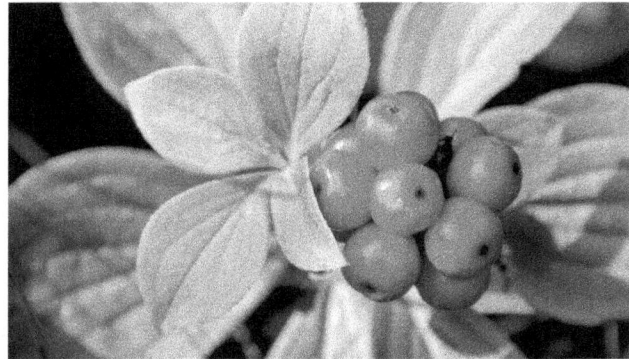

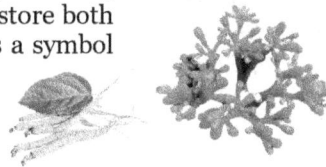

Dosage:
- **Standardized Extract:** 200-400 mg daily.
- **Tincture:** 2-4 mL (40-80 drops), 2-3 times daily.
- **Capsules:** 500-1,000 mg of dried root, 1-2 times daily.
- **Tea:** 1-2 tsp of dried root per cup of water, 1-2 times daily.

Safety:
- **Internal Use:** High doses or prolonged use may cause headaches.
- **Children:** Not recommended for young children.
- **Allergy Risk:** Those with sensitivities to ginseng or related plants should use cautiously.
- **Drug Interactions:** May interact with anticoagulants, diabetes medications, or stimulants.

Preparation Methods:
- **Edible Flowers:** Ginseng flowers are edible.
- **Teas & Infusions:** Boosts energy, supports immune health, and enhances mental clarity.
- **Decoctions:** Improves vitality and reduces fatigue.
- **Tinctures:** Aids in reducing stress, improving focus, and promoting immune function.
- **Syrups:** Boosts energy, supports respiratory health, and enhances endurance.
- **Salves & Balms:** Promotes skin rejuvenation, reduces inflammation, and improves circulation.
- **Poultices:** Aids swelling, irritation, and healing of wounds.
- **Topical:** Dilute ginseng in a carrier oil before application.

GOLDENROD

Latin: Solidago canadensis

Vital Parts: Flowers, Leaves, Stems
Harvest Season: Late Summer to Early Autumn

Description: Goldenrod is known for its diuretic and anti-inflammatory properties. It is commonly used to support kidney and urinary tract health, reduce inflammation, and alleviate seasonal allergies.

Native: Goldenrod is native to North America and parts of Europe, commonly found in meadows, prairies, and open fields.

Cultivation: Goldenrod thrives in well-drained, moderately fertile soil and full sun. It is drought-tolerant and often grown in wildflower gardens. The aerial parts (flowers and leaves) are used in herbal medicine.

Ancient Usage: Goldenrod, sometimes called the "sunbeam herb," has been used for centuries to support kidney health and reduce inflammation. Native American tribes used goldenrod to treat wounds, sore throats, and urinary infections. In European herbal medicine, it was valued for promoting detoxification and relieving seasonal allergies. Folklore connected goldenrod with good fortune, often believing that its appearance could indicate hidden treasures or positive changes ahead.

Medicinal Benefits:
- **Urinary Health:** Acts as a natural diuretic, flushing out toxins - alleviating UTIs and kidney stones.
- **Anti-Inflammatory:** Aids arthritis and gout.
- **Respiratory Support:** Eases symptoms of colds, allergies, and sinus congestion by reducing mucus and calming inflammation.
- **Digestive Health:** Soothes gastrointestinal inflammation and helps alleviate bloating and cramping.
- **Skin Health:** Treats minor wounds, burns, and skin irritations by promoting healing.
- **Immune Support:** Helps the body fight infections.
- **Detoxification:** Supports kidney and liver health.

Goldenrod is a tall, upright perennial herb that can grow up to 180 cm (6 feet) tall, with slender, branching stems and narrow, lance-shaped leaves. It produces dense clusters of small, bright yellow flowers arranged in plume-like spikes. The plant is commonly found in open fields and meadows.

Dosage:
- **Standardized Extract:** 200-500 mg daily.
- **Tincture:** 2-4 mL (40-80 drops), 2-3 times daily.
- **Tea:** 1-2 tsp per cup of water, 2-3 times daily.
- **Capsules:** 500-1,000 mg of dried herb, 1-2 times daily.

Safety:
- **Children:** Safe in small amounts for older children for respiratory and urinary support.
- **Allergy Risk:** Individuals allergic to plants in the Asteraceae family (e.g., daisies) should use cautiously.
- **Drug Interactions:** May enhance the effects of diuretics or blood pressure medications.

Preparation Methods:
- **Edible Flowers:** Goldenrod flowers are edible.
- **Teas & Infusions:** Supports urinary health, reduces inflammation, and alleviates seasonal allergies.
- **Decoctions:** Addresses respiratory issues, soothes sore throats, and promotes kidney health.
- **Tinctures:** Aids in reducing inflammation, supporting urinary tract health, and alleviating allergies.
- **Syrups:** Soothes coughs and respiratory discomfort.
- **Salves & Balms:** Relieves pain, inflammation. and skin irritations.
- **Poultices:** Reduces swelling, soothes bruises, and promotes wound healing.

GOTU KOLA

Latin: Centella asiatica

Vital Parts: Leaves, Stems
Harvest Season: Late Spring to Early Autumn

Description: Gotu kola is celebrated for its ability to support brain health, promote wound healing, and improve circulation.

Native: Gotu kola is native to tropical and subtropical regions of Asia, including India and Sri Lanka, and has been used in Ayurvedic and traditional Chinese medicine for centuries.

Cultivation: Gotu kola thrives in moist, well-drained soil and partial shade. It is often grown in tropical and subtropical climates. The leaves are harvested and used in herbal medicine, typically in teas and tinctures.

Ancient Usage: Gotu kola, often called the "herb of longevity," has been used in traditional Ayurvedic and Chinese medicine for its ability to enhance memory, promote mental clarity, and support wound healing. Ancient healers used it to improve circulation and treat skin conditions like eczema and psoriasis. In Southeast Asian folklore, it was believed to promote a long life, with stories of sages consuming gotu kola to extend their vitality and spiritual well-being.

Gotu kola is a low-growing, creeping perennial herb with slender, green stems and fan-shaped, rounded leaves with scalloped edges. The plant typically grows close to the ground, spreading horizontally. It produces small, pink to reddish flowers in clusters near the leaf bases.

Medicinal Benefits:
- **Cognitive Support:** Enhances memory, focus, and clarity.
- **Skin Health:** Aids in wound healing, reduces scarring, and improves skin elasticity.
- **Circulatory Health:** Improves blood flow and helps manage varicose veins.
- **Anti-Inflammatory:** Aids in arthritis and eczema.
- **Digestive Health:** Soothes inflammation, alleviating symptoms of gastritis.
- **Immune Support:** Aids in detoxification, helps fight infections, and promotes overall well-being.
- **Energy and Vitality:** Enhances physical and mental stamina while reducing fatigue.

Dosage:
- **Standardized Extract:** 200-500 mg daily.
- **Tincture:** 2-4 mL (40-80 drops), 2-3 times daily.
- **Tea:** 1-2 tsp per cup of water, 2-3 times daily.
- **Capsules:** 500-1,000, 1-2 times daily.

Safety:
- **Internal Use:** High doses may cause headaches.
- **Children:** Safe in small amounts for older children for skin conditions and cognitive support.
- **Allergy Risk:** Individuals with sensitivities to gotu kola or related plants should test a small amount before use.
- **Drug Interactions:** May interact with sedatives, diuretics, or blood sugar-lowering medications.

Preparation Methods:
- **Edible Flowers:** Gotu kola flowers are edible.
- **Teas & Infusions:** Supports cognitive health, reduces stress, and promotes circulation.
- **Decoctions:** Supports wound healing and improves blood flow.
- **Tinctures:** Aids in enhancing memory, reducing anxiety, and supporting skin repair.
- **Syrups:** Supports immune health, calms the nervous system, and promotes wellness.
- **Salves & Balms:** Reduces inflammation, improves circulation, and promotes the healing wounds and scars.
- **Poultices:** Reduces swelling, and irritation, and supports wound healing.

HAWTHORN

Latin: *Crataegus monogyna*

Vital Parts: Berries, Leaves, Flowers
Harvest Season: Late Summer to Early Autumn

Description: Hawthorn is renowned for its heart-supporting properties. It is commonly used to promote cardiovascular health by improving circulation, regulating blood pressure, and strengthening the heart muscle.

Native: Hawthorn is native to Europe, North America, and parts of Asia.

Cultivation: Hawthorn thrives in well-drained soil and full sun to partial shade. The berries, leaves, and flowers are used in herbal medicine, often as teas, tinctures, and capsules to support heart health and reduce anxiety.

Ancient Usage: Hawthorn, sometimes known as the "heart herb," has been used in European herbal medicine for centuries to support cardiovascular health. Ancient Greek and Roman healers used hawthorn berries to strengthen the heart, improve circulation, and reduce high blood pressure. In medieval folklore, hawthorn was considered a protective plant believed to guard homes, often associated with fairies and magical boundaries symbolizing hope and renewal.

Medicinal Benefits:
- **Heart Health:** Improves circulation, high blood pressure, angina, and congestive heart failure (CHF).
- **Blood Pressure Regulation:** Helps normalize blood pressure.
- **Antioxidant Properties:** Reduces the risk of chronic conditions.
- **Digestive Health:** Soothes mild digestive issues, including bloating and indigestion.
- **Stress and Anxiety Relief:** Calms the nervous system and reduces stress and anxiety.
- **Anti-Inflammatory:** Reduces inflammation in the cardiovascular system and other parts of the body.
- **Immune Support:** Boosts immunity with its antioxidant-rich profile.

Hawthorn is a dense, deciduous shrub or small tree that can grow up to 7.5 meters (25 feet) tall, with thorny branches and small, deeply lobed green leaves. It produces clusters of white to pale pink flowers in spring, followed by bright red, berry-like fruits known as haws.

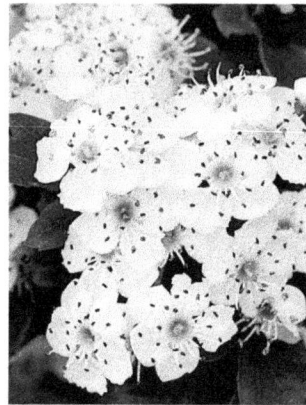

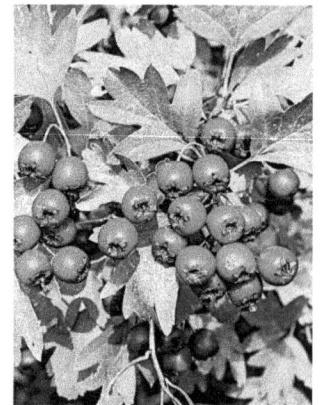

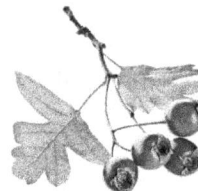

Dosage:
- **Standardized Extract:** 300-600 mg daily.
- **Tincture:** 2-4 mL (40-80 drops), 2-3 times daily.
- **Tea:** 1-2 tsp per cup of water, 2-3 times daily.
- **Capsules:** 500-1,000 mg of dried herb, 1-2 times daily.

Safety:
- **Internal Use:** High doses may cause digestive upset.
- **Children:** Safe for older children for mild digestive issues.
- **Allergy Risk:** Those with sensitivities to Rosaceae-family plants (e.g., apples, cherries) should use cautiously.
- **Drug Interactions:** May interact with medications for blood pressure, heart conditions, or anticoagulants.

Preparation Methods:
- **Edible Flowers:** Hawthorn flowers are edible.
- **Teas & Infusions:** Supports heart health, improves circulation, and reduces stress.
- **Decoctions:** Strengthens the cardiovascular system, reduces inflammation, and supports digestion.
- **Tinctures:** Aids in regulating blood pressure, improving heart function, and reducing anxiety.
- **Syrups:** Supports respiratory health, boosts immunity, and promotes cardiovascular wellness.
- **Salves & Balms:** Reduces inflammation, improves circulation, and soothes skin.
- **Poultices:** Reduces swelling, bruises, and promotes healing.

HIBISCUS

Latin: Hibiscus sabdariffa

Vital Parts: Flowers, Calyces, Leaves
Harvest Season: Late Summer to Early Fall

Description: Hibiscus is known for its ability to lower blood pressure, support cardiovascular health, and promote hydration. It is rich in antioxidants and vitamin C, making it beneficial for immune support.

Native: Hibiscus is native to tropical and subtropical regions of Africa and Asia.

Cultivation: Hibiscus prefers warm, humid climates with well-drained soil and full sun. The calyces (outer flower parts) are harvested and used in herbal medicine, typically prepared as teas and infusions.

Ancient Usage: Hibiscus, often referred to as the "flower of beauty," has been valued in traditional medicine for its ability to support heart health, lower blood pressure, and improve digestion. Ancient Egyptians used hibiscus to cool the body, relieve fever, and promote hydration. In Ayurvedic medicine, hibiscus flowers were used to nourish the skin and hair and balance hormones. Folklore saw hibiscus as a symbol of passion and strength, with its vibrant flowers often featured in ceremonies and offerings.

Hibiscus is a large, bushy perennial plant that can grow up to 2.5 meters (8 feet) tall, with sturdy, woody stems and broad, heart-shaped leaves with serrated edges. It produces large, showy flowers in a variety of colors, including red, pink, and yellow, with a prominent central stamen.

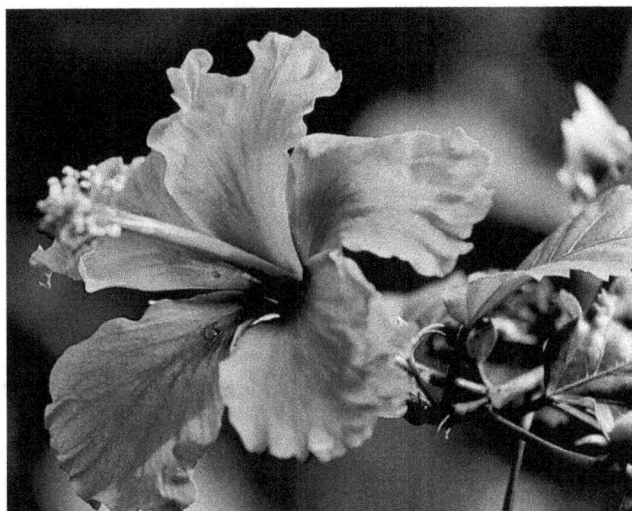

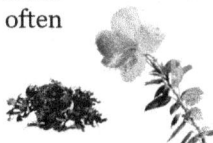

Medicinal Benefits:

- **Heart Health:** Lowers blood pressure and cholesterol.
- **Antioxidant Properties:** Rich in vitamin C, it combats oxidative stress and boosts immunity.
- **Weight Management:** Regulates metabolism and supports fat loss.
- **Digestive Aid:** Eases indigestion, relieves constipation, and promotes regularity.
- **Liver Health:** Enhances liver detoxification and function.
- **Anti-Inflammatory:** Aids joint and tissue health.
- **Skin Health:** Hydrates and rejuvenates the skin; combats signs of aging.

Dosage:

- **Standardized Extract:** 200-500 mg daily.
- **Tincture:** 2-4 mL (40-80 drops), 2-3 times daily .
- **Tea:** 1-2 tsp of dried flowers per cup of water, 2-3 times daily.
- **Capsules:** 500-1,000 mg, 1-2 times daily.

Safety:
- **Internal Use:** Excessive consumption may lower blood pressure.
- **Children:** Safe for children to boost immunity.
- **Drug Interactions:** May interact with blood pressure and diuretic medications.

Preparation Methods:

- **Edible Flowers:** Hibiscus flowers are edible and have a tart, cranberry flavor.
- **Teas & Infusions:** Supports immune health, aids digestion, and promotes hydration.
- **Decoctions:** Rich in antioxidants, helps regulate blood pressure, and reduces inflammation.
- **Tinctures:** Supports cardiovascular health, enhances circulation, and aids in **stress relief.**
- **Syrups:** Boosts immunity, soothes sore throats, and provides a vitamin C-rich tonic.
- **Salves & Balms:** Soothes irritated skin, reduces inflammation, and hydrates dry skin.
- **Poultices:** Helps cool the skin, reduces swelling, and soothes minor burns and insect bites.

HOLY BASIL

Latin: Ocimum sanctum

Vital Parts: Leaves, Flowers, Stems
Harvest Season: Late Spring to Early Autumn

Description: Holy basil, also known as Tulsi, is revered for its adaptogenic properties, helping the body manage stress and support overall wellness.

Native: Holy basil is native to India and other regions of Southeast Asia and is a key herb in Ayurvedic medicine.

Cultivation: Holy basil thrives in warm, well-drained soil with full sun. The leaves and flowers are harvested for herbal preparations, including teas, tinctures, and essential oils.

Ancient Usage: Holy basil, also known as the "queen of herbs," has been revered in Ayurvedic medicine for its powerful adaptogenic and spiritual properties. It was used to promote resilience to stress, support the immune system, and balance the body's energy. Holy basil was considered sacred in Hindu culture, often planted around homes and temples to purify the environment and protect against negative energies. In folklore, it symbolized divine protection, health, and spiritual well-being.

Holy basil is an aromatic, bushy annual or perennial herb that grows up to 60 cm (24 inches) tall, with branching stems and oval, toothed green or purple-tinged leaves. It produces small, tubular purple or pink flowers in elongated clusters known for their strong, clove-like aroma.

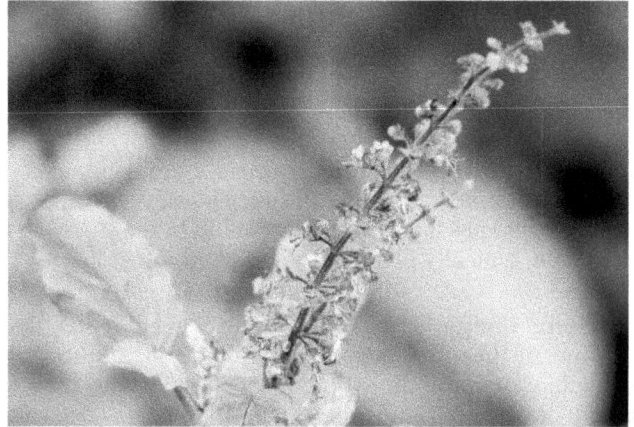

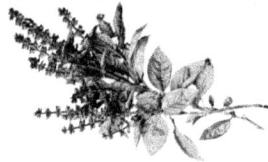

Medicinal Benefits:
- **Stress Relief:** Reduces anxiety and fatigue.
- **Immune Support:** Fights bacterial, viral, and fungal infections.
- **Respiratory Health:** Relieves coughs, colds, asthma, and bronchitis.
- **Cognitive Support:** Enhances mental clarity, focus, and memory.
- **Digestive Health:** Soothes indigestion, bloating, and gas.
- **Anti-Inflammatory:** Aids in arthritis and inflammatory bowel diseases.
- **Blood Sugar Regulation:** Beneficial for individuals with diabetes.
- **Heart Health:** Reduces cholesterol levels and improves circulation.
- **Skin Health:** Treats acne, wounds, and other skin irritations.

Dosage:
- **Standardized Extract:** 300-600 mg daily.
- **Tincture:** 2-4 mL (40-80 drops), 2-3 times daily
- **Tea:** 1-2 tsp per cup of water, 2-3 times daily.
- **Capsules:** 500-1,000 mg, 1-2 times daily.

Safety:
- **Internal Use:** Excessive use may cause nausea.
- **Children:** Safe for children for respiratory and digestive issues.
- **Allergy Risk:** Individuals sensitive to mint-family plants (Lamiaceae) should use cautiously.
- **Drug Interactions:** May enhance the effects of blood sugar-lowering medications and anticoagulants.

Preparation Methods:
- **Edible Flowers:** Holy basil flowers are edible.
- **Teas & Infusions:** Reduces stress, supports immunity, and promotes respiratory health.
- **Decoctions:** Aids respiratory issues, reduces inflammation, and supports digestive health.
- **Tinctures:** Bbalances stress, boosts energy, and improves mental clarity.
- **Syrups:** Soothes coughs, calms sore throats, and promotes immune health.
- **Salves & Balms:** Treats minor skin irritations, reduces inflammation, and promotes healing.
- **Poultices:** Soothes insect bites, reduces swelling, and supports wound healing.

HOPS

Zodiac: ♍ Virgo

Latin: *Humulus lupulus*

Vital Parts: Flowers (Cones)
Harvest Season: Late Summer to Early Autumn

Description: Hops are best known for their calming and sleep-promoting properties. They are commonly used to reduce anxiety, improve sleep quality, and alleviate restlessness.

Native: Hops are native to Europe, North America, and parts of Asia.

Cultivation: Hops thrive in well-drained soil and full sun, often requiring support structures for their climbing vines. The flowers (or cones) are harvested and used in herbal medicine, typically in teas, tinctures, and capsules to promote relaxation.

Ancient Usage: Hops, often called the "sleep herb," has been used for centuries for its calming and sedative properties. Ancient European herbalists used hops to treat insomnia, anxiety, and digestive issues. It was also valued for its antimicrobial qualities and was used to preserve food and beverages, particularly beer. In folklore, hops were associated with restful sleep and protection, often placed under pillows to ward off nightmares and promote peaceful rest.

Hops is a fast-growing, perennial climbing vine that can reach up to 6 meters (20 feet) in height, with rough, hairy stems and deeply lobed, serrated leaves. The plant produces papery, cone-shaped flowers (called hop cones) on female plants, which are pale green and highly aromatic.

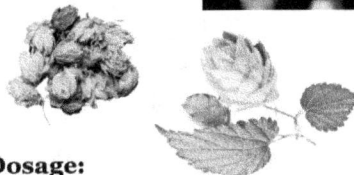

Medicinal Benefits:
- **Sleep Aid:** Promotes restful sleep and alleviates insomnia.
- **Stress and Anxiety Relief:** Reduces stress, nervous tension, and anxiety.
- **Digestive Support:** Eases indigestion, bloating, and loss of appetite.
- **Anti-Inflammatory:** Benefits arthritis and muscle pain.
- **Menopausal Symptom Relief:** Helps alleviate symptoms of hot flashes and mood swings.
- **Antimicrobial Properties:** Supports immune health by inhibiting the growth of certain bacteria and fungi.
- **Skin Health:** Soothes wounds, rashes, and skin irritations.

Dosage:
- **Standardized Extract:** 200-400 mg daily.
- **Tincture:** 2-4 mL (40-80 drops), 2-3 times daily.
- **Tea:** 1-2 tsp per cup of water, 2-3 times daily.
- **Capsules:** 500-1,000 mg of dried hops powder, 1-2 times daily.

Safety:
- **Internal Use:** Excessive use may cause drowsiness or mild stomach discomfort.
- **Drug Interactions:** May enhance the effects of sedatives, antidepressants, and alcohol.
- **Allergy Risk:** Individuals allergic to plants in the Cannabaceae family should test in small amounts before use.

Preparation Methods:
- **Edible Cones:** Hops flowers (cones) are edible but have a strong bitter taste.
- **Teas & Infusions:** Promotes relaxation, improves sleep quality, and reduces stress.
- **Decoctions:** Supports digestion, eases bloating, and acts as a mild sedative.
- **Tinctures:** Helps with anxiety, restlessness, and nervous system support.
- **Syrups:** Aids in sleep, soothes the nervous system, and reduces tension.
- **Salves & Balms:** Relieves muscle aches, soothes inflamed skin, and supports wound healing.
- **Poultices:** Eases pain, reduces swelling, and promotes relaxation of tense muscles.

Planet: Mercury

HOREHOUND

Zodiac: ♊ Gemini

Latin: *Marrubium vulgare*

Vital Parts: Leaves, Flowers
Harvest Season: Late Spring to Early Summer

Description: Horehound is traditionally used to support respiratory health by soothing coughs and reducing mucus buildup. It has expectorant and anti-inflammatory properties, making it a common remedy for bronchitis, colds, and sore throat.

Native: Horehound is native to Europe, North Africa, and parts of Asia and has naturalized in North America.

Cultivation: Horehound thrives in dry, well-drained soil and full sun. The aerial parts (leaves and flowers) are harvested and used in herbal medicine.

Ancient Usage: Horehound, known as the "cough herb," has been used since ancient times to relieve ailments such as coughs, colds, and bronchitis. The Greeks and Romans used horehound as a remedy to clear mucus and soothe sore throats. In medieval Europe, it was also employed to improve digestion and reduce inflammation. Folklore held that horehound offered protection against dark magic and was often planted near homes to ward off evil.

Horehound is a low-growing, perennial herb that reaches up to 60 cm (24 inches) in height, with square stems covered in fine hairs and wrinkled, grayish-green, oval leaves. The plant produces small, white, tubular flowers that form in dense whorls around the leaf nodes.

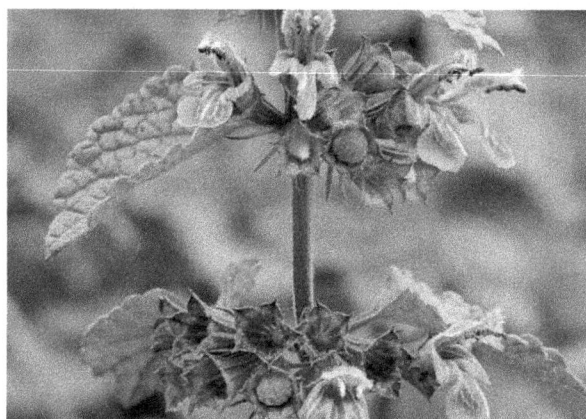

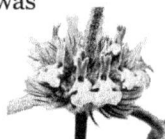

Medicinal Benefits:
- **Respiratory Support:** Relieves coughs, congestion, and bronchial irritation.
- **Digestive Aid:** Stimulates appetite, alleviates indigestion, and reduces bloating.
- **Liver Health:** Promotes liver detoxification and bile production.
- **Immune Booster:** Helps the body resist infections and colds.
- **Blood Sugar Regulation:** Traditionally used for managing diabetes symptoms.
- **Anti-Inflammatory:** Reduces inflammation, providing relief for conditions like arthritis and muscle pain.
- **Wound Healing:** Supports healing of cuts, abrasions, and minor skin irritations.

Dosage:
- **Standardized Extract:** 300-600 mg daily.
- **Tincture:** 2-4 mL (40-80 drops), 2-3 times daily.
- **Tea:** 1-2 tsp per cup of water, 2-3 times daily.
- **Capsules:** 500-1,000 mg of dried herb, 1-2 times daily.

Safety:
- **Internal Use:** Excessive consumption may cause mild stomach upset.
- **Allergy Risk:** Those with sensitivities to plants in the mint family (Lamiaceae) should use cautiously.
- **Drug Interactions:** May enhance the effects of diuretics and blood sugar medications.

Preparation Methods:
- **Edible Leaves:** Horehound leaves are edible but have a strong bitter taste.
- **Teas & Infusions:** Supports respiratory health, soothes coughs, and aids digestion.
- **Decoctions:** Acts as an expectorant, relieves congestion, and boosts immunity.
- **Tinctures:** Aids in digestion, stimulates appetite, and helps clear mucus from the lungs.
- **Syrups:** Traditionally used for coughs, sore throats, and respiratory relief.
- **Salves & Balms:** Soothes skin irritations, minor cuts, and insect bites.
- **Poultices:** Reduces swelling, eases chest congestion, and supports wound healing.

HORSETAIL

Latin: *Equisetum arvense*

Vital Parts: Stems, Shoots
Harvest Season: Spring to Early Summer

Description: Horsetail is valued for its high silica content, which supports bone health, hair, skin, and nail strength. It also has diuretic properties, making it useful for promoting kidney and urinary tract health.

Native: Horsetail is native to Europe, Asia, and North America, typically found in moist, sandy soils.

Cultivation: Horsetail thrives in damp, well-drained soil and partial to full sun. The aerial parts are harvested and used in herbal medicine, typically as teas, tinctures, and capsules to support bone health, urinary health, and skin repair.

Ancient Usage: Horsetail, sometimes known as "shavegrass," has been valued since ancient times for its high silica content, which supports bone, hair, and nail health. Roman and Greek physicians, including Dioscorides, recommended horsetail to promote wound healing and strengthen bones. It was used as a diuretic to support kidney function and reduce inflammation. In folklore, horsetail symbolized endurance and regeneration, often seen as a plant that could restore vitality to both the body and the land.

Medicinal Benefits:
- **Bone and Joint Health:** Supports bone strength and helps manage osteoporosis.
- **Wound Healing:** Speeds healing of cuts, scrapes, and burns when applied topically.
- **Urinary Health:** Acts as a natural diuretic, alleviating bladder infections, UTIs, and kidney stones.
- **Hair and Nail Health:** Strengthens brittle hair and nails and prevents hair breakage.
- **Skin Health:** Helps manage acne, eczema, and other inflammatory skin conditions.
- **Digestive Health:** Eases gastrointestinal inflammation and diarrhea.
- **Respiratory Support:** Soothes coughs and bronchitis.

Horsetail is a perennial, reed-like herb that can grow up to 1 meter (3 feet) tall, with jointed, hollow, green stems and whorls of thin, needle-like leaves at regular intervals along the stem. The plant reproduces via spores rather than flowers, producing small cone-like structures at the tips of fertile stems. Its distinctive segmented appearance resembles bamboo.

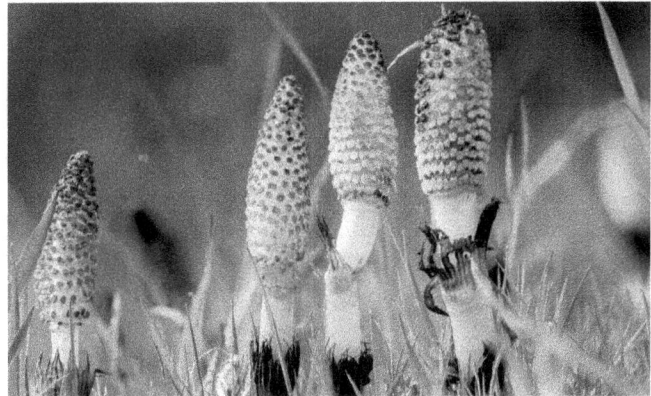

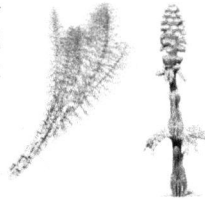

Dosage:
- **Standardized Extract:** 300-600 mg daily.
- **Tincture:** 2-4 mL (40-80 drops), 2-3 times daily.
- **Tea:** 1-2 tsp per cup of water, 2-3 times daily.
- **Capsules:** 500-1,000 mg, 1-2 times daily.

Safety:
- **Internal Use:** Excessive use may deplete thiamine (vitamin B1).
- **Children:** Safe for skin and urinary issues.
- **Allergy Risk:** Individuals sensitive to horsetail species should use cautiously.
- **Drug Interactions:** May interact with diuretics, anticoagulants, and lithium.

Preparation Methods:
- **Edible Shoots:** Young horsetail shoots are edible when cooked.
- **Teas & Infusions:** Supports bone health, strengthens hair and nails, and aids kidney function.
- **Decoctions:** Rich in silica, promotes skin elasticity, and supports urinary tract health.
- **Tinctures:** Aids in wound healing, improves connective tissue strength, and supports joint health.
- **Syrups:** Strengthens the immune system, soothes coughs, and supports respiratory health.
- **Salves & Balms:** Promotes wound healing, reduces inflammation, and nourishes the skin.
- **Poultices:** Helps with joint pain, bruises, and speeds up healing.

HYSSOP

Latin: Hyssopus officinalis

Vital Parts: Leaves, Flowers, Stems
Harvest Season: Late Spring to Early Summer

Description: Hyssop is known for its antimicrobial and expectorant properties. It is used to alleviate respiratory conditions, including coughs, bronchitis, and colds.

Native: Hyssop is native to southern Europe, the Middle East, and parts of central Asia.

Cultivation: Hyssop prefers well-drained, slightly alkaline soil and full sun. The leaves and flowers are harvested for herbal use, often prepared as teas, infusions, or tinctures.

Ancient Usage: Hyssop, often called the "purification herb," has been used since biblical times for its cleansing and protective properties. Ancient Hebrew and Christian traditions used hyssop in purification rituals to ward off evil and purify sacred spaces. Greek and Roman herbalists valued it for treating respiratory ailments, including coughs and colds. In medieval Europe, hyssop was believed to promote both physical and spiritual health, symbolizing protection and renewal.

Medicinal Benefits:
- **Respiratory Health:** Clears congestion, soothes coughs, and alleviates symptoms of colds, bronchitis, and asthma.
- **Digestive Aid:** Relieves bloating, gas, and indigestion by stimulating digestive enzymes.
- **Anti-Inflammatory:** Reduces swelling and irritation, particularly in respiratory and digestive tracts.
- **Immune Support:** Combats infections and supports overall immunity.
- **Wound Healing:** Applied topically to clean wounds and promote faster healing.
- **Nervous System Support:** Acts as a mild sedative, calming anxiety and tension.

Hyssop is a bushy, perennial herb that grows up to 60 cm (24 inches) tall, with woody, square stems and narrow, lance-shaped, dark green leaves. It produces spikes of small, fragrant blue to violet flowers, though pink or white varieties also occur.

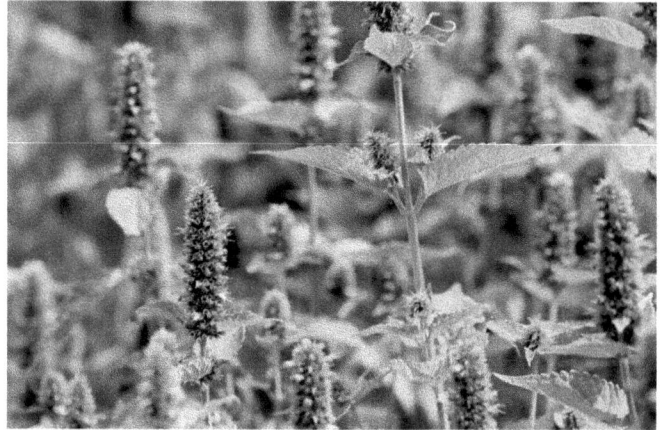

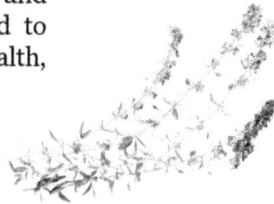

Dosage:
- **Standardized Extract:** 200-400 mg daily.
- **Tincture:** 2-4 mL (40-80 drops), 2-3 times daily.
- **Tea:** 1-2 tsp per cup of water, 2-3 times daily.
- **Capsules:** 500-1,000 mg, 1-2 times daily.

Safety:
- **Internal Use:** Excessive use may cause nausea.
- **Allergy Risk:** Individuals sensitive to mint-family plants (Lamiaceae) should use cautiously.
- **Essential Oil:** Highly concentrated and should be used only in diluted forms for external applications.

Preparation Methods:
- **Edible Leaves & Flowers:** Hyssop leaves and flowers are edible, with a minty, bitter taste.
- **Teas & Infusions:** Supports respiratory health, soothes coughs, and aids digestion.
- **Decoctions:** Acts as an expectorant, clears congestion, and boosts immunity.
- **Tinctures:** Aids in digestion, relieves bloating, and helps with respiratory issues.
- **Syrups:** Traditionally used for coughs, sore throats, and cold relief.
- **Salves & Balms:** Soothes skin irritations, minor cuts, and insect bites.
- **Poultices:** Reduces swelling, eases muscle pain, and supports wound healing.

JUNIPER

Latin: Juniperus communis

Vital Parts: Berries, Needles, Bark
Harvest Season: Late Summer to Early Winter

Description: Juniper is known for its diuretic, detoxifying, and antimicrobial properties. It is often used to promote kidney and urinary tract health.

Native: Juniper is native to Europe, North America, and parts of Asia, thriving in diverse climates from temperate forests to arid regions.

Cultivation: Juniper thrives in well-drained, sandy soil and full sun. The berries are harvested and used in herbal medicine, typically as tinctures, teas, and essential oils.

Ancient Usage: Juniper, known as the "guardian herb," has been revered since ancient times for its protective and detoxifying properties. Ancient Egyptians used juniper in their embalming practices, while the Greeks and Romans used its berries to purify air and ward off illness. It was also employed as a diuretic to cleanse the body of toxins. Folklore held that juniper branches could protect homes from negative forces, often hung above doorways to ward off evil spirits.

Juniper is a hardy, evergreen shrub or small tree that can grow up to 10 meters (33 feet) tall, with thin, needle-like, sharp green leaves and reddish-brown bark. It produces small, yellow flowers, followed by round, blue-purple, berry-like cones that are aromatic and resinous.

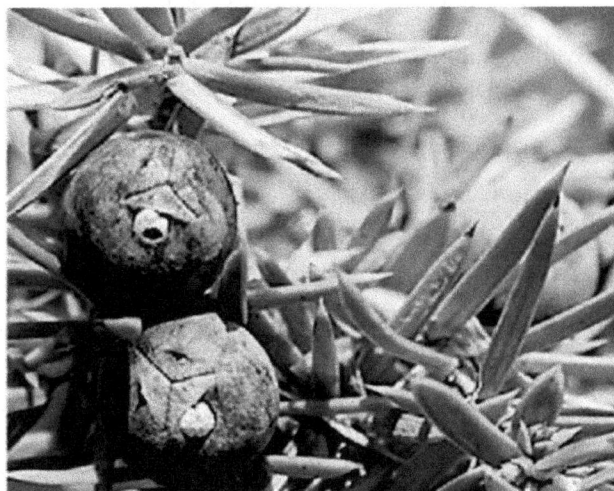

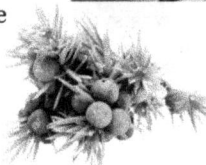

Medicinal Benefits:

- **Detoxification Support:** Eliminates toxins from the body.
- **Digestive Aid:** Stimulates digestion, reduces bloating, and relieves indigestion.
- **Anti-Inflammatory:** Helps reduce joint pain, arthritis, and muscle soreness.
- **Urinary Tract Health:** Supports bladder and kidney health, helping with infections and fluid retention.
- **Respiratory Support:** Eases symptoms of colds and coughs.
- **Circulatory Boost:** Improves blood flow, reduces swelling, and supports heart health.
- **Antimicrobial & Immune Support:** Naturally fights bacteria and infections.

Dosage:
- **Standardized Extract:** 300-600 mg daily.
- **Tincture:** 2-4 mL (40-80 drops), 2-3 times daily.
- **Tea:** 1-2 tsp per cup of water, 1-2 times daily.
- **Capsules:** 500-1,000 mg, 1-2 times daily.

Safety:
- **Internal Use:** Excessive consumption may irritate the kidneys.
- **Allergy Risk:** Individuals with sensitivities to coniferous plants should use cautiously.
- **Drug Interactions:** May interact with diuretics, blood pressure medications, and blood-thinning drugs.

Preparation Methods:
- **Edible Berries:** Juniper berries are edible and have a strong, piney flavor.
- **Teas & Infusions:** Supports kidney health, aids digestion, and acts as a mild diuretic.
- **Decoctions:** Detoxifies the body, relieves bloating, and promotes urinary tract health.
- **Tinctures:** Supports digestion, reduces inflammation, and helps fight infections.
- **Syrups:** Used for respiratory relief, immune support, and digestive balance.
- **Salves & Balms:** Soothes sore muscles, reduces joint pain, and promotes circulation.
- **Poultices:** Helps with wounds, swelling, and relieving aches and pains.

JAPANESE HONEYSUCKLE

Latin: *Lonicera japonica*

Vital Parts: Flowers, Leaves, Stems
Harvest Season: Late Spring to Early Autumn

Description: Japanese Honeysuckle is recognized for its antimicrobial, anti-inflammatory, and soothing properties. It is commonly used to support respiratory health.

Native: Japanese Honeysuckle is native to East Asia, particularly Japan, China, and Korea. It has since spread to many other regions due to its vigorous growth and adaptability to various climates.

Cultivation: Japanese Honeysuckle thrives in well-drained, moderately fertile soil and full to partial sun. The flowers and leaves are harvested for use in herbal medicine, typically prepared as teas, tinctures, or essential oils.

Description: Japanese Honeysuckle, often called the "flower of tranquility," has been valued in traditional medicine for centuries for its calming and healing properties. In ancient China, it was used to clear heat, detoxify the body. The flowers were often brewed into teas to treat colds, coughs, and fever. In Japan, it was also believed to bring peace and harmony to the home, with its sweet fragrance used in rituals to calm the mind and spirit. Folklore suggests that the vine was symbolic of strong relationships, offering protection and unity.

Japanese Honeysuckle is a fast-growing, fragrant, semi-evergreen vine that can reach up to 10 meters (33 feet) in length. It features glossy, oval, dark green leaves and produces clusters of highly aromatic, tubular, white to yellow flowers that bloom in late spring to summer. These flowers give way to small, dark purple to black berries.

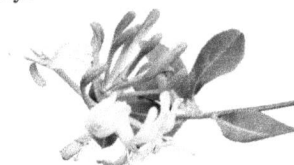

Medicinal Benefits:
- **Respiratory Health:** Treats colds, coughs, bronchitis, and the flu.
- **Anti-Inflammatory:** Reduces arthritis and muscle soreness.
- **Immune System Support:** Prevents and treats colds, infections, and flu-like symptoms.
- **Antimicrobial:** Fights bacteria in the respiratory system and urinary tract.
- **Skin Health:** Soothes skin irritations, rashes, eczema, and burns.
- **Antioxidant:** Protects the body from oxidative stress and cellular damage.
- **Calming & Relaxation:** Reduces anxiety, promotes relaxation, and improves sleep quality.
- **Detoxification:** Eliminates toxins in the respiratory and urinary systems.
- **Fever Reduction:** Contains cooling and anti-inflammatory effects.

Dosage:
- **Standardized Extract:** 300-500 mg daily.
- **Tincture:** 2-4 mL (40-80 drops), 2-3 times daily.
- **Tea:** 1-2 tsp of dried flowers, 1-2 times daily.
- **Capsules:** 500-1,000 mg of dried powder, 1-2 times daily.

Safety:
- **Internal Use:** Excessive use may cause mild digestive upset
- **Children:** Safe for children for skin conditions.

Preparation Methods:
- **Edible Flowers:** Japanese honeysuckle flowers are edible.
- **Teas & Infusions:** Supports immune health, soothes sore throats, and alleviates respiratory infections.
- **Decoctions:** Addresses fever, reduces inflammation, and promotes detoxification.
- **Tinctures:** Aids in combating infections, reducing inflammation, and supporting respiratory health.
- **Syrups:** Soothes coughs, calms sore throats, and promotes respiratory wellness.
- **Salves & Balms:** Treats minor skin irritations, reduces inflammation, and promotes healing of wounds.
- **Poultices:** Reduces swelling, soothes irritation, and supports wound healing.

KAVA KAVA

Latin: Piper methysticum

Vital Parts: Roots
Harvest Season: Late Summer to Early Autumn

Description: Kava kava is renowned for its calming and anxiolytic properties. It is commonly used to reduce anxiety, promote relaxation, and improve sleep quality.

Native: Kava kava is native to the Pacific Islands, particularly in regions such as Fiji, Vanuatu, and Hawaii, where it has traditional cultural significance.

Cultivation: Kava kava thrives in warm, humid climates with well-drained, fertile soil and partial shade. The roots are harvested and used in herbal medicine, typically prepared as teas and tinctures.

Ancient Usage: Kava kava, often called the "peace herb," has been a cornerstone of traditional Pacific Island cultures for its calming and socializing effects. Islanders used kava in ceremonies to promote peace, relaxation, and community bonding. It was also employed to reduce anxiety, ease muscle tension, and promote restful sleep. Folklore viewed kava as a sacred plant that connected individuals with their ancestors and spiritual harmony.

Medicinal Benefits:

- **Anxiety & Stress Relief:** Calms the nervous system, reduces tension, and promotes relaxation.
- **Sleep Support:** Reduces insomnia and promotes sleep.
- **Muscle Relaxation:** Eases muscle tension, spasms, and body discomfort.
- **Mood Enhancement:** Promotes a sense of well-being and aids mild depression.
- **Pain Relief:** Aids headaches, muscle pain, and nerve discomfort.
- **Cognitive Function:** Improves mental clarity and focus.
- **Social Anxiety Support:** Promotes relaxation and confidence.

Kava kava is a tropical, bushy perennial plant that grows up to 3 meters (10 feet) tall, with thick, green, heart-shaped leaves and smooth, jointed stems. It produces small, pale, spike-like flowers, although these rarely develop into fruit.

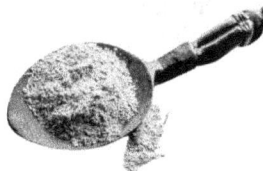

Dosage:

- **Standardized Extract:** 200-400 mg daily.
- **Tincture:** 2-4 mL (40-80 drops), 2-3 times daily.
- **Tea:** 1-2 tsp of dried root per cup of water, 1-2 times daily.
- **Capsules:** 500-1,000 mg, 1-2 times daily.

Safety:

- **Internal Use:** Excessive use may cause liver toxicity.
- **Children:** Generally not recommended for children.
- **Allergy Risk:** Individuals with sensitivities to kava or related plants should use cautiously.
- **Drug Interactions:** May interact with sedatives, antidepressants, and alcohol.

Preparation Methods:

- **Edible Root:** Kava kava root is used to make calming beverages.
- **Teas & Infusions:** Promotes relaxation, reduces stress, and enhances sleep.
- **Decoctions:** Supports muscle relaxation, eases anxiety, and soothes the nervous system.
- **Tinctures:** Helps with stress, mood, and tension.
- **Syrups:** Calms the mind, supports restful sleep, and reduces nervous energy.
- **Salves & Balms:** Eases muscle tension, soothes pain, and reduces inflammation.
- **Poultices:** Helps with muscle aches, joint discomfort, and relaxation therapy.

Planet: Venus

LADY'S MANTLE

Zodiac: ♎ Libra

Latin: Alchemilla vulgaris

Vital Parts: Leaves, Flowers
Harvest Season: Late Spring to Early Summer

Description: Lady's mantle is known for its astringent and anti-inflammatory properties. It is commonly used to support women's reproductive health.

Native: Lady's mantle is native to Europe and Asia and has naturalized in parts of North America.

Cultivation: Lady's mantle thrives in well-drained, moist soil and partial shade. The leaves and flowers are harvested for herbal preparations, including teas, tinctures, and infusions, to support reproductive and digestive health.

Ancient Usage: Lady's mantle, sometimes referred to as "the alchemist's plant," has been used in European herbal medicine to support women's reproductive health. It was traditionally used to reduce menstrual cramps, support fertility, and aid recovery after childbirth. Medieval herbalists believed the plant had magical properties, particularly its ability to collect morning dew, which was considered a potent elixir. Folklore associated lady's mantle with protection and healing, symbolizing feminine strength and balance.

Medicinal Benefits:
- **Menopausal Support:** Alleviates hot flashes, night sweats, mood swings, and other menopausal symptoms.
- **Hormonal Balance:** Supports menstrual health, reduces cramps, and eases PMS.
- **Anti-Inflammatory:** Reduces inflammation, providing relief for joint pain and arthritis.
- **Nervous System Support:** Calms the nervous system, reduces anxiety, and promotes relaxation.
- **Muscle Relaxation:** Eases tension and spasms, particularly in the uterus.
- **Bone Health:** Reduces the risk of osteoporosis.

Lady's mantle is a low-growing, perennial herb with rounded, lobed, fan-shaped green leaves that have serrated edges and a velvety texture. The plant grows up to 60 cm (24 inches) tall and produces clusters of small, yellow-green, star-shaped flowers.

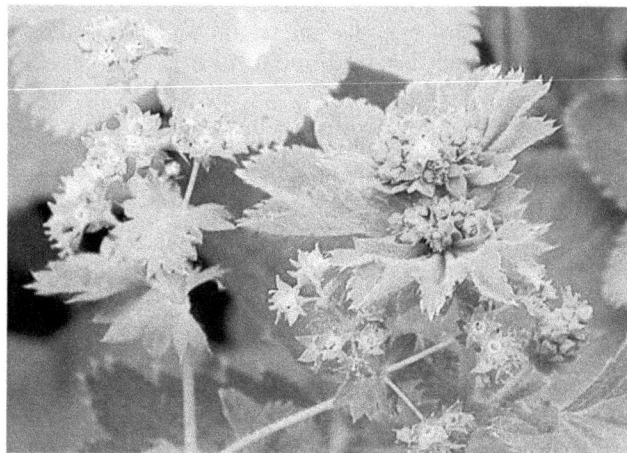

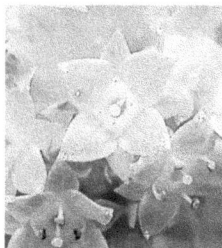

Dosage:
- **Standardized Extract:** 300-600 mg daily.
- **Tincture:** 2-4 mL (40-80 drops), 2-3 times daily.
- **Tea:** 1-2 tsp per cup of water, 2-3 times daily.
- **Capsules:** 500-1,000 mg, 1-2 times daily.

Safety:
- **Internal Use:** Excessive consumption may cause mild stomach upset.
- **Bleeding Disorders:** May promote blood clotting. Avoid if you have a bleeding disorder.
- **Drug Interactions:** May interact with anticoagulants or blood-thinning medications.

Preparation Methods:
- **Edible Leaves & Flowers:** The leaves and flowers are edible.
- **Teas & Infusions:** Supports menstrual health, relieves cramps, and aids digestion.
- **Decoctions:** Promotes wound healing.
- **Tinctures:** Balances hormones and eases menopause symptoms.
- **Syrups:** Soothes sore throats, supports immune health, and aids digestion.
- **Salves & Balms:** Helps with skin irritations wounds, and healing.
- **Poultices:** Reduces swelling, cuts, and helps with bruises and rashes.

LAVENDER

Latin: *Lavandula angustifolia*

Vital Parts: Flowers, Leaves
Harvest Season: Mid-Summer to Early Autumn

Description: Lavender is widely known for its calming and soothing effects. It is commonly used to reduce anxiety, promote relaxation, and improve sleep quality.

Native: Lavender is native to the Mediterranean region.

Cultivation: Lavender thrives in well-drained, sandy soil and full sun. The flowers are harvested and used in herbal preparations, including teas, essential oils, and topical applications, to promote relaxation, sleep, and skin care.

Ancient Usage: Lavender, often called the "calming herb," has been used for centuries to promote relaxation, improve sleep, and reduce anxiety. The Romans used lavender in their baths and homes to purify the air and calm the mind. Ancient Egyptians employed it in embalming rituals and perfumes. In folklore, lavender was believed to offer protection and peace, often hung in doorways to ward off negative energies.

Lavender is a fragrant, bushy perennial herb that grows up to 1 meter (3 feet) tall, with woody stems and narrow, gray-green, lance-shaped leaves. It produces spikes of small, purple to violet flowers, which are highly aromatic.

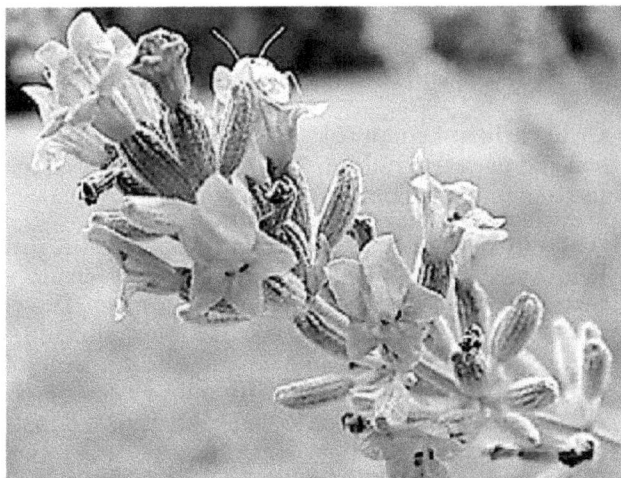

Medicinal Benefits:
- **Stress Relief:** Reduces stress, anxiety, and tension.
- **Sleep Aid:** Promotes restful sleep and helps alleviate insomnia.
- **Skin Health:** Soothes burns, cuts, rashes, and irritation.
- **Pain Relief:** Eases headaches, migraines, and muscle tension when applied topically or inhaled.
- **Anti-Inflammatory:** Reduces inflammation, making it useful for joint pain and muscle soreness.
- **Antimicrobial Properties:** Supports the healing of wounds and infections.
- **Digestive Aid:** Relieves indigestion, bloating, and nausea.
- **Respiratory Support:** Opens airways and soothes coughs and congestion when inhaled.

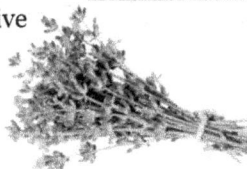

Dosage:
- **Standardized Extract:** 200-400 mg daily.
- **Tincture:** 2-4 mL (40-80 drops), 2-3 times daily.
- **Tea:** 1-2 tsp of dried flowers per cup of water, 2-3 times daily.
- **Capsules:** 500-1,000 mg, 1-2 times daily.

Safety:
- **Internal Use:** Excessive consumption may cause nausea or gastrointestinal discomfort.
- **Drug Interactions:** May enhance the effects of sedatives or medications that affect the nervous system.

Preparation Methods:
- **Edible Flowers:** Lavender flowers are widely edible.
- **Teas & Infusions:** Reduces stress, promotes relaxation, and soothes digestive discomfort.
- **Decoctions:** Aids respiratory health, inflammation, and supports restful sleep.
- **Tinctures:** Aids in relieving anxiety, promoting relaxation, and supporting balance.
- **Syrups:** Soothes coughs and sore throats.
- **Salves & Balms:** Treats burns, soothes skin irritations, and reduces inflammation.
- **Poultices:** Reduces swelling, promotes wound healing, and soothes irritation.
- **Topical Only:** Lavender essential oil should not be ingested.

LEMON BALM

Latin: Melissa officinalis

Vital Parts: Leaves, Flowers
Harvest Season: Late Spring to Early Autumn

Description: Lemon balm is known for its calming and mood-enhancing properties. It is commonly used to alleviate anxiety, reduce stress, and promote sleep.

Native: Lemon balm is native to southern Europe, western Asia, and the Mediterranean region.

Cultivation: Lemon balm thrives in well-drained, fertile soil and partial to full sun. The leaves are harvested for use in herbal medicine.

Ancient Usage: Lemon balm, also known as the "herb of happiness," has been used since ancient Greece to uplift mood, soothe nerves, and promote digestion. The Greek physician Dioscorides recommended it for reducing stress and relieving insomnia. In medieval Europe, lemon balm was used to strengthen the heart and promote longevity. Folklore held that planting lemon balm attracted harmony and prosperity.

Lemon balm is a bushy perennial herb that can grow up to 90 cm (3 feet) tall, with square stems and heart-shaped, serrated green leaves that emit a lemony fragrance when crushed. It produces small, white to pale yellow flowers in clusters near the leaf bases.

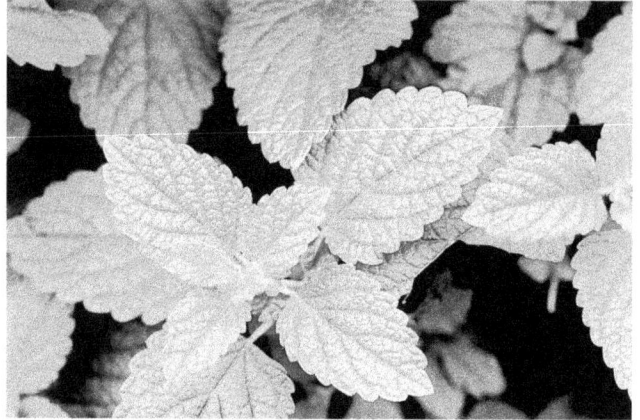

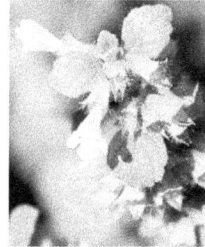

Medicinal Benefits:
- **Stress and Anxiety Relief:** Reduces stress, nervous tension, and anxiety.
- **Sleep Support:** Promotes relaxation and improves sleep quality.
- **Digestive Health:** Relieves indigestion, bloating, and gas by soothing the digestive tract and stimulating digestive enzymes.
- **Cognitive Support:** Enhances focus, memory, and mental clarity.
- **Antiviral Properties:** Effective against herpes simplex, often used topically to treat cold sores.
- **Immune Support:** Boosts immunity with its antimicrobial and antioxidant properties.
- **Pain Relief:** Reduces tension headaches, menstrual cramps, and other mild pain.
- **Heart Health:** Lowers blood pressure and reduces palpitations.

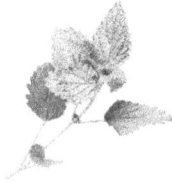

Dosage:
- **Standardized Extract:** 300-600 mg daily.
- **Tincture:** 2-4 mL (40-80 drops), 2-3 times daily.
- **Tea:** 1-2 tsp per cup of water, 2-3 times daily.
- **Capsules:** 500-1,000 mg, 1-2 times daily.

Safety:
- **Internal Use:** High doses may cause stomach upset.
- **Children:** Safe for children for calming effects or digestive issues.
- **Allergy Risk:** Individuals sensitive to mint-family plants (Lamiaceae) should use cautiously.
- **Drug Interactions:** May enhance the effects of sedatives, thyroid medications, and drugs for anxiety and depression.

Preparation Methods:
- **Edible Leaves & Flowers:** Lemon balm leaves and flowers are edible, with a mild citrusy flavor.
- **Teas & Infusions:** Calms the nervous system, reduces stress, and promotes restful sleep.
- **Decoctions:** Supports digestion, eases bloating, and boosts immune function.
- **Tinctures:** Helps with anxiety, mood balance, and cognitive function.
- **Syrups:** Soothes sore throats, supports relaxation, and aids digestion.
- **Salves & Balms:** Eases skin irritation, soothes cold sores, and promotes healing.
- **Poultices:** Reduces swelling, cools insect bites, and relieves headaches.

LICORICE

Latin: *Glycyrrhiza glabra*

Vital Parts: Roots, Rhizomes
Harvest Season: Late Autumn

Description: Licorice is prized for its anti-inflammatory, soothing, and immune-supporting properties. It is commonly used to relieve sore throats, coughs, and respiratory issues.

Native: Licorice is native to southern Europe, the Middle East, and parts of Asia.

Cultivation: Licorice thrives in deep, well-drained, sandy soil and full sun. The roots are harvested and used in herbal medicine, typically prepared as teas, tinctures, and capsules.

Ancient Usage: Licorice, sometimes called the "sweet root," has been used for thousands of years to soothe the respiratory and digestive systems. Ancient Egyptians included it in healing tonics and believed it had rejuvenating properties. Traditional Chinese medicine valued licorice as a harmonizing herb, often added to formulas to enhance their effectiveness. In folklore, licorice was associated with balance and healing, believed to restore physical and emotional well-being.

Licorice is a tall, perennial legume that grows up to 1.5 meters (5 feet) tall, with upright stems and pinnate leaves composed of small, oval leaflets. It produces clusters of pale violet to blue flowers, which develop into flat, brown seed pods.

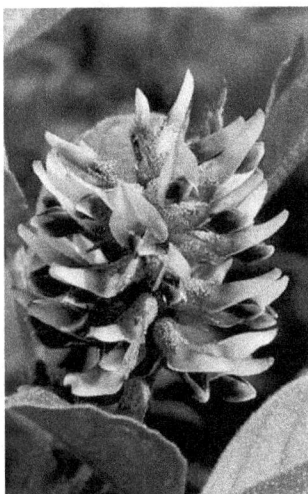

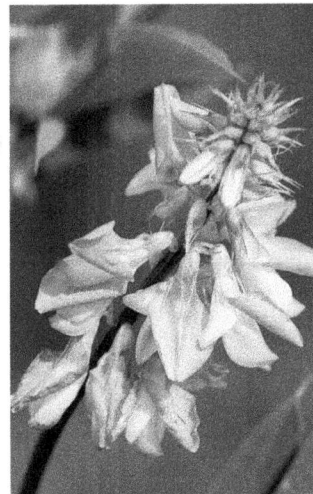

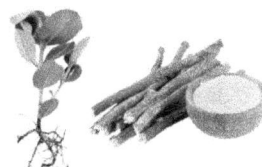

Medicinal Benefits:
- **Digestive Health:** Alleviates indigestion, heartburn, and gastritis. Aids ulcers and acid reflux.
- **Respiratory Support:** Soothes coughs, bronchitis, and sore throats.
- **Anti-Inflammatory:** Aids in arthritis and IBD.
- **Immune Support:** Enhances the immune system and combats viral infections, including colds and herpes.
- **Adrenal Support:** Combats stress and fatigue.
- **Skin Health:** Treats eczema, psoriasis, and skin rashes.
- **Hormonal Balance:** Mimics the effects of cortisol.

Dosage:
- **Standardized Extract:** 200-500 mg of (DGL) daily.
- **Tincture:** 2-4 mL (40-80 drops), 2-3 times daily.
- **Tea:** 1-2 tsp of dried root per cup of water, 2-3 times daily.
- **Capsules:** 500-1,000 mg of root powder, 1-2 times daily.

Safety:
- **Children:** Safe in small amounts.
- **Allergy Risk:** Individuals allergic to legumes should use cautiously.
- **Drug Interactions:** May interact with medications for blood pressure, diuretics, corticosteroids, and heart conditions.

Preparation Methods:
- **Teas & Infusions:** Soothes sore throats, supports digestive health, and boosts immunity.
- **Decoctions:** Relieves respiratory congestion and inflammation.
- **Tinctures:** Aids in balancing hormones, soothing digestive discomfort, and alleviating respiratory issues.
- **Syrups:** Soothes coughs, calms sore throats, and supports respiratory wellness.
- **Salves & Balms:** Treats skin irritations and soothes dry and itchy skin.
- **Poultices:** Reduces swelling, irritation, and promotes healing of minor wounds and rashes.

LINDEN

Latin: *Tilia cordata*

Vital Parts: Flowers, Leaves, Bark
Harvest Season: Late Spring to Early Summer

Description: Linden is known for its calming and sedative properties. It is commonly used to reduce anxiety, promote relaxation, and improve sleep quality.

Native: Linden is native to Europe, North America, and parts of Asia, commonly found in temperate regions.

Cultivation: Linden thrives in moist, well-drained soil and full sun to partial shade.

Ancient Usage: Linden, often referred to as the "tree of peace," has been revered in European traditions for its calming and anti-inflammatory properties. Ancient Slavic and Germanic peoples saw the linden tree as sacred, gathering beneath its branches for community meetings and rituals. Linden flowers were used to reduce fevers, ease respiratory ailments, and promote restful sleep. In folklore, linden was believed to offer protection and symbolize justice, love, and peace.

Linden is a large, deciduous tree that can grow up to 20 meters (65 feet) tall, with a broad, spreading canopy and heart-shaped green leaves with serrated edges. It produces clusters of small, fragrant, pale yellow flowers accompanied by long, bract-like structures.

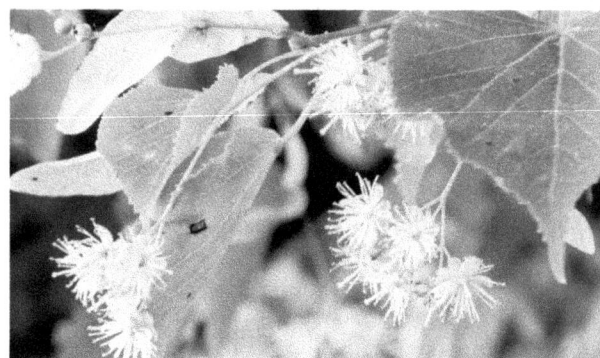

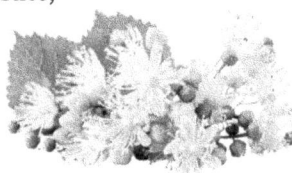

Medicinal Benefits:
- **Calming & Stress Relief:** Soothes the nervous system, reduces anxiety, and promotes relaxation.
- **Sleep Support:** Aids in relieving insomnia and encourages restful sleep.
- **Heart Health:** Supports cardiovascular function, helps lower blood pressure, and improves circulation.
- **Respiratory Support:** Eases congestion, soothes coughs, and supports lung health.
- **Digestive Aid:** Relieves bloating, indigestion, and stomach discomfort.
- **Anti-Inflammatory:** Reduces joint pain and muscle soreness.
- **Immune Support:** Helps fight infections and colds.

Dosage:
- **Standardized Extract:** 300-600 mg daily.
- **Tincture:** 2-4 mL (40-80 drops), 2-3 times daily.
- **Tea:** 1-2 tsp cup of water, 2-3 times daily.
- **Capsules:** 500-1,000 mg of dried flowers, 1-2 times daily.

Safety:
- **Internal Use:** Excessive use may strain the heart.
- **Children:** Safe for children for colds, coughs, or restlessness.
- **Allergy Risk:** Individuals with sensitivities to tree pollen should use cautiously.
- **Drug Interactions:** May enhance the effects of sedatives or blood pressure medications.

Preparation Methods:
- **Edible Flowers & Leaves:** Linden flowers and leaves are edible with a mild, sweet flavor.
- **Teas & Infusions:** Calms the nervous system, eases stress, and supports sleep.
- **Decoctions:** Reduces inflammation, soothes coughs, and aids heart health.
- **Tinctures:** Helps with anxiety, promotes relaxation, and supports immune function.
- **Syrups:** Soothes sore throats, relieves coughs, and enhances respiratory health.
- **Salves & Balms:** Moisturizes skin, reduces irritation, and soothes minor burns.
- **Poultices:** Eases headaches, reduces swelling, and relieves joint pain.

LION'S MANE

Latin: Hericium erinaceus

Vital Parts: Fruiting Body
Harvest Season: Late Summer to Autumn

Description: Lion's mane is renowned for its neuroprotective properties and ability to support cognitive health.

Native: Lion's mane is native to North America, Europe, and Asia, typically found on hardwood trees in forests.

Cultivation: Reishi grows well on logs or wood-based substrates. It prefers a cool, humid environment and can take several months to grow, but it can be cultivated indoors or in shaded outdoor areas.

Ancient Usage: Lion's mane, often called the "nerve mushroom," has been used in traditional Chinese and Japanese medicine to support brain health, improve memory, and promote nerve regeneration. It was believed to enhance mental clarity and protect against age-related cognitive decline. Buddhist monks consumed it to aid concentration during meditation. Folklore regarded lion's mane as a symbol of wisdom and longevity, with its shaggy appearance likened to the strength of a lion.

Lion's mane is a distinctive, edible mushroom with a white, shaggy, cascading structure that resembles a lion's mane. It grows on hardwood trees and logs, forming rounded clusters of long, hair-like spines.

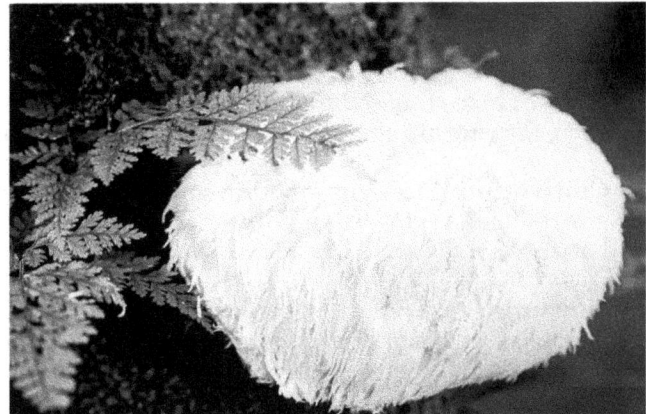

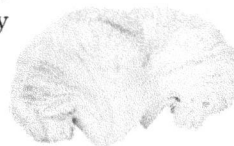

Medicinal Benefits:
- **Brain Health:** Supports brain cell regeneration, enhances memory, and improves focus.
- **Nervous System Repair:** Promotes healing of nerve damage.
- **Mood Enhancement:** Reduces depression and anxiety.
- **Digestive Health:** Aids in the prevention of ulcers and gastritis.
- **Immune Support:** Promotes gut health and increases white blood cells.
- **Anti-Inflammatory:** Supports arthritis and autoimmune disorders.
- **Antioxidant Properties:** Contributes to longevity and wellness.

Dosage:
- **Standardized Extract:** 500-1,000 mg daily.
- **Tincture:** 2-4 mL (40-80 drops), 2-3 times daily.
- **Capsules:** 500-1,000 mg, 1-2 times daily.
- **Tea:** 1-2 tsp of dried mushroom per cup of water, 1-2 times daily.

Safety:
- **Allergy Risk:** Although rare, allergic reactions may occur.
- **Drug Interactions:** May enhance the effects of medications for blood sugar or nerve-related conditions.
- **Moderation:** Excessive consumption may cause mild digestive discomfort.

Preparation Methods:
- **Edible Mushroom:** Lion's mane can be sautéed, roasted, or added to soups.
- **Teas & Infusions:** Supports cognitive health, inflammation, and immunity.
- **Decoctions:** Promotes nerve regeneration and digestive health.
- **Tinctures:** Supports brain function, reduces anxiety, and aids nerve repair.
- **Capsules:** Supports brain and nervous system health.
- **Salves & Balms:** Treats wounds, inflammation, and soothes skin irritations.
- **Poultices:** Reduces swelling, soothes irritation, and promotes healing.

MACA ROOT

Latin: Lepidium meyenii

Vital Parts: Root

Harvest Season: Late Autumn to Winter

Description: Maca is an adaptogenic root known for its ability to enhance energy, stamina, and hormonal balance. It is commonly used to improve libido, fertility, and overall vitality.

Native: Maca is native to the high Andes Mountains of Peru, thriving in extreme conditions at high altitudes.

Cultivation: Maca grows best in cold, high-altitude environments with well-drained, rocky soil. The root is harvested and used in herbal medicine.

Ancient Usage: Maca, sometimes referred to as the "Peruvian ginseng," has been used for thousands of years to boost energy, endurance, and fertility. Warriors consumed maca before battles to enhance strength and stamina. It was also valued for balancing hormones and improving reproductive health. Folklore saw maca as a sacred plant that promoted vitality and prosperity in both physical and spiritual realms.

Maca is a low-growing, hardy perennial plant that forms a short, rosette of scalloped green leaves. Its most notable feature is the underground, fleshy, turnip-like root, which comes in various colors such as yellow, red, and black. The plant produces small, white flowers.

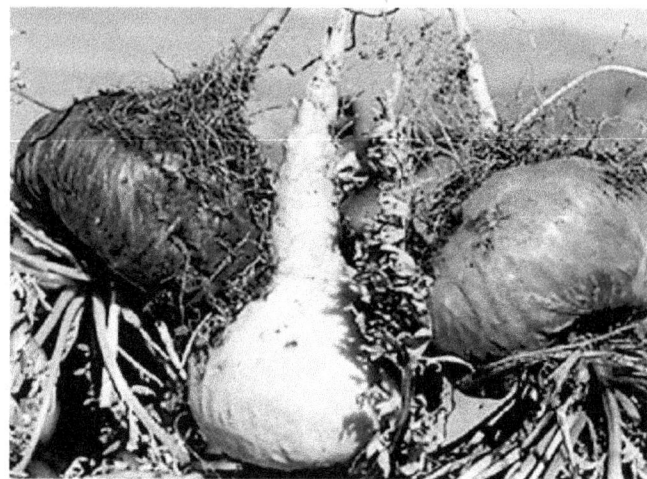

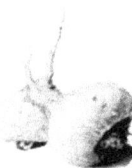

Medicinal Benefits:

- **Energy and Stamina:** Enhances physical and mental energy levels.
- **Hormonal Balance:** Alleviates symptoms of PMS, menopause, and low libido.
- **Fertility Support:** Boosts fertility by improving sperm quality and regulating ovulation.
- **Stress Reduction:** Acts as an adaptogen, helping the body manage stress and promote resilience.
- **Cognitive Support:** Improves memory, focus, and mental clarity.
- **Bone Health:** Supports bone density and strength.
- **Immune Support:** Combats oxidative stress.

Dosage:

- **Standardized Extract:** 1,000-1,500 mg daily.
- **Tincture:** 2-4 mL (40-80 drops), 2-3 times daily.
- **Capsules:** 500-1,000 mg, 1-2 times daily.
- **Tea:** 1-2 tsp of per cup of water, 1-2 times daily.

Safety:

- **Internal Use:** High doses may cause mild digestive discomfort or hormonal changes.
- **Allergy Risk:** Those sensitive to cruciferous vegetables (e.g., broccoli, kale) should use cautiously.
- **Drug Interactions:** May interact with medications that affect hormones or thyroid function.

Preparation Methods:

- **Edible Root:** Maca root is edible and commonly consumed in powdered form.
- **Teas & Infusions:** Supports energy, hormonal balance, and endurance.
- **Decoctions:** Enhances stamina, reduces stress, and promotes overall vitality.
- **Tinctures:** Boosts libido, balances hormones, and improves mood.
- **Syrups:** Provides sustained energy, supports adrenal health, and enhances resilience.
- **Salves & Balms:** Nourishes the skin, promotes circulation, and supports muscle recovery.
- **Poultices:** Helps with inflammation, muscle fatigue, and joint pain relief.

MAITAKE

Latin: *Grifola frondosa*

Vital Parts: Fruiting Body
Harvest Season: Late Summer to Early Autumn

Description: Maitake is valued for its immune-enhancing and anti-inflammatory properties. It is commonly used to support immune system function.

Native: Maitake is native to northeastern Japan and parts of North America, often found at the base of oak and other hardwood trees.

Cultivation: Maitake mushrooms thrive in cool, humid environments with moderate to indirect light. They grow best on hardwood substrates like oak, elm, or other deciduous trees, but can also be cultivated on sawdust or wood chips. Maitake prefers slightly acidic, moist, and well-drained soil.

Ancient Usage: Maitake, often called the "dancing mushroom," has been prized in traditional Japanese and Chinese medicine for its immune-boosting and adaptogenic properties. It was believed to promote longevity, balance energy, and protect against illness. Legends say that those who found maitake mushrooms would dance with joy due to their rarity and healing power. Folklore associated maitake with abundance and protection, symbolizing resilience in the face of adversity.

Medicinal Benefits:
- **Immune System Support:** Helps the body fight infections.
- **Blood Sugar Regulation:** Improves insulin sensitivity.
- **Heart Health:** Helps lower cholesterol, supports healthy blood pressure, and improves circulation.
- **Anti-Inflammatory:** Eases joint pain and muscle discomfort.
- **Cognitive Support:** Protects brain function, enhances mental clarity, and supports memory.
- **Hormonal Balance:** Supports adrenal health and aids in regulating hormones naturally.
- **Energy & Vitality:** Boosts stamina, reduces fatigue, and supports overall vitality.

Dosage:
- **Standardized Extract:** 500-1,000 mg daily.
- **Tincture:** 2-4 mL (40-80 drops), 2-3 times daily.
- **Capsules:** 500-1,000 mg, 1-2 times daily.
- **Tea:** 1-2 tsp per cup of water, 1-2 times daily.

Safety:
- **Internal Use:** Excessive intake may cause mild digestive upset.
- **Children:** Safe in small amounts for culinary uses.
- **Drug Interactions:** Maitake may enhance the effects of blood sugar-lowering and blood pressure medications.

Maitake is a large, clustered, edible mushroom that grows at the base of hardwood trees. It has overlapping, fan-shaped, grayish-brown caps with a soft, slightly ridged texture.

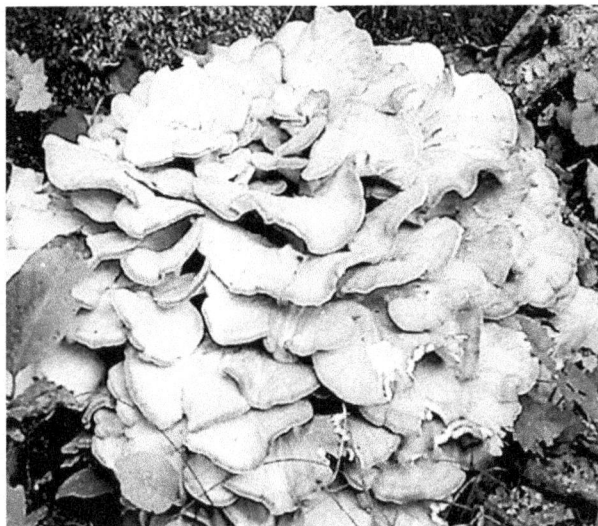

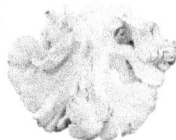

Preparation Methods:
- **Edible Mushroom:** Maitake is highly nutritious and can be eaten fresh, cooked, or dried.
- **Teas & Infusions:** Supports immune function, boosts energy, and aids digestion.
- **Decoctions:** Enhances vitality, regulates blood sugar, and supports cardiovascular health.
- **Tinctures:** Strengthens the immune system, balances hormones, and promotes overall well-being.
- **Syrups:** Provides immune support, aids respiratory health, and boosts energy.
- **Salves & Balms:** Soothes inflammation, supports skin health, and aids in wound healing.
- **Poultices:** Reduces swelling, eases joint pain, and promotes circulation.

MARSHMALLOW

Latin: Althaea officinalis

Vital Parts: Roots, Leaves, Flowers
Harvest Season: Late Summer to Early Autumn

Description: Marshmallow is known for its soothing and mucilaginous properties. It is used to relieve irritation in the throat, digestive tract, and urinary system.

Native: Marshmallow is native to Europe, North Africa, and parts of Asia, typically found in marshy or moist areas.

Cultivation: Marshmallow thrives in moist, rich, well-drained soil and full sun to partial shade. The roots, leaves, and flowers are harvested for herbal medicine.

Ancient Usage: Marshmallow, known as the "soothing herb," has been used since ancient Egyptian times to reduce inflammation and ease throat, digestive, and respiratory discomfort. Egyptians used marshmallow root to treat wounds and sore throats and considered it a sacred plant. In medieval Europe, marshmallow was used in remedies to soothe coughs, ulcers, and skin irritations. Folklore viewed marshmallow as a nurturing and protective plant, symbolizing comfort and healing.

Marshmallow is a tall, herbaceous perennial that grows up to 1.5 meters (5 feet) tall, with erect stems and soft, velvety, lobed green leaves. It produces pale pink to white, funnel-shaped flowers along the stem.

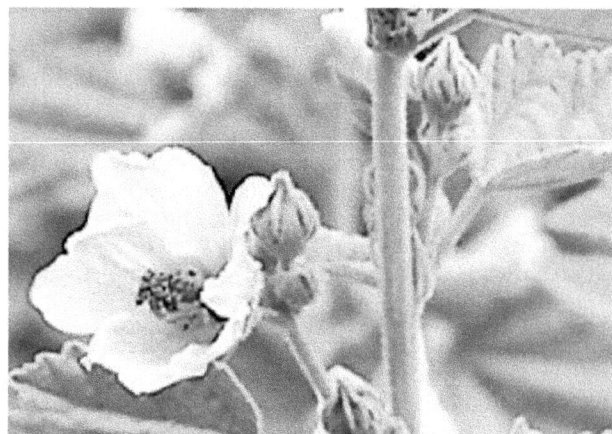

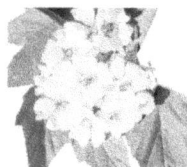

Medicinal Benefits:
- **Digestive Health:** Soothes the stomach lining and alleviates gastritis, acid reflux, and ulcers.
- **Respiratory Support:** Eases dry coughs, bronchitis, and sore throats.
- **Urinary Health:** Provides relief for UTIs and hydration.
- **Skin Health:** Soothes inflammation and promotes healing.
- **Oral Health:** Relieves canker sores, gum inflammation, and other oral irritations.
- **Anti-Inflammatory:** Supports the digestive and respiratory tracts.

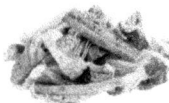

Dosage:
- **Standardized Extract:** 300-600 mg daily.
- **Tincture:** 2-4 mL (40-80 drops), 2-3 times daily.
- **Tea:** 1-2 tsp per cup of cold water, 2-3 times daily.
- **Capsules:** 500-1,000 mg of dried root powder, 1-2 times daily.

Safety:
- **Children:** Safe for children in small amounts for coughs or digestive upset.
- **Drug Interactions:** May interfere with the absorption of medications; take marshmallow preparations at least 2 hours apart from other drugs.

Preparation Methods:
- **Edible Flowers:** Marshmallow flowers are edible.
- **Teas & Infusions:** Soothes sore throats, supports digestion, and alleviates urinary discomfort.
- **Decoctions:** Relieves respiratory congestion, calms inflammation, and promotes digestive health.
- **Tinctures:** Aids in soothing mucous membranes, reduces inflammation, and supports respiratory wellness.
- **Syrups:** Soothes coughs, calms sore throats, and supports immune health.
- **Salves & Balms:** Treats dry skin, reduces inflammation, and promotes healing of minor wounds.
- **Poultices:** Soothes burns, swelling, wounds, and rashes.

MEADOWSWEET

Latin: *Filipendula ulmaria*

Vital Parts: Flowers, Leaves, Stems
Harvest Season: Late Spring to Early Summer

Description: Meadowsweet is known for its anti-inflammatory and pain-relieving properties. It is commonly used to relieve headaches, joint pain, and symptoms of colds and flu.

Native: Meadowsweet is native to Europe and Asia and is commonly found in damp meadows and along riverbanks.

Cultivation: Meadowsweet thrives in moist, well-drained soil and full sun to partial shade. The aerial parts (flowers and leaves) are harvested and used in herbal medicine.

Ancient Usage: Meadowsweet, often called the "queen of the meadow," has been used in European herbal medicine for centuries to relieve pain, reduce inflammation, and support digestive health. The Druids revered meadowsweet as one of their sacred herbs, using it in rituals and healing practices. It was a key ingredient in early pain-relieving remedies, as its natural salicylates inspired the development of modern aspirin. Folklore associated meadowsweet with protection and peace, often used to purify homes and promote harmony.

Meadowsweet is a perennial herb that grows up to 1.5 meters (5 feet) tall, with reddish, ridged stems and serrated, pinnate leaves that have a downy underside. It produces clusters of small, creamy-white, fragrant flowers arranged in dense, plume-like spikes.

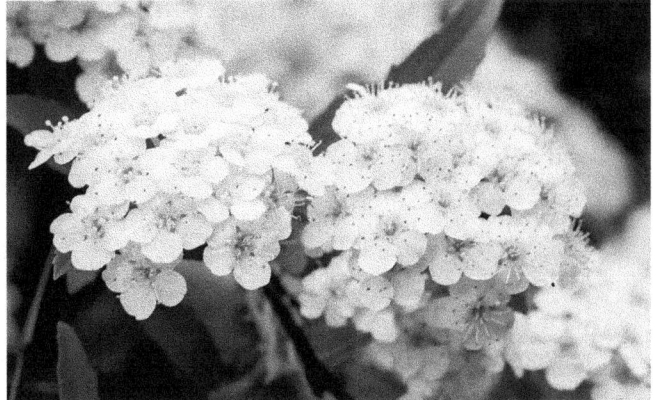

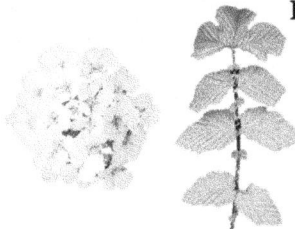

Medicinal Benefits:

- **Pain Relief:** Eases headaches, joint pain, and muscle soreness.
- **Anti-Inflammatory:** Supports arthritis, gout, and digestive discomfort.
- **Digestive Aid:** Soothes acid reflux, heartburn, and nausea.
- **Fever Reducer:** Helps lower fevers and eases colds and flu.
- **Urinary Tract Support:** Supports kidney and bladder health while reducing fluid retention.
- **Heart Health:** Supports circulation, helps regulate blood pressure, and protects cardiovascular function.
- **Antimicrobial & Immune Support:** Helps fight infections.

Dosage:

- **Standardized Extract:** 200-400 mg daily.
- **Tincture:** 2-4 mL (40-80 drops), 2-3 times daily.
- **Tea:** 1-2 tsp per cup of water, 2-3 times daily.
- **Capsules:** 500-1,000 mg, 1-2 times daily.

Safety:
- **Internal Use:** Excessive intake may irritate sensitive stomachs.
- **Aspirin Sensitivity:** Avoid use if allergic to aspirin or salicylates.
- **Drug Interactions:** May interact with blood-thinning medications.

Preparation Methods:

- **Edible Flowers & Leaves:** Meadowsweet flowers and leaves are edible, with a mild and sweet aroma.
- **Teas & Infusions:** Supports digestion, relieves heartburn, and reduces inflammation.
- **Decoctions:** Eases joint pain, soothes headaches, and supports urinary tract health.
- **Tinctures:** Helps with acid reflux, alleviates pain, and promotes respiratory health.
- **Syrups:** Soothes sore throats, relieves coughs, and reduces fever.
- **Salves & Balms:** Eases muscle aches, soothes irritated skin, and promotes healing.
- **Poultices:** Reduces swelling, calms skin rashes, and relieves minor wounds or burns.

MILK THISTLE

Latin: *Silybum marianum*

Vital Parts: Seeds, Leaves
Harvest Season: Late Summer to Early Autumn

Description: Milk thistle is valued for its liver-supporting and detoxifying properties. It is commonly used to protect the liver from toxins and improve digestion.

Native: Milk thistle is native to the Mediterranean region but has spread to other temperate regions worldwide.

Cultivation: Milk thistle thrives in well-drained, nutrient-poor soil and full sun. The seeds are harvested and used in herbal medicine to support liver health.

Ancient Usage: Milk thistle, sometimes referred to as the "liver protector," has been used since ancient times to support liver health and detoxification. The ancient Greeks and Romans used it to treat liver and gallbladder conditions, including jaundice and hepatitis. In medieval Europe, milk thistle was believed to offer protection against poison and was used to promote recovery from excessive drinking. Folklore saw the plant's white-veined leaves as a sign of divine blessing, linked to legends of the Virgin Mary.

Milk thistle is a tall, biennial or annual herb that can grow up to 2 meters (6 feet) tall, with spiny, green leaves marbled with white veins. It produces large, thistle-like purple flowers surrounded by sharp, protective bracts.

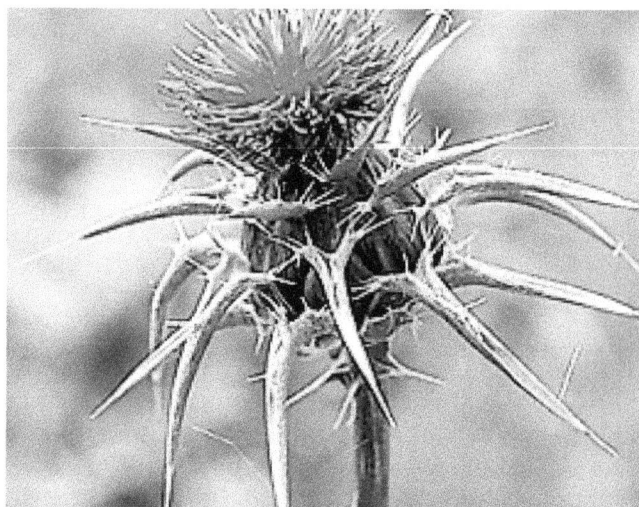

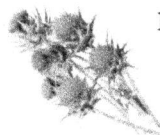

Medicinal Benefits:
- **Liver Support:** Protects the liver from toxins, alcohol, and medications.
- **Detoxification:** Enhances liver function and promotes bile production.
- **Antioxidant Properties:** Neutralizes free radicals, reducing oxidative stress.
- **Digestive Health:** Alleviates bloating and indigestion.
- **Blood Sugar Regulation:** Reduces blood sugar levels in those with type 2 diabetes.
- **Skin Health:** Manages acne and eczema.
- **Immune Support:** Possesses anti-inflammatory and antioxidant effects.

Dosage:
- **Standardized Extract:** 300-600 mg daily.
- **Tincture:** 2-4 mL (40-80 drops), 2-3 times daily.
- **Capsules:** 500-1,000 mg, 1-2 times daily.
- **Tea:** 1-2 tsp per cup of water, 1-2 times daily.

Safety:
- **Internal Use:** Overuse may cause nausea and diarrhea.
- **Children:** Safe in small amounts for liver support.
- **Allergy Risk:** Those allergic to the Asteraceae family (e.g., daisies, ragweed) should use cautiously.
- **Drug Interactions:** May interact with anticoagulants, statins, and cancer drugs.

Preparation Methods:
- **Teas & Infusions:** Supports liver health, aids digestion, and promotes detoxification.
- **Decoctions:** Addresses liver inflammation, supporting kidney health, and reducing oxidative stress.
- **Tinctures:** Aids in liver detoxification, promotes digestive wellness, and reduces inflammation.
- **Syrups:** Supports liver function, soothes digestive discomfort, and boosts immunity.
- **Salves & Balms:** Treats minor skin irritations, soothes inflammation, and promotes healing of wounds.
- **Poultices:** Reduces swelling, soothes irritation, and promotes woun healing.
- **Topical:** Always test milk thistle preparations on a small area of skin to ensure no irritation occurs before broader application.

MOTHERWORT

Latin: Leonurus cardiaca

Vital Parts: Leaves, Flowers
Harvest Season: Late Spring to Early Summer

Description: Motherwort is known for its calming and heart-supporting properties. It is used to reduce anxiety, promote emotional balance, and support heart health.

Native: Motherwort is native to Europe and Asia and has been naturalized in parts of North America.

Cultivation: Motherwort thrives in well-drained, moderately fertile soil and full sun to partial shade. The aerial parts (leaves and flowers) are harvested for use in herbal medicine.

Ancient Usage: Motherwort, often called the "herb of the mother," has been used since ancient Greece to support women's reproductive and emotional health. It was traditionally used to ease menstrual pain, calm anxiety, and promote recovery after childbirth. Medieval herbalists valued motherwort for its ability to soothe the heart, both physically and emotionally. Folklore regarded the plant as a symbol of maternal care and protection, believed to offer peace and strength to those in need.

Motherwort is a tall, perennial herb that grows up to 1.5 meters (5 feet) tall, with square, branching stems and deeply lobed, serrated green leaves. It produces small, pale purple to pink, tubular flowers arranged in whorls around the upper leaf nodes.

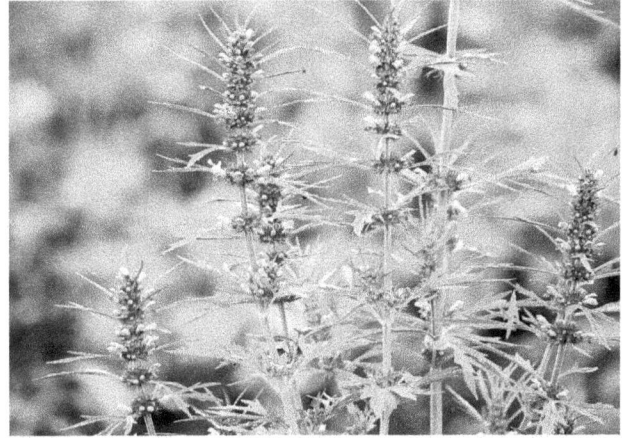

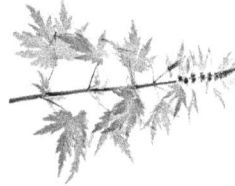

Medicinal Benefits:
- **Heart Health:** Regulates blood pressure and improves circulation.
- **Stress & Anxiety Relief:** Calms the nervous system, reduces tension, and promotes relaxation.
- **Hormonal Balance:** Supports menstrual health, eases PMS symptoms, and regulates cycles.
- **Menopausal Support:** Reduces hot flashes, mood swings, and emotional imbalances.
- **Digestive Aid:** Soothes bloating and stomach discomfort.
- **Anti-Inflammatory:** Reduces muscle tension, joint pain, and overall inflammation.
- **Uterine Tonic:** Strengthens the uterus, supports fertility, and may aid postpartum recovery.

Dosage:
- **Standardized Extract:** 300-600 mg daily.
- **Tincture:** 2-4 mL (40-80 drops), 2-3 times daily.
- **Tea:** 1-2 tsp per cup of water, 2-3 times daily.
- **Capsules:** 500-1,000 mg, 1-2 times daily.

Safety:
- **Internal Use:** Excessive intake may cause stomach discomfort.
- **Allergy Risk:** Individuals with sensitivities to plants in the mint family (Lamiaceae) should use cautiously.
- **Drug Interactions:** May interact with sedatives or medications affecting heart function.

Preparation Methods:
- **Edible Leaves & Flowers:** Motherwort leaves and flowers are edible but have a bitter taste.
- **Teas & Infusions:** Supports heart health, stress, and eases menstrual discomfort.
- **Decoctions:** Calms the nervous system, balances hormones, and supports digestion.
- **Tinctures:** Aids anxiety, promotes well-being, and regulates heartbeat.
- **Syrups:** Aids in relaxation and supports hormonal balance.
- **Salves & Balms:** Relieves muscle tension, cramps, and promotes circulation.
- **Poultices:** Reduces swelling, soothes irritated skin, and aids minor wounds.

MYRRH

Latin: *Commiphora myrrha*

Vital Parts: Resin
Harvest Season: Late Autumn to Winter

Description: Myrrh is known for its antimicrobial, anti-inflammatory, and wound-healing properties. It is commonly used to support oral health, promote skin healing, and combat infections.

Native: Myrrh is native to arid regions of northeastern Africa and the Arabian Peninsula.

Cultivation: Myrrh thrives in dry, rocky soil and full sun. The resin is harvested and used in herbal medicine, typically in tinctures, essential oils, and topical applications to support skin healing, immune function, and oral health.

Ancient Usage: Myrrh, often called the "sacred resin," has been valued since ancient times for its antiseptic and spiritual properties. The ancient Egyptians used myrrh in embalming rituals and to treat wounds and infections. In biblical times, it was one of the gifts given to the Christ child, symbolizing healing and divinity. Folklore regarded myrrh as a protector against negative forces, often burned as incense to purify the air and promote spiritual connection.

Myrrh is a small, thorny, drought-tolerant tree that grows up to 5 meters (16 feet) tall, with rough, gray bark and small, oval, green leaves. It produces clusters of small, pale yellow flowers. The tree exudes an aromatic resin from cuts in the bark, which hardens into reddish-brown, tear-shaped pieces used for medicinal and spiritual purposes.

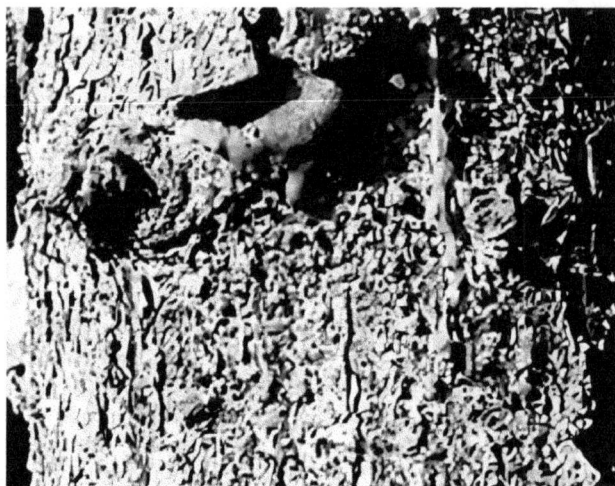

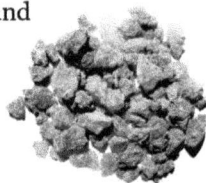

Medicinal Benefits:
- **Immune Support:** Helps fight infections.
- **Oral Health:** Supports gum health, reduces inflammation, and helps with mouth sores.
- **Digestive Aid:** Soothes indigestion, bloating, and supports gut health.
- **Respiratory Health:** Clears congestion, soothes coughs, and supports lung function.
- **Anti-Inflammatory:** Reduces joint pain and muscle soreness.
- **Wound Healing:** Promotes tissue repair, recovery, and prevents infections.
- **Circulatory Support:** Enhances blood flow and supports cardiovascular health.

Dosage:
- **Standardized Extract:** 200-500 mg daily.
- **Tincture:** 2-4 mL (40-80 drops), 2-3 times daily.
- **Capsules:** 500-1,000 mg, 1-2 times daily.
- **Tea:** 1-2 tsp per cup of water, 1-2 times daily.

Safety:
- **Children:** Safe in small amounts for external use.
- **Allergy Risk:** Individuals with sensitivities to resins should use cautiously.
- **Drug Interactions:** May interact with blood-thinning and diabetes medications.

Preparation Methods:
- **Teas & Infusions:** Supports immune function, soothes sore throats, and aids digestion.
- **Decoctions:** Promotes oral health, and reduces inflammation.
- **Tinctures:** Helps with wound healing, supports respiratory health, and aids in digestive balance.
- **Syrups:** Soothes coughs, relieves congestion, and boosts immunity.
- **Salves & Balms:** Promotes wound healing, reduces inflammation, and supports skin health.
- **Poultices:** Helps with infections, relieves muscle pain, and promotes faster healing of wounds.

NETTLE

Latin: *Urtica dioica*

Vital Parts: Leaves, Stems, Roots
Harvest Season: Spring to Early Summer

Description: Nettle is known for its anti-inflammatory and nutrient-rich properties. It is commonly used to support joint health, reduce allergy symptoms, and promote healthy skin and hair.

Native: Nettle is native to Europe, Asia, and North America, typically found in nutrient-rich soils near rivers and forests.

Cultivation: Nettle thrives in moist, well-drained soil and partial to full sun. The leaves and roots are harvested for herbal medicine.

Ancient Usage: Nettle, sometimes called the "herb of strength," has been used in traditional medicine to support blood health, reduce inflammation, and improve kidney function. Ancient Greeks used nettle to treat arthritis and stimulate circulation. In medieval Europe, nettle was a key remedy for anemia and skin conditions. Folklore associated nettle with protection and endurance, believing that the plant warded off danger and energized the body.

Nettle is a tall, perennial herb that can grow up to 1.5 meters (5 feet) tall, with square, hairy stems and deeply serrated, heart-shaped green leaves. The plant is covered in fine stinging hairs that release an irritant upon contact. It produces small, greenish flowers arranged in drooping clusters along the upper stems.

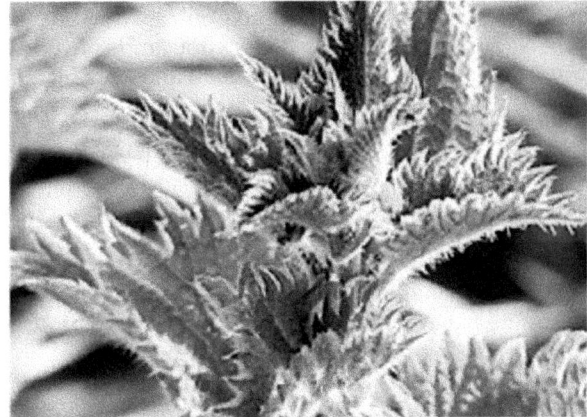

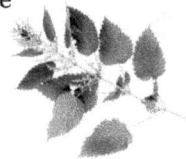

Medicinal Benefits:
- **Energy & Vitality:** Combats fatigue and supports wellness.
- **Allergy Relief:** Reduces allergies and hay fever.
- **Hormonal Balance:** Eases PMS and helps with menopausal transitions.
- **Anti-Inflammatory:** Reduces joint pain, muscle soreness, and arthritis.
- **Kidney & Urinary Tract Support:** Acts as a natural diuretic, promoting kidney health and detoxification.
- **Immune Boosting:** Contains high levels of vitamins and antioxidants.
- **Hair & Skin Health:** Reduces dandruff, and improves eczema and acne.

Dosage:
- **Standardized Extract:** 300-600 mg daily.
- **Tincture:** 2-4 mL (40-80 drops), 2-3 times daily.
- **Tea:** 1-2 tsp per cup of water, 2-3 times daily.
- **Capsules:** 500-1,000 mg, 1-2 times daily.

Safety:
- **Internal Use:** Prolonged use may cause stomach upset.
- **Children:** Safe for children for allergy relief and mild skin conditions.
- **Allergy Risk:** Individuals sensitive to plants in the Urticaceae family should use cautiously.
- **Drug Interactions:** May interact with blood pressure, diuretic, and anticoagulant medications.

Preparation Methods:
- **Edible Leaves & Seeds:** Nettle leaves and seeds are edible and best consumed cooked or dried.
- **Teas & Infusions:** Supports energy levels, boosts iron intake, and aids in allergy relief.
- **Decoctions:** Strengthens the immune system, supports kidney function, and reduces inflammation.
- **Tinctures:** Helps with joint pain, balances hormones, and supports adrenal health.
- **Syrups:** Provides mineral-rich nourishment, supports respiratory health, and boosts vitality.
- **Salves & Balms:** Soothes skin irritations, eases joint pain, and reduces inflammation.
- **Poultices:** Relieves muscle soreness, helps with eczema, and promotes wound healing.

ONION

Latin: Allium cepa.

Vital Parts: Bulbs, Leaves (Scapes), Flowers
Harvest Season: Late Summer to Early Autumn

Description: Onion is known for its powerful antimicrobial, anti-inflammatory, and antioxidant properties.

Native: Onions are native to Central Asia, but they have been cultivated worldwide for thousands of years, particularly in the Mediterranean and Asia Minor regions.

Cultivation: Onions thrive in well-drained, fertile soil with good sunlight. They are typically grown in a temperate climate and require moderate care, including regular watering and occasional fertilization.

Ancient Usage: Onion has a long history of use in ancient cultures, particularly in Egypt, Greece, and Rome. The ancient Egyptians considered onions to be a symbol of eternity, and they were often used in burial rituals to honor the dead. They believed onions could provide strength and vitality, and they were included in the diets of workers building the pyramids. In Greek and Roman times, onions were used to treat a variety of ailments, including headaches, indigestion, and respiratory issues. Folklore held that onions could ward off evil spirits and were placed around the home for protection.

Onion is a bulbous perennial plant known for its distinctive, pungent flavor and aroma. It typically grows to a height of 30 to 91 cm (12 to 36 inches) tall, with hollow, cylindrical green leaves that resemble grass. The plant produces a spherical cluster of small, white or purple flowers that bloom atop a tall, slender stalk. The underground bulb, composed of layered, fleshy scales, is the edible part of the plant and varies in size and color, ranging from white to yellow to red.

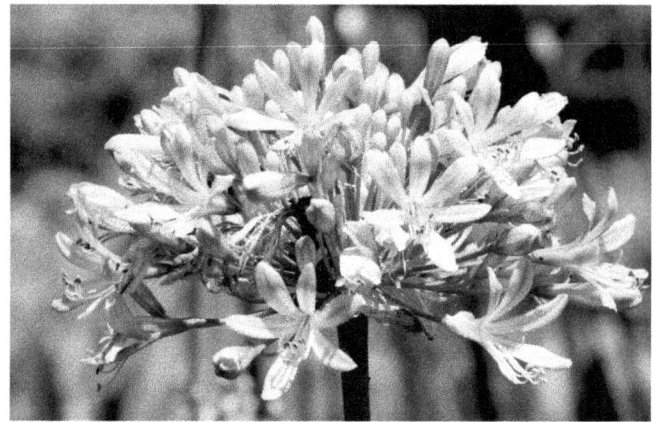

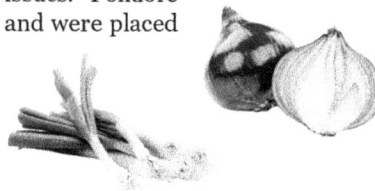

Medicinal Benefits:
- **Immune Support:** Helps the body fight off infections.
- **Anti-Inflammatory:** Supports arthritis and joint pain.
- **Heart Health:** Lowers blood pressure and reduces cholesterol.
- **Respiratory Health:** Aids coughs, colds, and asthma.
- **Digestive Health:** Aids digestion, and can help prevent constipation.
- **Blood Sugar Regulation:** Beneficial for diabetes.
- **Skin Health:** Helps treat skin conditions like acne and eczema.

Dosage:
- **Standardized Extract:** 300-500 mg daily.
- **Tincture:** 2-4 mL (40-80 drops), 2-3 times daily.
- **Tea:** 1-2 tsp or a bulb per cup of water, 2-3 times daily.
- **Capsules:** 500-1,000 mg of dried onion powder, 1-2 times daily.

Safety:
- **Internal Use:** Excessive intake may lead to bloating, heartburn, or diarrhea.
- **Drug Interactions:** Caution is advised for individuals on medication for blood pressure, blood sugar, or blood thinners.

Preparation Methods:
- **Teas & Infusions:** Supports respiratory health, eases coughs, and promotes digestion.
- **Decoctions:** Supports heart health, reduces inflammation, and improves circulation.
- **Tinctures:** Aids in fighting infections, boosts the immune system, and promotes digestive health.
- **Syrups:** Soothes sore throats, calms coughs, and supports respiratory health.
- **Salves & Balms:** Reduces muscle aches, inflammation, and minor skin irritations.
- **Poultices:** Reduces pain and inflammation in sore muscles, swollen joints, and minor cuts.

OREGANO

Latin: *Origanum vulgare*

Oregano is a low-growing, bushy perennial herb that can reach up to 60 cm (24 inches) tall, with woody stems and small, oval, dark green leaves. It produces highly aromatic clusters of small, pink to purple flowers that bloom at the tips of the stems.

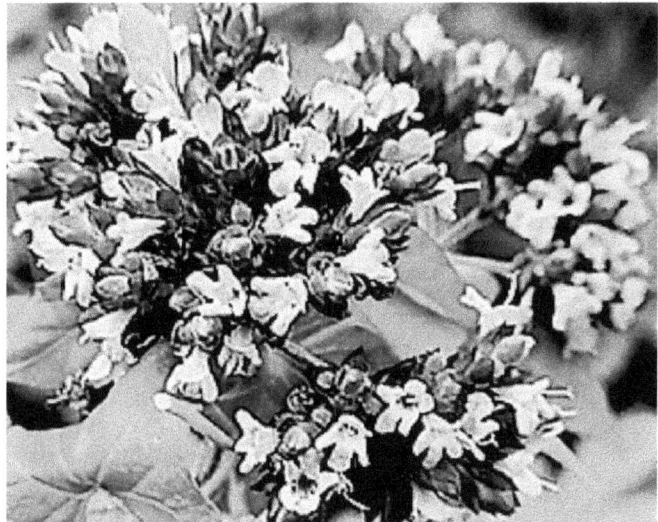

Vital Parts: Leaves, Flowers, Oil
Harvest Season: Late Spring to Early Autumn

Description: Oregano is known for its potent antimicrobial, antioxidant, and anti-inflammatory properties. It is commonly used to support respiratory health, improve digestion, and combat infections.

Native: Oregano is native to the Mediterranean region and parts of western Asia.

Cultivation: Oregano thrives in well-drained, moderately fertile soil and full sun. The leaves are harvested for use in herbal medicine, often prepared as teas, tinctures, and essential oils.

Ancient Usage: Oregano, often referred to as the "joy of the mountains," has been used for centuries to support respiratory and digestive health. The ancient Greeks used it as a remedy for infections and to promote digestive comfort. In Roman culture, oregano symbolized happiness and protection, frequently used in food and medicine. Folklore believed that oregano could ward off evil spirits and bring peace to households.

Medicinal Benefits:
- **Immune Support:** Strengthens the immune system and helps combat bacterial, viral, and fungal infections.
- **Respiratory Health:** Clears congestion, soothes coughs, and supports respiratory function.
- **Digestive Aid:** Relieves bloating, indigestion, and intestinal discomfort.
- **Antimicrobial Properties:** Fights bacteria, fungi, and parasites, both internally and externally.
- **Anti-Inflammatory:** Reduces inflammation, benefiting conditions like arthritis and sore muscles.
- **Antioxidant Support:** Protects cells from oxidative stress, reducing the risk of chronic diseases.
- **Skin Health:** Treats acne, fungal infections, and minor wounds with its antimicrobial properties.

Dosage:
- **Standardized Extract:** 300-600 mg daily.
- **Tincture:** 2-4 mL (40-80 drops), 2-3 times daily.
- **Tea:** 1-2 tsp per cup of water, 2-3 times daily.
- **Capsules:** 500-1,000 mg of dried herb, 1-2 times daily.

Safety:
- **Internal Use:** Medicinal oregano oil should be diluted, doses should be used cautiously.
- **Drug Interactions:** May interact with blood-thinning medications, antidiabetics, and immunosuppressants.
- **Allergy Risk:** Individuals allergic to plants in the Lamiaceae family (e.g., mint, thyme) should use cautiously.

Preparation Methods:
- **Edible Flowers:** Oregano flowers are edible and can be added into dishes.
- **Teas & Infusions:** Supports digestion, boosts immunity, and soothes respiratory discomfort.
- **Decoctions:** Treats coughs, clears congestion, and supports the immune system.
- **Tinctures:** Combats infections, supports digestion, and boosts immunity.
- **Syrups:** Soothes sore throats and coughs while supporting respiratory health.
- **Salves & Balms:** Treats fungal infections, reduces inflammation, and promotes healing of minor cuts.
- **Poultices:** Reduces swelling, soothes irritation, and treats minor infections.

PARSLEY

Latin: Petroselinum crispum

Vital Parts: Leaves, Stems, Roots, Seeds
Harvest Season: Spring to Early Autumn

Description: Parsley is known for its detoxifying, diuretic, and anti-inflammatory properties. It is commonly used to support kidney function, promote digestion, and provide antioxidant benefits. Parsley is rich in vitamins and minerals, including vitamin C and iron.

Native: Parsley is native to the Mediterranean region. The herb thrives in temperate climates, in coastal areas with well-drained soil and moderate humidity.

Cultivation: Parsley thrives in moist, fertile soil with full sun to partial shade. The leaves and roots are harvested for use in herbal medicine.

Ancient Usage: Parsley, known as the "herb of death and renewal," has a rich history in both culinary and medicinal traditions. The ancient Greeks associated parsley with both mourning and victory, often placing it on graves and crowning winners of athletic games. Medicinally, it was used to support kidney health, improve digestion, and reduce inflammation. Folklore believed parsley could protect against misfortune, and planting it was thought to ensure good luck and prosperity.

Parsley is a low-growing, biennial herb with smooth, branching stems and bright green, deeply divided, curly or flat leaves. It grows up to 60 cm (24 inches) tall and produces small, yellow-green flowers in umbrella-shaped clusters (umbels).

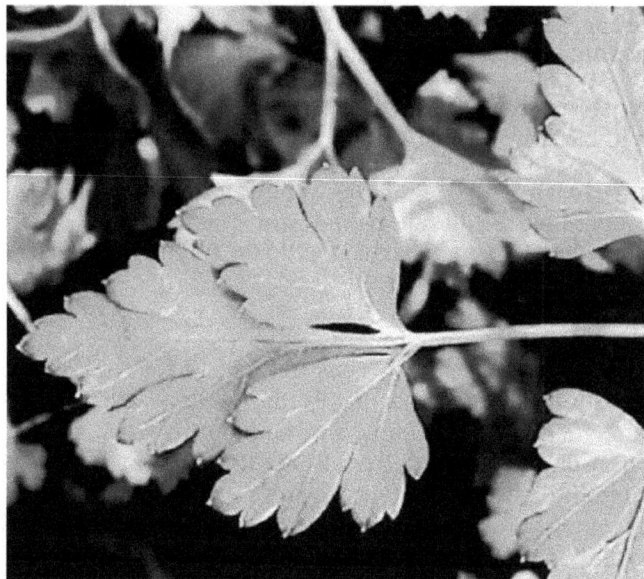

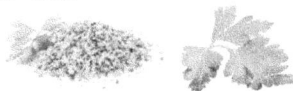

Medicinal Benefits:
- **Digestive Support:** Aids digestion, reduces bloating, and relieves gas.
- **Kidney & Urinary Tract Health:** Supports kidney function and reduces fluid retention.
- **Detoxification:** Supports liver health and removes toxins.
- **Heart Health:** Improves circulation, blood pressure, and cardiovascular wellness.
- **Anti-Inflammatory:** Reduces joint pain, muscle soreness, and inflammation.
- **Immune Support:** Rich in antioxidants and vitamin C.
- **Hormonal Balance:** Supports menstrual health and eases PMS.

Dosage:
- **Standardized Extract:** 200-400 mg daily.
- **Tincture:** 2-4 mL (40-80 drops), 2-3 times daily.
- **Tea:** 1-2 tsp per cup of water, 2-3 times daily.
- **Capsules:** 500-1,000 mg, 1-2 times daily.

Safety:
- **Internal Use:** Excessive use may cause digestive discomfort.
- **Allergy Risk:** Individuals allergic to plants in the Apiaceae family (e.g., celery, carrots) should use cautiously.
- **Drug Interactions:** May interact with diuretics and blood-thinning medications.

Preparation Methods:
- **Edible Leaves & Stems:** Parsley leaves and stems are edible, and are rich in vitamins.
- **Teas & Infusions:** Supports kidney health, aids digestion, and reduces bloating.
- **Decoctions:** Promotes detoxification and supports urinary tract health.
- **Tinctures:** Regulates menstrual cycles, supports liver function, and boosts circulation.
- **Syrups:** Supports immune health, and aids digestion.
- **Salves & Balms:** Soothes inflammation and promotes skin healing.
- **Poultices:** Relieves swelling and detoxifies the skin.

PASSIONFLOWER

Latin: Passiflora incarnata

Vital Parts: Leaves, Flowers, Stems
Harvest Season: Late Spring to Early Autumn

Description: Passionflower is renowned for its calming and anxiety-reducing properties. It is commonly used to alleviate insomnia, stress, and nervous tension.

Native: Passionflower is native to the southeastern United States and parts of Central and South America.

Cultivation: Passionflower thrives in well-drained soil and full sun to partial shade. The aerial parts (leaves, flowers, and stems) are harvested for herbal medicine, often prepared as teas and tinctures.

Ancient Usage: Passionflower, sometimes known as the "flower of tranquility," has been used for centuries to calm the mind, improve sleep, and reduce anxiety. Native American tribes used it to treat insomnia, nervous tension, and seizures. Spanish explorers named it "passionflower" for its resemblance to symbols of Christ's crucifixion, seeing it as a sacred plant. Folklore regarded it as a plant of peace, believed to enhance spiritual balance and protect against nightmares.

Passionflower is a climbing, perennial vine with thin, green stems and deeply lobed, dark green leaves. It produces large, intricate flowers with a crown of white and purple filaments surrounding a central structure of stamens and pistils.

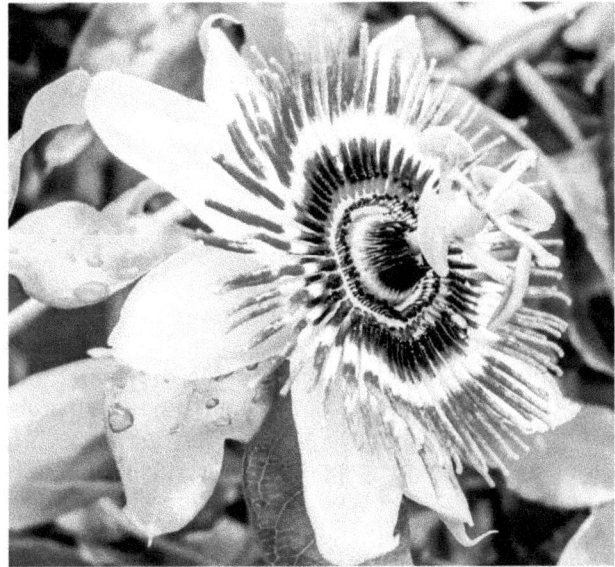

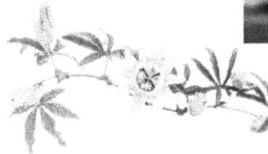

Medicinal Benefits:

- **Stress and Anxiety Relief:** Reduces nervous tension and anxiety.
- **Sleep Support:** Enhances relaxation and sleep quality.
- **Pain Relief:** Eases headaches, muscle tension, and mild pain.
- **Digestive Health:** Relieves cramping and bloating.
- **Nervous System Support:** Helps calm symptoms of nervous restlessness.
- **Menstrual Health:** Alleviates menstrual cramps and tension.
- **Cardiovascular Health:** Promotes relaxation and reduces heart palpitations.

Dosage:
- **Standardized Extract:** 300-600 mg daily.
- **Tincture:** 2-4 mL (40-80 drops), 2-3 times daily.
- **Tea:** 1-2 tsp per cup of water, 2-3 times daily.
- **Capsules:** 500-1,000 mg of dried herb, 1-2 times daily.

Safety:
- **Internal Use:** Excessive use may cause drowsiness.
- **Children:** Used as a remedy for restlessness or sleep disturbances.
- **Allergy Risk:** Individuals with sensitivities to Passiflora species should use cautiously.
- **Drug Interactions:** May interact with sedatives, antidepressants, and anti-anxiety medications.

Preparation Methods:
- **Edible Flowers:** Passionflower flowers are edible and can be used fresh.
- **Teas & Infusions:** Promotes relaxation, reduces anxiety, and supports restful sleep.
- **Decoctions:** Alleviates nervous tension, reduces inflammation, and supports digestive health.
- **Tinctures:** Aids in calming the nervous system, relieving stress, and improving sleep quality.
- **Syrups:** Soothes coughs, calms nervous tension, and supports respiratory health.
- **Salves & Balms:** Treats skin irritations, inflammation, and promotes healing.
- **Poultices:** Reduces swelling, soothes irritation, and promotes wound healing.

PEPPERMINT

Latin: Mentha × piperita

Vital Parts: Leaves
Harvest Season: Spring to Autumn

Description: Peppermint is well-known for its digestive-supporting and soothing properties. It is commonly used to relieve bloating, gas, and indigestion. Peppermint has cooling effects, making it effective for headaches and tension.

Native: Peppermint is a natural hybrid of water mint and spearmint, originally cultivated in Europe and now grown worldwide.

Cultivation: Peppermint thrives in moist, well-drained soil and partial to full sun. The leaves are harvested and used in herbal medicine.

Ancient Usage: Peppermint, sometimes called the "breath of freshness," has been used for centuries to support digestion, ease headaches, and relieve respiratory conditions. Ancient Egyptians used peppermint for indigestion, while Greek and Roman physicians praised its ability to soothe stomach pain and improve concentration. In medieval Europe, peppermint was often hung in homes to purify the air and repel pests. Folklore saw peppermint as a symbol of vitality and protection, believed to promote mental clarity and health.

Peppermint is a fast-growing, perennial herb that can reach up to 90 cm (3 feet) tall, with square stems and lance-shaped, dark green leaves covered in fine hairs. The plant produces spikes of small, pale purple flowers at the tops of the stems.

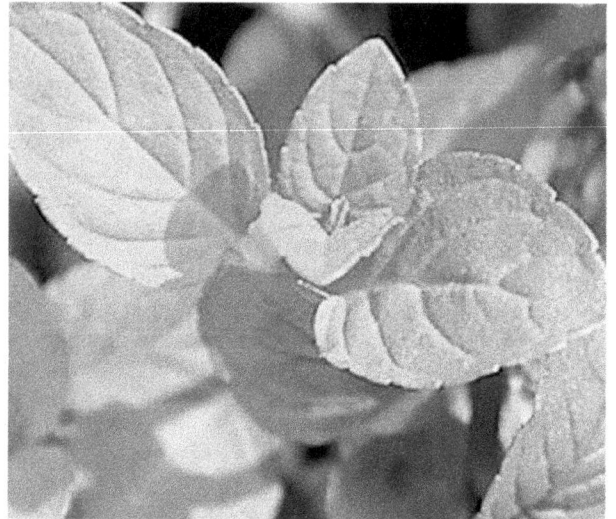

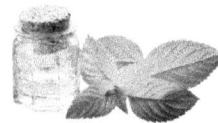

Medicinal Benefits:
- **Digestive Support:** Relieves bloating, gas, and nausea.
- **Respiratory Health:** Soothes congestion, coughs, and lung function.
- **Pain Relief:** Eases headaches, migraines, and muscle tension.
- **Energy & Focus:** Refreshes the mind, boosts mental clarity, and reduces fatigue.
- **Anti-Inflammatory:** Reduces muscle soreness, joint pain, and inflammation.
- **Immune Support:** Helps fight infections and colds.
- **Stress & Anxiety Relief:** Calms the nervous system and eases tension.

Dosage:
- **Standardized Extract:** 200-500 mg daily.
- **Tincture:** 2-4 mL (40-80 drops), 2-3 times daily.
- **Tea:** 1-2 tsp per cup of water daily.
- **Capsules:** 500-1,000 mg, 1-2 times daily.

Safety:
- **Internal Use:** Excessive consumption may cause heartburn.
- **Children:** Safe for older children; avoid undiluted oil due to its potential to cause respiratory distress.
- **Allergy Risk:** Individuals with sensitivities to mint-family plants (Lamiaceae) should use cautiously.
- **Drug Interactions:** May interact with antacids or medications for acid reflux.

Preparation Methods:
- **Edible Leaves & Stems:** Peppermint leaves and stems are edible, with a refreshing flavor.
- **Teas & Infusions:** Supports digestion, headaches, and nausea.
- **Decoctions:** Clears respiratory passages, eases congestion, and relieves bloating.
- **Tinctures:** Helps with digestive issues, reduces stress, and boosts mental clarity.
- **Syrups:** Soothes sore throats, relieves coughs, and supports respiratory health.
- **Salves & Balms:** Cools irritated skin, relieves muscle tension, and reduces inflammation.
- **Poultices:** Eases headaches, relieves joint pain, and soothes insect bites.

PLANTAIN

Latin: Plantago major

Vital Parts: Leaves, Seeds
Harvest Season: Spring to Autumn

Description: Plantain is known for its anti-inflammatory and wound-healing properties. It is commonly used to soothe skin irritations, promote healing of wounds and cuts, and alleviate respiratory conditions.

Native: Plantain is native to Europe and Asia but has naturalized in many parts of North America.

Cultivation: Plantain thrives in a variety of soils and full sun to partial shade. The leaves are harvested for herbal use, often prepared as teas, infusions, and poultice.

Ancient Usage: Plantain, often called the "healer of wounds," has been used for centuries to soothe skin irritations, promote wound healing, and support digestion. Ancient herbalists, including the Romans, valued it for treating cuts, insect bites, and inflammation. Native American tribes used plantain to relieve pain, draw out toxins, and soothe sore throats. In folklore, plantain was seen as a protector against physical harm, often carried as a charm for health and resilience.

Plantain is a low-growing, perennial herb with a rosette of broad, oval leaves that have prominent veins running lengthwise. It produces tall, slender flower spikes with small, inconspicuous greenish-brown flowers.

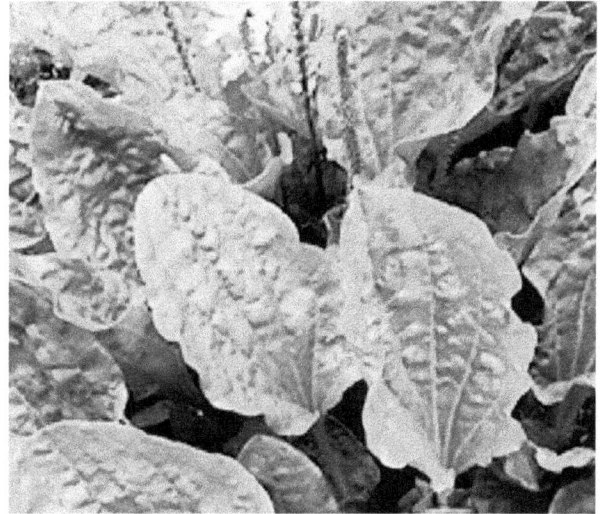

Medicinal Benefits:
- **Wound Healing:** Speeds recovery from cuts, burns, and insect bites.
- **Digestive Support:** Soothes indigestion, relieves bloating, and helps with ulcers and acid reflux.
- **Anti-Inflammatory:** Reduces swelling, joint pain, and muscle soreness.
- **Respiratory Health:** Eases coughs, soothes sore throats, and supports lung function.
- **Detoxification:** Supports kidney and liver health.
- **Skin Soothing:** Helps with eczema, rashes, and irritated skin conditions.
- **Urinary Tract Support:** Acts as a natural diuretic, helping with UTIs and fluid retention.

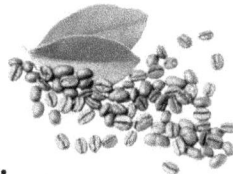

Dosage:
- **Standardized Extract:** 200-400 mg daily.
- **Tincture:** 2-4 mL (40-80 drops), 2-3 times daily.
- **Tea:** 1-2 tsp per cup of water, 2-3 times daily.
- **Capsules:** 500-1,000 mg, 1-2 times daily.

Safety:
- **Children:** Safe for children, particularly for treating minor skin conditions or coughs.
- **Allergy Risk:** Individuals with sensitivities to related plants should test a small amount before widespread use.

Preparation Methods:
- **Edible Leaves & Seeds:** Plantain leaves and seeds are edible.
- **Teas & Infusions:** Supports respiratory health, soothes sore throats, and aids digestion.
- **Decoctions:** Reduces inflammation, promotes wound healing, and supports urinary tract health.
- **Tinctures:** Helps with skin conditions, soothes digestive issues, and supports immune function.
- **Syrups:** Relieves coughs, soothes irritation, and promotes lung health.
- **Salves & Balms:** Heals cuts, burns, and insect bites while reducing skin inflammation.
- **Poultices:** Draws out toxins, soothes stings and rashes, and speeds wound healing.

POMEGRANATE

Latin: *Punica granatum*

Vital Parts: Seeds (Arils), Peel, Flowers, Bark
Harvest Season: Late Summer to Autumn

Description: Pomegranate is rich in antioxidants and has anti-inflammatory, cardiovascular-supporting, and immune-enhancing properties. It is commonly used to promote heart health, improve circulation, and protect against oxidative stress.

Native: Pomegranate is native to the Middle East, North Africa, and parts of South Asia.

Cultivation: Pomegranate thrives in well-drained, sandy soil and full sun. The fruit and seeds are harvested for use in herbal medicine, often consumed fresh or as juice, powders, or extracts to support heart health and reduce inflammation.

Ancient Usage: Pomegranate, sometimes known as the "fruit of life," has been revered since ancient times for its antioxidant-rich seeds and symbolism of fertility and renewal. In ancient Persia and Egypt, it was considered a sacred fruit used in rituals and offerings. The Greeks associated it with the myth of Persephone and the cycles of life and death. In folklore, pomegranate was believed to promote abundance and prosperity, often planted near homes to ensure longevity and wealth.

Pomegranate is a small, deciduous tree or large shrub that can grow up to 6 meters (20 feet) tall, with thorny branches and glossy, lance-shaped leaves. It produces large, red to orange, funnel-shaped flowers, which develop into round, thick-skinned fruits containing numerous juicy, red arils surrounding edible seeds.

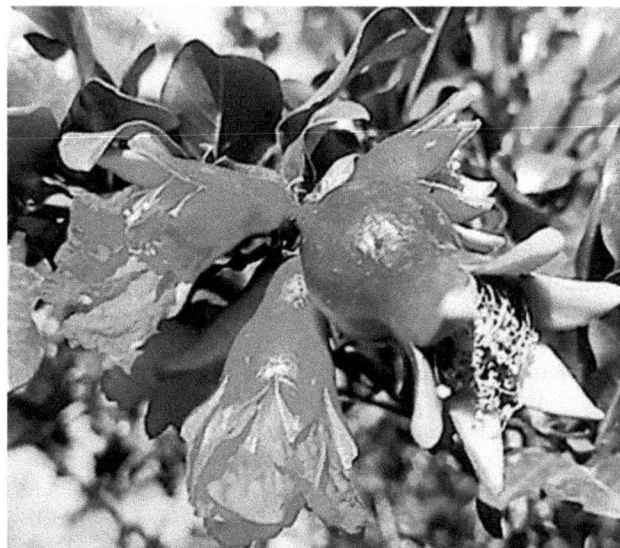

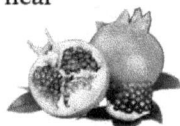

Medicinal Benefits:
- **Heart Health:** Improves circulation and regulates blood pressure.
- **Antioxidant Power:** Combats oxidative stress and supports cellular health.
- **Hormonal Balance:** Supports estrogen levels and menopause.
- **Digestive Aid:** Promotes gut health, eases bloating, and supports digestion.
- **Immune Support:** Contains high vitamin C and antimicrobial properties.
- **Anti-Inflammatory:** Reduces joint pain and muscle soreness.
- **Skin & Anti-Aging:** Aids collagen production, hydrates the skin, and reduces signs of aging.

Dosage:
- **Standardized Extract:** 300-600 mg daily.
- **Tincture:** 2-4 mL (40-80 drops), 2-3 times daily.
- **Tea:** 1-2 tsp per cup of water, 1-2 times daily.
- **Capsules:** 500-1,000 mg, 1-2 times daily.

Safety:
- **Children:** Safe for children to support immune health and digestion.
- **Allergy Risk:** Those with fruit allergies should test small amounts.
- **Drug Interactions:** May interfere with blood thinners and blood pressure medications.

Preparation Methods:
- **Edible Seeds & Peel:** Pomegranate seeds are edible and the peel has medicinal uses.
- **Teas & Infusions:** Supports heart health, boosts immunity, and aids digestion.
- **Decoctions:** Supports gut health and promotes detoxification.
- **Tinctures:** Aids in hormonal balance, enhances circulation, and provides antioxidant protection.
- **Syrups:** Strengthens the immune system, soothes sore throats, and supports cardiovascular health.
- **Salves & Balms:** Nourishes the skin, promotes collagen production, and protects against dryness.
- **Poultices:** Aids with skin infections, swelling, and healing.

RED CLOVER

Latin: Trifolium pratense

Vital Parts: Leaves, Flowers
Harvest Season: Late Spring to Early Autumn

Description: Red clover is known for its hormone-balancing and detoxifying properties. It is commonly used to support women's health, particularly during menopause, to alleviate symptoms such as hot flashes and hormonal imbalances.

Native: Red clover is native to Europe, Asia, and North Africa but is widely cultivated in North America.

Cultivation: Red clover thrives in fertile, well-drained soil and full sun. The flowers are harvested for herbal use, often prepared as teas, tinctures, and capsules

Ancient Usage: Red clover, often called the "blood purifier," has been used in traditional herbal medicine to support detoxification, improve circulation, and balance hormones. Native American tribes and European herbalists used it to treat skin conditions, respiratory issues, and menopausal symptoms. In medieval Europe, red clover was considered a plant of good fortune, believed to protect against illness and bring prosperity. Folklore held that finding a four-leaf clover could ward off evil and grant wishes.

Red clover is a short-lived, perennial herb that grows up to 90 cm (3 feet) tall, with branching stems and trifoliate (three-part) leaves marked by a pale V-shaped pattern. It produces rounded clusters of small, pink to purple flowers.

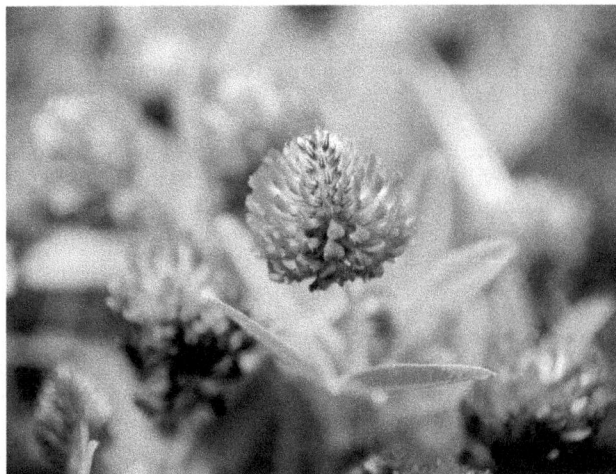

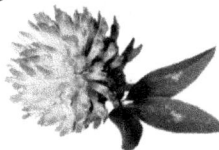

Medicinal Benefits:
- **Hormonal Balance:** Aids PMS, menopause, and menstrual irregularities.
- **Menopausal Support:** Reduces hot flashes, night sweats, and mood swings.
- **Detoxification:** Aids in the removal of toxins.
- **Respiratory Health:** Eases coughs, congestion, and supports lung function.
- **Bone Health:** Helps maintain bone density and reduces the risk of osteoporosis.
- **Heart Health:** Supports circulation, improves blood flow, and promotes cardiovascular wellness.
- **Skin Healing:** Soothes eczema, psoriasis, and other skin irritations.

Dosage:
- **Standardized Extract:** 200-400 mg daily.
- **Tincture:** 2-4 mL (40-80 drops), 2-3 times daily.
- **Tea:** 1-2 tsp per cup of water, 2-3 times daily.
- **Capsules:** 500-1,000 mg, 1-2 times daily.

Safety:
- **Internal Use:** Prolonged use in may affect hormone-sensitive conditions.
- **Children:** Safe for soothing skin conditions or mild respiratory complaints.
- **Allergy Risk:** Individuals allergic to the legume family (Fabaceae) should use cautiously.
- **Drug Interactions:** May interact with anticoagulants, hormone replacement therapy, and birth control pills.

Preparation Methods:
- **Edible Flowers & Leaves:** Red clover flowers and leaves are edible and mildly sweet.
- **Teas & Infusions:** Supports hormonal balance, detoxification, and aids respiratory health.
- **Decoctions:** Purifies the blood and reduces inflammation.
- **Tinctures:** Helps with menopause, circulation, and supports skin health.
- **Syrups:** Soothes coughs, strengthens the immune system, and promotes lung health.
- **Salves & Balms:** Nourishes the skin, soothes eczema, aids minor irritations.
- **Poultices:** Reduces swelling, and speeds up wound healing.

RED RASPBERRY

Latin: Rubus idaeus

Vital Parts: Leaves, Berries
Harvest Season: Spring to Early Summer

Description: Red raspberry is valued for its hormone-regulating and uterine-supporting properties. It is used to promote reproductive health, ease menstrual cramps, and support pregnancy.

Native: Red raspberry is native to Europe and parts of Asia and North America.

Cultivation: Red raspberries grow best in well-drained, loamy soil with full sun and regular moisture, thriving in USDA Zones 3-9. Plant bare-root canes in early spring, provide trellising for support, prune regularly, and harvest ripe berries in late summer when they easily detach from the plant.

Ancient Usage: Red raspberry, sometimes referred to as the "mother's herb," has been used for centuries to support women's reproductive health. Native American tribes used the leaves to ease childbirth, regulate menstruation, and promote fertility. European herbalists valued raspberry leaf tea for its ability to strengthen the uterus and reduce labor pain. Folklore associated the plant with protection and fertility, believing it brought strength and vitality to families.

Medicinal Benefits:
- **Women's Health Support:** Supports fertility and eases menstrual discomfort.
- **Pregnancy & Labor Aid:** Aids with smoother pregnancy and childbirth.
- **Hormonal Balance:** Reduces PMS and eases menopause discomfort.
- **Digestive Aid:** Soothes indigestion and relieves bloating.
- **Anti-Inflammatory:** Reduces muscle soreness and joint pain.
- **Immune Support:** Helps fight infections.
- **Heart Health:** Improves blood flow and regulates blood pressure.
- **Skin & Wound Healing:** Soothes skin irritations, rashes, and wounds.
- **Respiratory Health:** Soothes sore throats and coughs.

Red raspberry is a deciduous, thorny shrub that can grow up to 2 meters (6 feet) tall, with arching canes and compound, serrated green leaves consisting of three to five leaflets. It produces small, white flowers that develop into red, juicy, aggregate fruits.

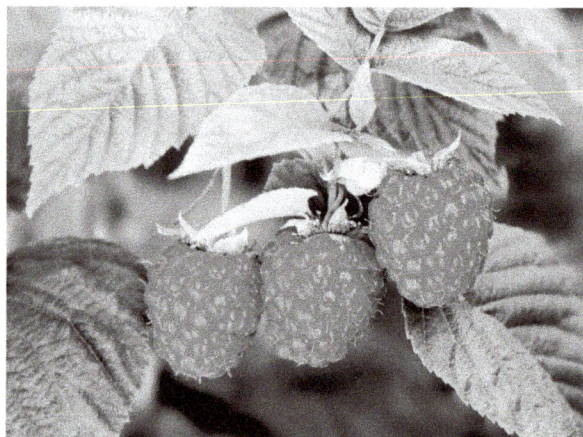

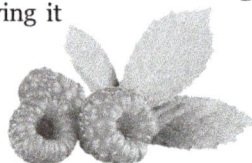

Dosage:
- **Standardized Extract:** 200-500 mg daily.
- **Tincture:** 2-4 mL (40-80 drops), 2-3 times daily.
- **Tea:** 1-2 tsp per cup of water, 2-3 times daily.
- **Capsules:** 500-1,000 mg of dried herb, 1-2 times daily.

Safety:
- **Internal Use:** Prolonged or excessive use may cause mild digestive upset.
- **Children:** Safe as a remedy for diarrhea or sore throats.
- **Allergy Risk:** Individuals allergic to plants in the Rosaceae family (e.g., strawberries, apples) should use cautiously.

Preparation Methods:
- **Edible Leaves & Berries:** Red raspberry leaves and berries are edible, rich in vitamins and antioxidants.
- **Teas & Infusions:** Supports reproductive health, strengthens the uterus, and aids digestion.
- **Decoctions:** Reduces inflammation, soothes sore throats, and supports immune health.
- **Tinctures:** Helps with menstrual cramps, balances hormones, and supports pregnancy wellness.
- **Syrups:** Provides vitamin C, boosts immunity, and soothes coughs.
- **Salves & Balms:** Soothes irritated skin, promotes healing, and reduces inflammation.
- **Poultices:** Helps with rashes, insect bites, and minor wounds.

REISHI

Latin: *Ganoderma lucidum*

Vital Parts: Fruiting Body and Spores

Harvest Season: Late Summer to Autumn

Description: Reishi is known for its immune-modulating, adaptogenic, and anti-inflammatory properties. It is commonly used to reduce stress, support immune function, and promote longevity.

Native: Reishi is native to East Asia and grows on decaying hardwood trees.

Cultivation: Reishi grows well on logs or wood-based substrates. It prefers a cool, humid environment and can take several months to grow, but it can be cultivated indoors or in shaded outdoor areas.

Ancient Usage: Reishi, often called the "mushroom of immortality," has been revered in traditional Chinese medicine for thousands of years to promote longevity and boost the immune system. Ancient Chinese emperors sought reishi for its ability to grant vitality and spiritual harmony. It was believed to balance the body's life force (qi) and protect against illness. In folklore, reishi was seen as a symbol of divine power and inner peace, often used in rituals.

Medicinal Benefits:
- **Immune Support:** Supports the body's ability to fight infections.
- **Stress and Anxiety Relief:** Promotes relaxation and mental clarity.
- **Liver Health:** Aids in detoxifying the liver.
- **Heart Health:** Regulates blood pressure and cholesterol.
- **Anti-Inflammatory:** Aids arthritis, autoimmune disorders, and chronic pain.
- **Antioxidant Properties:** Slows the aging process.
- **Sleep Aid:** Calms the nervous system and supports hormonal balance.
- **Cancer Support:** Inhibits tumor growth and supports the immune system.

Reishi is a large, woody mushroom with a distinctive, shiny, reddish-brown, kidney-shaped cap and a short, thick stem. It grows on hardwood trees and logs, often appearing in a shelf-like formation.

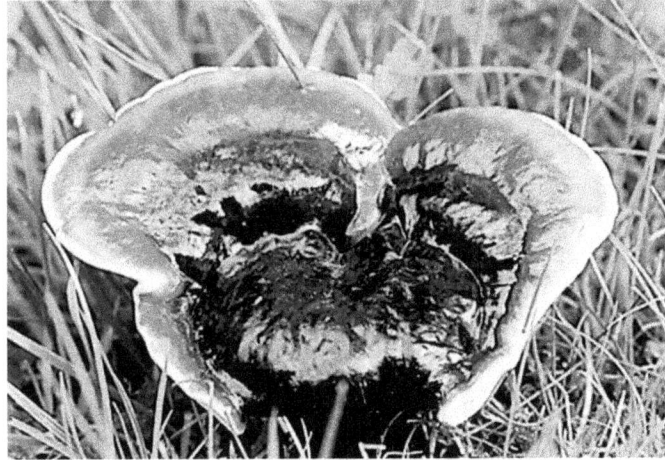

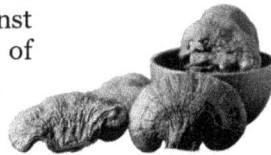

Dosage:
- **Standardized Extract:** 500-1,000 mg daily.
- **Tincture:** 2-4 mL (40-80 drops), 2-3 times daily.
- **Tea:** 1-2 tsp of dried mushroom per cup of water, 1-2 times daily.
- **Capsules:** 500-1,000 mg of dried mushroom extract, 1-2 times daily.

Safety:
- **Drug Interactions:** Reishi may interact with immunosuppressants, blood-thinning, and blood pressure medications.
- **Excessive Use:** Overuse may cause dry mouth, upset stomach, or dizziness.

Preparation Methods:
- **Teas & Infusions:** Supports immune health, reduces stress, and promotes relaxation.
- **Decoctions:** Provides immune support and liver detoxification.
- **Tinctures:** Reduces stress, and enhances immunity.
- **Powders:** Dried reishi is ground into a fine powder that can be added to smoothies, coffee, or capsules for convenient daily use.
- **Capsules:** Pre-made supplements provide a standardized dose of reishi's active compounds.
- **Syrups:** Soothes coughs, promotes relaxation, and supports respiratory health.

ROSEMARY

Latin: *Salvia rosmarinus*

Vital Parts: Leaves, Flowers
Harvest Season: Year-Round in Warm Climates

Description: Rosemary is a hardy, perennial herb that thrives in well-drained, sandy or loamy soil with full sun exposure. Rosemary is known for its cognitive-supporting and anti-inflammatory properties.

Native: Rosemary is native to the Mediterranean region, where it thrives in the warm, dry climates. It has been cultivated in Southern Europe, North Africa, and parts of Asia, where it is valued for its medicinal and culinary uses.

Cultivation: It is drought-tolerant once established. The needle-like leaves are harvested throughout the year and are most potent in the summer months when the plant's essential oils are at their peak.

Ancient Usage: Rosemary, known as the "herb of remembrance," has been used since ancient times to improve memory, stimulate circulation, and ward off illness. The Greeks and Romans used it in religious ceremonies, weddings, and funerals, believing it to promote clarity and protection. In medieval Europe, rosemary was often placed under pillows to prevent nightmares and hung in homes to purify the air. Folklore associated it with loyalty, courage, and mental clarity.

Rosemary is an aromatic, evergreen shrub that grows up to 1.5 meters (5 feet) tall, with woody stems and narrow, needle-like, dark green leaves with silvery undersides. It produces small, pale blue or lavender flowers clustered along the stems.

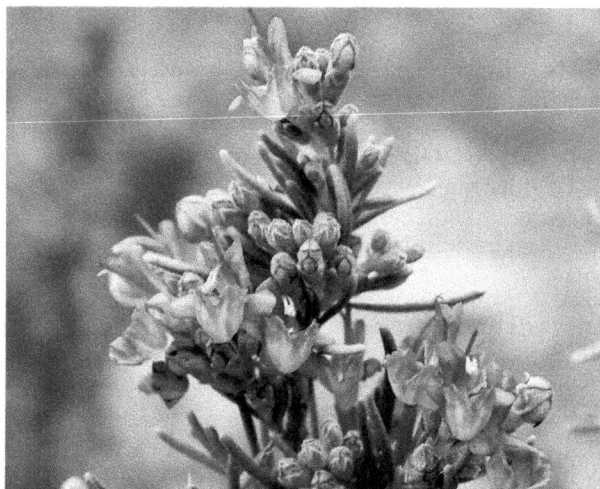

Medicinal Benefits:

- **Cognitive Support:** Enhances memory, focus, and mental clarity.
- **Digestive Health:** Eases indigestion, gas, and bloating.
- **Immune Support:** Helps the body fight infections.
- **Respiratory Health:** Alleviates symptoms of colds, bronchitis, and asthma.
- **Anti-Inflammatory:** Supports muscle and joint health.
- **Circulatory Health:** Improves blood circulation.
- **Hair and Scalp Health:** Stimulates hair growth and reduces dandruff.

Dosage:

- **Standardized Extract:** 200-400 mg daily.
- **Tincture:** 2-4 mL (40-80 drops), 2-3 times daily.
- **Tea:** 1-2 tsp of dried leaves per cup of water, 2-3 times daily.
- **Capsules:** 500-1,000 mg of dried herb, 1-2 times daily.

Safety:

- **Internal Use:** Excessive use may cause stomach upset.
- **Children:** Safe in small amounts for respiratory or digestive support.
- **Allergy Risk:** Those with sensitivities to plants in the mint family (Lamiaceae) should use cautiously.
- **Drug Interactions:** May interact with blood pressure medications, anticoagulants, and diuretics.

Preparation Methods:

- **Edible Flowers:** Rosemary flowers are edible.
- **Teas & Infusions:** Supports memory, boosts circulation, and aids digestion.
- **Decoctions:** Relieves respiratory issues and inflammation, and promotes hair health.
- **Tinctures:** Improves focus and circulation and reduces joint pain.
- **Syrups:** Soothes coughs, supports respiratory health, and boosts vitality.
- **Salves & Balms:** Reduces muscle pain, andvimproves circulation.
- **Poultices:** Reduces swelling, soothes insect bites, and promotes wound healing.

SAGE

Latin: *Salvia officinalis*

Vital Parts: Leaves, Flowers
Harvest Season: Spring to Early Summer

Description: Sage is valued for its cognitive-enhancing, antimicrobial, and anti-inflammatory properties. It is commonly used to improve memory and promote digestion.

Native: Sage is native to the Mediterranean region, where it flourishes in warm, dry climates along rocky hillsides and coastal landscapes. Historically, it has been cultivated across Europe, North Africa, and Western Asia, prized for its medicinal, culinary, and ceremonial uses.

Cultivation: Sage thrives in well-drained, sandy soil and full sun. The leaves are harvested for use in herbal medicine, prepared as teas, tinctures, and essential oils.

Ancient Usage: Sage, often called the "sacred herb," has been used for centuries to promote health, wisdom, and purification. The ancient Greeks and Romans used it to treat wounds, digestive problems, and respiratory conditions. Native American tribes used sage in smudging ceremonies to cleanse and protect against negative energies. Folklore associated sage with immortality and protection, believing that growing it in the home brought long life and peace.

Medicinal Benefits:
- **Cognitive Support:** Enhances memory, concentration, and clarity, and may help manage symptoms of Alzheimer's disease.
- **Hormonal Balance:** Reduces hot flashes, night sweats, and hormonal imbalances.
- **Digestive Health:** Relieves indigestion, bloating, and gas.
- **Respiratory Support:** Eases colds, coughs, and sore throats.
- **Oral Health:** Reduces gum inflammation, treats mouth sores, and combats bad breath.
- **Skin Health:** Treats minor wounds, acne, and rashes.
- **Immune Support:** Boosts immunity and fights infections.

Sage is a woody-stemmed, evergreen perennial herb that grows up to 1 meter (3 feet) tall, with gray-green, oval, velvety leaves. It produces spikes of tubular, purple to blue flowers in the upper portions of the plant.

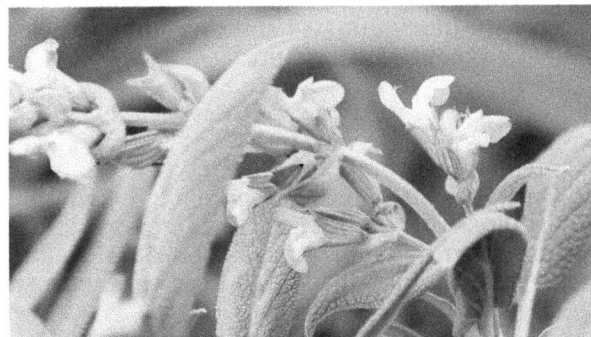

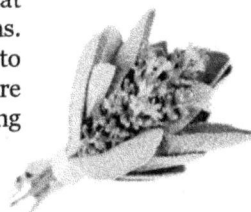

Dosage:
- **Standardized Extract:** 300-600 mg daily.
- **Tincture:** 2-4 mL (40-80 drops), 2-3 times daily.
- **Tea:** 1-2 tsp per cup of water, 2-3 times daily.
- **Capsules:** 500-1,000 mg, 1-2 times daily.

Safety:
- **Internal Use:** Prolonged doses may cause side effects.
- **Children:** Safe for sore throats and digestive issues.
- **Allergy Risk:** Those with sensitivities to mint-family plants (Lamiaceae) should use cautiously.
- **Drug Interactions:** May interact with medications for blood sugar, seizures, or blood pressure.

Preparation Methods:
- **Edible Leaves & Flowers:** Sage leaves and flowers are edible, with a strong, earthy flavor.
- **Teas & Infusions:** Supports digestion, reduces inflammation, and soothes sore throats.
- **Decoctions:** Enhances memory, relieves cold symptoms, and balances hormones.
- **Tinctures:** Helps with menopausal symptoms, supports oral health, and reduces stress.
- **Syrups:** Soothes coughs, boosts immunity, and supports respiratory health.
- **Salves & Balms:** Aids in wound healing, reduces inflammation, and soothes skin conditions.
- **Poultices:** Draws out infections, relieves muscle pain, and calms skin irritations.

SHIITAKE

Latin: Lentinula edodes

Vital Parts: Fruiting Body
Harvest Season: Spring to Autumn

Description: Shiitake mushrooms are known for their immune-boosting, antioxidant, and cardiovascular-supporting properties. They are commonly used to enhance immune system function, improve heart health, and promote overall vitality.

Native: Shiitake is native to East Asia and grows naturally on decaying hardwood trees.

Cultivation: Shiitake mushrooms grow well on hardwood logs or sawdust-based substrates. They require moderate humidity and temperatures between 55°F to 75°F (13°C to 24°C). They're relatively easy to grow at home and can be grown indoors or outdoors.

Ancient Usage: Shiitake, sometimes known as the "elixir of life," has been used in traditional Chinese and Japanese medicine to boost immunity, improve circulation, and support longevity. Ancient healers believed shiitake mushrooms could protect against disease and enhance vitality. They were often reserved for royalty due to their rarity and powerful health benefits. In folklore, shiitake was seen as a symbol of strength and prosperity and thought to promote health.

Shiitake is a large, edible mushroom with a broad, brown, umbrella-shaped cap and a white, firm stem. The cap surface is slightly cracked or scaly, and the underside has gills that release spores. It grows on decaying hardwood trees.

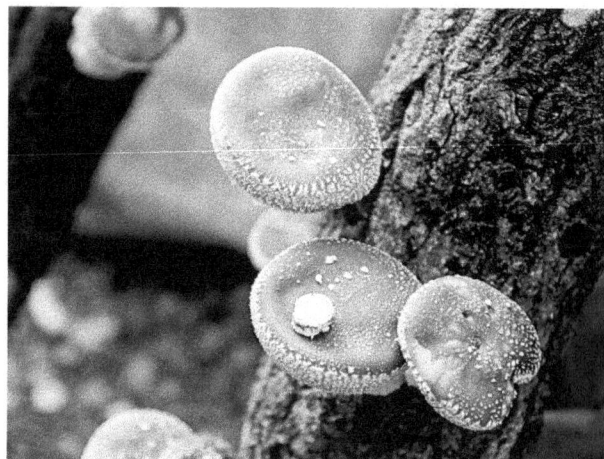

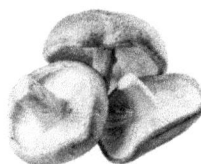

Medicinal Benefits:
- **Immune Support:** Stimulates the activity of white blood cells.
- **Cardiovascular Health:** Reduces cholesterol levels and blood pressure.
- **Anti-Inflammatory:** Benefits arthritis and chronic pain.
- **Cancer Support:** Lentinan, a compound in shiitake, can enhance cancer treatment by boosting immune response.
- **Antiviral and Antibacterial Properties:** Contains compounds that inhibit the growth of viruses and bacteria.
- **Skin Health:** Promotes healthy skin, as it is high in antioxidants.
- **Digestive Health:** Acts as a prebiotic, supporting gut health.

Dosage:
- **Standardized Extract:** 500-1,000 mg daily.
- **Tincture:** 2-4 mL (40-80 drops), 2-3 times daily
- **Tea:** 1-2 tsp per cup of water, 1-2 times daily.
- **Capsules:** 500-1,000 mg, 1-2 times daily.

Safety:
- **Internal Use:** Excessive intake may cause mild digestive upset.
- **Allergy Risk:** Some individuals may experience skin irritation.
- **Drug Interactions:** May enhance the effects of blood-thinning medications.
- **Children:** Safe in small amounts, particularly in culinary uses.

Preparation Methods:
- **Edible Uses:** Shiitake mushrooms are commonly used in cooking and can be sautéed, grilled, or used as a meat substitute in vegetarian dishes.
- **Teas & Infusions:** Supports immune health and improves digestion.
- **Decoctions:** Provides immune support and reduces inflammation.
- **Tinctures:** Supports immune function, cardiovascular health, and overall vitality.
- **Powders:** Dried shiitake can be added to soups, smoothies, or capsules for convenient daily use.
- **Syrups:** Soothes coughs and supports respiratory health.
- **Salves & Balms:** Promotes wound healing and soothes skin irritations.

SKULLCAP

Latin: Scutellaria lateriflora

Vital Parts: Leaves, Flowers, Stems
Harvest Season: Late Spring to Early Autumn

Description: Skullcap is known for its calming and nervine properties. It is commonly used to reduce anxiety, promote relaxation, and improve sleep.

Native: Skullcap is native to North America and is often found in moist woodlands and riverbanks.

Cultivation: Skullcap thrives in moist, well-drained soil and partial shade. The aerial parts (leaves and flowers) are harvested and used in herbal medicine.

Ancient Usage: Skullcap, sometimes known as the "calming herb," has been used for centuries to ease anxiety, nervous tension, and insomnia. Native American tribes used it to promote relaxation and support women's health, particularly for menstrual and childbirth-related pain. In early American herbal medicine, skullcap was valued for calming hysteria and seizures. Folklore associated it with protection against mental distress and was believed to promote peace and emotional balance.

Skullcap is a low-growing, perennial herb that reaches up to 60 cm (24 inches) tall, with square stems and lance-shaped, serrated green leaves. It produces small, tubular blue to violet flowers that bloom in clusters along the upper stems.

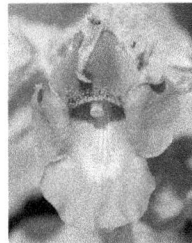

Medicinal Benefits:
- **Nervous System Support:** Reduces anxiety, stress, and nervous tension.
- **Sleep Aid:** Promotes relaxation and improves sleep quality caused by stress or insomnia.
- **Anti-Spasmodic:** Relieves muscle tension, spasms, and cramps.
- **Pain Relief:** Alleviates headaches, nerve pain, and joint discomfort.
- **Seizure Management:** Supports individuals with mild seizures and tremors.
- **Immune Support:** Contains antioxidants that combat oxidative stress and help boost overall immunity.

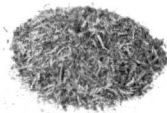

Dosage:
- **Standardized Extract:** 200-400 mg daily.
- **Tincture:** 2-4 mL (40-80 drops), 2-3 times daily.
- **Tea:** 1-2 tsp per cup of water, 2-3 times daily.
- **Capsules:** 500-1,000 mg, 1-2 times daily.

Safety:
- **Internal Use:** Excessive use may cause dizziness or drowsiness.
- **Children:** Safe in small doses for calming effects or mild pain relief.
- **Allergy Risk:** Individuals sensitive to mint-family plants (Lamiaceae) should use cautiously.
- **Drug Interactions:** May enhance the effects of sedatives, antidepressants, or antianxiety medications.

Preparation Methods:
- **Teas & Infusions:** Calms the nervous system, eases anxiety, and promotes restful sleep.
- **Decoctions:** Reduces inflammation and muscle tension.
- **Tinctures:** Used for stress relief, insomnia, nervous exhaustion, and cognitive function.
- **Powders:** Supports daily stress and anxiety.
- **Capsules:** Standardized extract provides convenient support for relaxation and nervous system balance.
- **Syrups:** Helps ease tension headaches and nervous agitation.
- **Salves & Balms:** Applied for nerve pain, muscle spasms, and soothing irritated skin.

SLIPPERY ELM

Latin: *Ulmus rubra*

Vital Parts: Inner Bark
Harvest Season: Late Winter to Early Spring

Description: Slippery elm is known for its soothing and mucilaginous properties. It is commonly used to relieve sore throats, coughs, and digestive irritation. Slippery elm also supports gut health by promoting the healing of mucous membranes.

Native: Slippery elm is native to North America, particularly in the eastern and central regions.

Cultivation: Slippery elm thrives in well-drained, fertile soil and full sun. The inner bark is harvested and used in herbal medicine, often prepared as teas, lozenges, and powders to soothe inflammation and support respiratory and digestive health.

Ancient Usage: Slippery elm, often called the "soothing bark," has been used by Native American tribes to treat digestive issues, sore throats, and wounds. The inner bark was prepared as a poultice to soothe inflamed skin and as a tea to ease coughs and gastrointestinal irritation. Early settlers adopted slippery elm to treat fevers and promote healing in cases of colds and ulcers. Folklore held that slippery elm could protect against illness, symbolizing nurturing and protection.

Medicinal Benefits:
- **Digestive Health:** Alleviates acid reflux, ulcers, colitis, and irritable bowel syndrome (IBS).
- **Respiratory Support:** Provides relief from sore throats, coughs, and bronchitis.
- **Urinary Health:** Reduces irritation and inflammation associated with UTIs.
- **Skin Health:** Treats burns, wounds and boils.
- **Nutritional Support:** Offers nourishment for recovering from illness.
- **Anti-Inflammatory:** Eases inflammation, supporting holistic wellness.

Dosage:
- **Standardized Extract:** 300-600 mg daily.
- **Tincture:** 2-4 mL (40-80 drops), 2-3 times daily.
- **Tea:** 1-2 tsp per cup of hot water, 2-3 times daily.
- **Capsules:** 500-1,000 mg daily.

Safety:
- **Children:** Safe for children, especially for soothing sore throats or digestive issues.
- **Allergy Risk:** Those allergic to elm trees should use cautiously.
- **Sustainability:** Overharvesting has impacted wild populations of slippery elm; opt for sustainably sourced products to ensure preservation.

Slippery elm is a medium-sized, deciduous tree that can grow up to 20 meters (65 feet) tall, with rough, gray-brown bark and large, ovate, toothed leaves with a sandpaper-like texture. It produces small, inconspicuous reddish flowers that develop into flat, round seed pods. The inner bark is mucilaginous and has been used to soothe the digestive tract and throat.

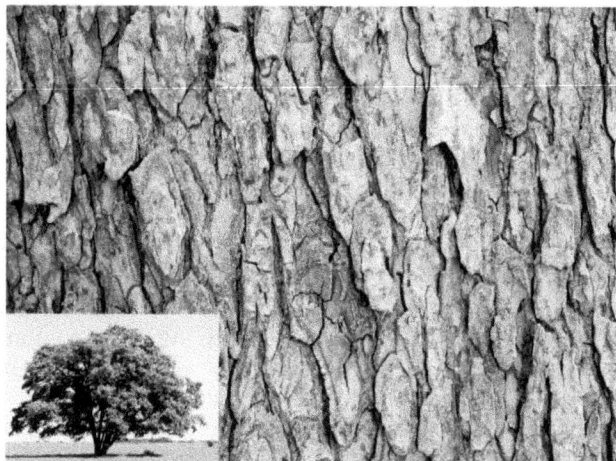

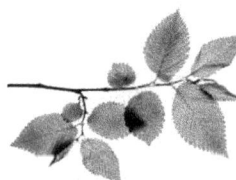

Preparation Methods:
- **Edible Inner Bark:** The inner bark is edible and has a soothing, mucilaginous texture.
- **Teas & Infusions:** Coats the throat, soothes digestion, and relieves inflammation.
- **Decoctions:** Supports respiratory health, eases sore throats, and promotes gut healing.
- **Tinctures:** Helps with acid reflux, soothes irritated tissues, and supports digestion.
- **Syrups:** Relieves coughs, soothes sore throats, and supports mucous membranes.
- **Salves & Balms:** Aids wounds, burns, and irritated skin.
- **Poultices:** Reduces infections, swelling, and promotes wound healing.

SPOTTED BEE BALM

Latin: Monarda punctata

Vital Parts: Leaves, Flowers

Harvest Season: Late Summer to Early Autumn

Description: Spotted bee balm is valued for its antimicrobial, expectorant, and digestive-supporting properties. It is commonly used to relieve respiratory congestion, promote digestion, and combat infections.

Native: Spotted bee balm is native to North America and is commonly found in prairies, meadows, and sandy soils.

Cultivation: Spotted bee balm thrives in well-drained, sandy soil and full sun. The leaves and flowers are harvested for use in herbal medicine.

Ancient Usage: Spotted bee balm, sometimes called "horsemint," has been used for its antimicrobial and respiratory-supporting properties. Native American tribes used it to treat colds, coughs, and fevers. It was also valued for its ability to ease digestive discomfort. In folklore, bee balm was seen as a protector of the home, believed to attract positive energy and ward off illness.

Spotted bee balm is a perennial herb that grows up to 90 cm (3 feet) tall, with square stems and narrow, lance-shaped green leaves. It produces showy, pink to lavender flowers with darker purple spots, arranged in tiers around the stem.

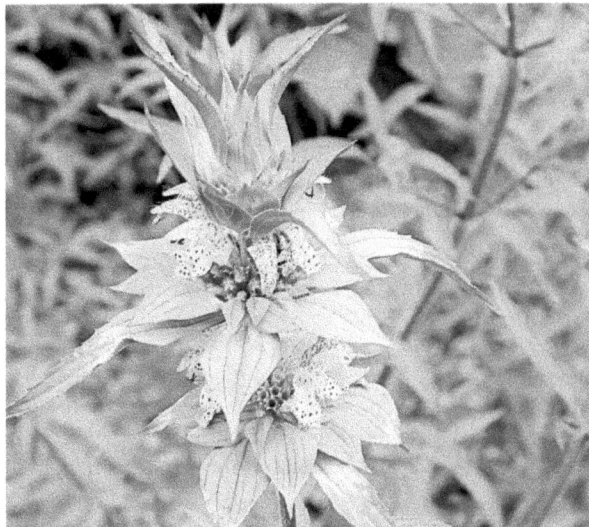

Medicinal Benefits:

- **Respiratory Support:** Relieves congestion, clears mucus, and eases symptoms of colds, bronchitis, and asthma.
- **Digestive Health:** Soothes indigestion, bloating, and gas by relaxing the digestive tract and stimulating digestive enzymes.
- **Antimicrobial Properties:** Fights bacterial, fungal, and viral infections.
- **Anti-Inflammatory:** Aids in sore throats and arthritis.
- **Pain Relief:** Alleviates minor headaches, muscle tension, and menstrual cramps.
- **Skin Health:** Treats minor wounds, insect bites, and rashes.

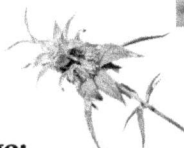

Dosage:

- **Standardized Extract:** 200-400 mg daily.
- **Tincture:** 2-4 mL (40-80 drops), 2-3 times daily.
- **Tea:** 1-2 tsp per cup of water, 2-3 times daily.
- **Capsules:** 500-1,000 mg, 1-2 times daily.

Safety:

- **Internal Use:** Excessive use may cause stomach upset.
- **Children:** Safe for older children for respiratory and digestive support.
- **Allergy Risk:** Those with sensitivities to the mint-family (Lamiaceae) should use cautiously.

Preparation Methods:

- **Edible Flowers:** Spotted bee balm flowers are edible.
- **Teas & Infusions:** Supports respiratory health, soothes sore throats, and aids digestion.
- **Decoctions:** Alleviates congestion, inflammation, and supports immune health.
- **Tinctures:** Aids in relieving colds, reducing stress, and promoting digestive wellness.
- **Syrups:** Soothes coughs, sore throats, and respiratory tract.
- **Salves & Balms:** Treats skin irritations and promotes healing.
- **Poultices:** Reduces swelling, soothes insect bites, and supports wound healing.

ST. JOHN'S WORT

Latin: *Hypericum perforatum*

Vital Parts: Flowers, Leaves, Stems
Harvest Season: Late Spring to Early Autumn

Description: St. John's wort is renowned for its mood-enhancing and antidepressant properties. It is commonly used to alleviate symptoms of mild to moderate depression, anxiety, and nervous tension.

Native: St. John's wort is native to Europe and Asia and has naturalized in many parts of North America.

Cultivation: St . John's wort thrives in well-drained, sandy soil and full sun. The flowers and aerial parts are commonly harvested for herbal use.

Ancient Usage: St. John's wort, often referred to as the "sunshine herb," has been used since ancient times to treat depression, anxiety, and nerve pain. The Greeks and Romans used it to ward off evil spirits and promote healing from wounds and burns. In medieval Europe, it was gathered on St. John's Day, believed to protect against curses and bring happiness. Folklore associated the herb with light and protection, symbolizing both physical and spiritual healing.

St. John's wort is a bushy, perennial herb that grows up to 1 meter (3 feet) tall, with branched stems and small, oval, dark green leaves. It produces clusters of bright yellow, five-petaled flowers with prominent stamens.

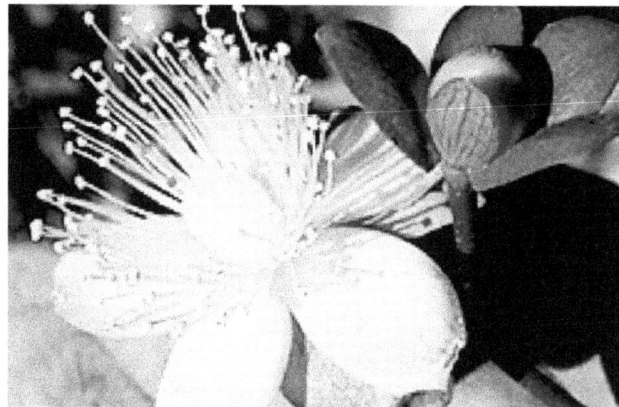

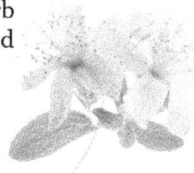

Medicinal Benefits:

- **Mood Support:** Alleviates depression, anxiety, and seasonal affective disorder (SAD).
- **Nerve Pain Relief:** Reduces sciatica, neuralgia, and shingles.
- **Wound Healing:** Treats minor cuts, burns, bruises, and skin irritations.
- **Anti-Inflammatory:** Helps manage arthritis, muscle pain, and skin conditions like eczema.
- **Antiviral Properties:** Fights cold sores and shingles.
- **Digestive Health:** Soothes the stomach and aids in relieving mild digestive complaints, including bloating and cramping.
- **Sleep Support:** Calms the nervous system and reduces restlessness.

Dosage:

- **Standardized Extract:** 300-600 mg daily.
- **Tincture:** 2-4 mL (40-80 drops), 2-3 times daily.
- **Tea:** 1-2 tsp per cup of water, 2-3 times daily.
- **Capsules:** 500-1,000 mg of dried herb, 1-2 times daily.

Safety:

- **Internal Use:** High doses may cause dizziness.
- **Children:** Not recommended for children.
- **Allergy Risk:** Those with sensitivities to Hypericum species should use cautiously.
- **Drug Interactions:** Can interact with antidepressants, birth control pills, blood thinners, and immunosuppressants.

Preparation Methods:

- **Teas & Infusions:** Supports mood balance, reduces anxiety, and aids digestive discomfort.
- **Decoctions:** Promotes nerve health, reduces inflammation, and supports overall relaxation.
- **Tinctures:** Aids in reducing symptoms of depression and nerve pain.
- **Syrups:** Supports respiratory health, calms nerves, and promotes relaxation.
- **Salves & Balms:** Relieves muscle pain, soothes nerve discomfort, and promotes the healing of wounds and burns.
- **Poultices:** Reduces swelling, soothes bruises, and supports wound healing.
- **Topical:** Test on a small area of skin to ensure no irritation occurs.

THYME

Latin: *Thymus vulgaris*

Vital Parts: Leaves, Stems
Harvest Season: Spring to Late Summer

Description: Thyme is known for its antimicrobial, anti-inflammatory, and expectorant properties, often used to support respiratory health and digestion.

Native: Thyme is native to the Mediterranean region, thriving in dry, rocky areas and sunny hillsides.

Cultivation: Thyme thrives in well-drained, sandy or loamy soil and prefers full sun. It is widely cultivated in gardens for both culinary and medicinal uses.

Ancient Usage: Thyme, often called the "herb of courage," has been used since ancient times to strengthen the body and protect against illness. The Greeks and Romans used thyme in baths and burned it as incense to purify spaces and enhance bravery. In medieval Europe, thyme was placed under pillows to prevent nightmares and worn by knights for courage in battle. Folklore regarded thyme as a protector against evil and a symbol of strength and vitality.

Thyme is a low-growing, woody perennial herb that reaches up to 30 cm (12 inches) tall, with small, narrow, gray-green leaves. It produces clusters of tiny, tubular pink to purple flowers at the tips of the stems.

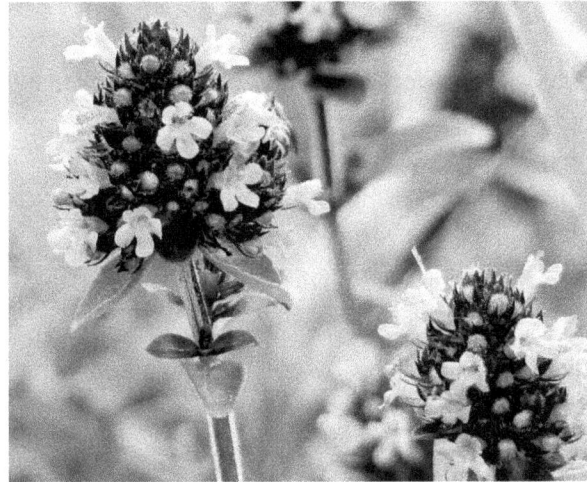

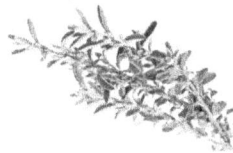

Medicinal Benefits:
- **Respiratory Health:** Clears mucus, relieves coughs, and alleviates bronchitis, asthma, and sinus congestion.
- **Digestive Aid:** Soothes indigestion, bloating, and cramping.
- **Immune Support:** Combats colds, flu, and infections.
- **Oral Health:** Treats gum inflammation, bad breath, and throat infections.
- **Antimicrobial Properties:** Fights bacterial and fungal infections, such as athlete's foot and fungal nail infections.
- **Anti-Inflammatory:** Aids arthritis and sore throats.
- **Skin Health:** Applied topically to treat acne, wounds, and skin irritations.

Dosage:
- **Standardized Extract:** 200-500 mg daily.
- **Tincture:** 2-4 mL (40-80 drops), 2-3 times daily.
- **Tea:** 1-2 tsp of dried herb per cup of water, 2-3 times daily.
- **Capsules:** 500-1,000 mg of dried herb, 1-2 times daily.

Safety:
- **Internal Use:** High doses may cause digestive upset in some individuals.
- **Children:** Safe for older children in small amounts for digestive support.
- **Allergy Risk:** Those with sensitivities to mint-family plants (Lamiaceae) should use cautiously.

Preparation Methods:
- **Edible Flowers:** Thyme flowers are edible.
- **Teas & Infusions:** Supports respiratory health, soothes sore throats, and aids digestion.
- **Decoctions:** Treats persistent coughs, bronchitis, or colds.
- **Tinctures:** Aids infections, immune, and digestive health.
- **Syrups:** Eases coughs, soothes respiratory irritation, and promotes throat health.
- **Salves & Balms:** Treats skin infections, wounds, and pain.
- **Poultices:** Soothes inflamed skin, insect bites, and minor wounds due.
- **Topical:** Combats fungal infections and acne.

Planet: Jupiter

TURMERIC

Zodiac: ⚹ Sagittarius

Latin: *Curcuma longa*

Vital Parts: Roots, Rhizomes
Harvest Season: Late Autumn to Early Winter

Description: Turmeric is known for its potent anti-inflammatory and antioxidant properties, often used to support joint health, digestion, and overall immune function.

Native: Turmeric is native to South Asia, particularly India, thriving in tropical and subtropical regions.

Cultivation: Turmeric thrives in warm, humid climates with well-drained, fertile soil and partial to full sunlight.

Ancient Usage: Turmeric, known as the "golden root," has been a cornerstone of Ayurvedic and traditional Chinese medicine for its anti-inflammatory and detoxifying properties. Ancient Indian healers used it to balance digestion, purify the blood, and heal wounds. It was also employed in religious ceremonies and rituals, symbolizing prosperity and protection. Folklore associated turmeric with spiritual strength and good fortune, often used to ward off negativity.

Turmeric is a tropical, perennial herb that grows up to 1 meter (3 feet) tall, with broad, lance-shaped green leaves and short, thick stems. It produces pale yellow to white flowers arranged on spikes. The plant's vibrant orange rhizome is highly valued for its culinary, medicinal, and anti-inflammatory properties.

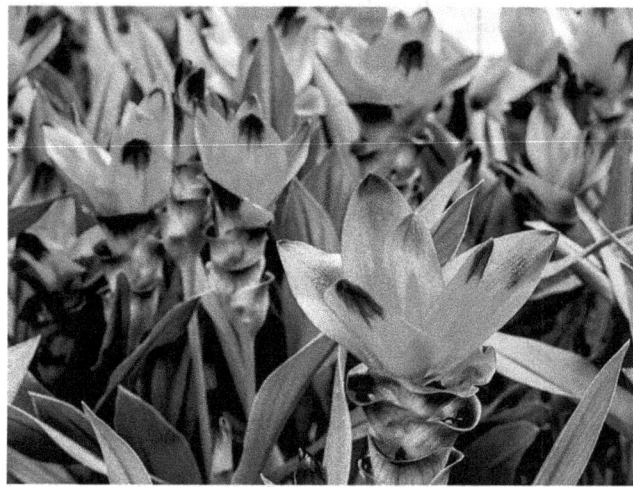

Medicinal Benefits:
- **Anti-Inflammatory:** Aids in arthritis and joint pain.
- **Antioxidant Properties:** Protects cells from oxidative stress.
- **Digestive Health:** Stimulates bile production, alleviating indigestion, bloating, and gas.
- **Immune Support:** Helps the body combat infections and chronic diseases.
- **Liver Health:** Promotes detoxification and supports healthy liver function.
- **Skin Health:** Manages acne, eczema, and other skin conditions.
- **Heart Health:** Improves circulation, cholesterol, and supports cardiovascular health.
- **Brain Health:** Enhances memory and focus.

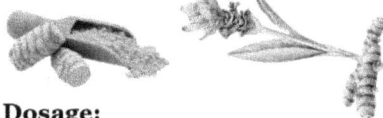

Dosage:
- **Standardized Extract:** 500-1,000 mg daily.
- **Tincture:** 2-4 mL (40-80 drops), 2-3 times daily.
- **Tea:** 1-2 tsp of powdered root per cup of water, 2-3 times daily.
- **Capsules:** 500-1,000 mg, 1-2 times daily.

Safety:
- **Internal Use:** High doses may cause stomach upset.
- **Children:** Safe for children in for boosting immunity and aiding digestion.
- **Allergy Risk:** Individuals with sensitivities to plants in the ginger family (Zingiberaceae) should use cautiously.
- **Drug Interactions:** May interact with anticoagulants, diabetes, and blood pressure medications.

Preparation Methods:
- **Edible Flowers:** Turmeric flowers are edible and add a mildly spicy flavor.
- **Teas & Infusions:** Enhances anti-inflammatory and immune-boosting effects.
- **Decoctions:** Reduces inflammation, supports digestion, and relieves joint pain.
- **Tinctures:** Manages inflammation, digestive issues, and immune support.
- **Syrups:** Turmeric decoction can be combined with honey to create a syrup for soothing sore throats, boosting immunity, and reducing respiratory inflammation.
- **Salves & Balms:** Treats skin conditions such as eczema, psoriasis, and wounds.
- **Poultices:** Reduces swelling, fights infection, and promotes healing.
- **Topical Only:** Turmeric can stain skin and clothing, and is often mixed with coconut oil to reduce staining.

Planet: Neptune

VALERIAN

Zodiac: ♓ Pisces

Latin: Valeriana officinalis

Vital Parts: Roots, Rhizomes
Harvest Season: Late Autumn

Description: Valerian is known for its calming and sedative properties, often used to promote relaxation, improve sleep, and reduce anxiety.

Native: Valerian is native to Europe and parts of Asia, often found in damp meadows, along riverbanks, and in woodland areas.

Cultivation: Valerian thrives in moist, well-drained soil and prefers full sun to partial shade. It is commonly cultivated in herbal gardens for medicinal and ornamental purposes.

Ancient Usage: Valerian, sometimes called the "herb of tranquility," has been used since ancient Greece to promote relaxation, reduce anxiety, and improve sleep. Hippocrates praised valerian for its calming effects and ability to ease nervous tension. In medieval Europe, it was used to relieve insomnia and hysteria and was often included in charms to protect against evil spirits. Folklore regarded valerian as a symbol of peace and comfort, believed to calm both the mind and spirit.

Medicinal Benefits:
- **Sleep Aid:** Promotes restful sleep and helps reduce insomnia.
- **Anxiety Relief:** Eases anxiety, nervousness, and restlessness with its natural sedative properties.
- **Muscle Relaxant:** Relieves tension, muscle spasms, and cramps.
- **Stress Reduction:** Helps manage stress and promotes relaxation.
- **Headache Relief:** Alleviates tension headaches and migraines caused by stress.
- **Digestive Health:** Soothes digestive upset, cramps, and irritable bowel syndrome (IBS).

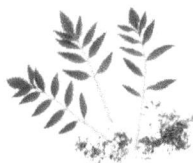

Valerian is a tall, perennial herb that can grow up to 1.5 meters (5 feet) tall, with hollow, ridged stems and pinnate leaves composed of multiple lance-shaped leaflets. It produces clusters of small, fragrant, white to pink flowers at the top of the plant.

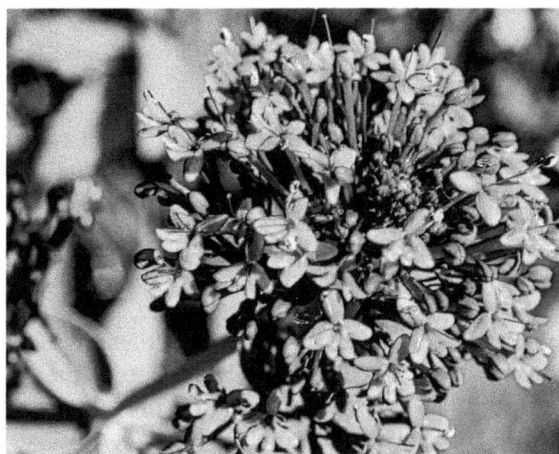

Dosage:
- **Standardized** Extract: 300-600 mg daily.
- **Tincture:** 2-4 mL (40-80 drops), 2-3 times daily.
- **Tea:** 1-2 tsp per cup of water, 1-2 times daily.
- **Capsules:** 500-1,000 mg of dried root, 1-2 times daily.

Safety:
- **Internal Use:** Excessive use may cause stomach discomfort.
- **Children:** Use cautiously.
- **Sedative Effects:** May cause drowsiness.
- **Drug Interactions:** May enhance the effects of sedatives, sleep aids, and depression medications.

Preparation Methods:
- **Teas & Infusions:** Promotes relaxation, reduces anxiety, and supports sleep.
- **Decoctions:** Valerian root is simmered in water to create a stronger decoction to aid insomnia, nervous tension, and mild muscle spasms.
- **Tinctures:** The root is preserved in alcohol or glycerin to create a tincture for fast-acting relief from stress, anxiety, or sleep disturbances.
- **Syrups:** Soothes the nervous system and promotes sleep.
- **Salves & Balms:** Eases muscle tension and joint pain.
- **Poultices:** Applied to sore muscles and joints to reduce tension and inflammation.
- **Topical:** Used topically to relieve pain and tension.

133

Planet: Venus

VIOLET

Zodiac: ♉ Taurus

Latin: Viola odorata

Vital Parts: Leaves, Flowers, Roots
Harvest Season: Early Spring to Late Summer

Description: Violet is known for its soothing and anti-inflammatory properties, often used to support skin health, respiratory irritation, and detoxification.

Native: Violet is native to temperate regions of Europe, Asia, and North America, often found in woodlands, meadows, and moist, shady areas.

Cultivation: Violet thrives in well-drained, moist soil and prefers partial to full shade. It is often grown in gardens for its ornamental flowers and medicinal uses.

Ancient Usage: Violet, often called the "flower of modesty," has been used for centuries to soothe respiratory ailments, skin conditions, and inflammation. Ancient Greeks used violets in remedies to relieve coughs and headaches, while early Europeans valued them for their ability to calm the mind and promote restful sleep. Violets were also associated with love and protection in folklore, often used in rituals to attract harmony and peace.

Violet is a low-growing, perennial herb with heart-shaped, dark green leaves and creeping stems. It produces small, fragrant, five-petaled flowers in shades of purple, blue, or white.

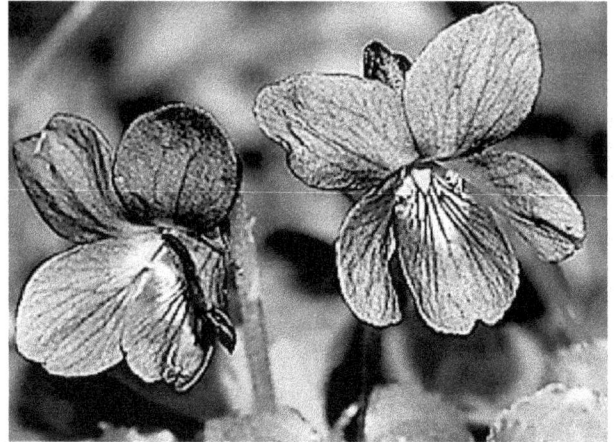

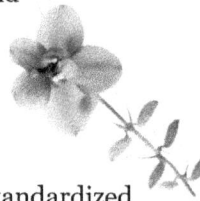

Medicinal Benefits:
- **Respiratory Support:** Eases coughs, bronchitis, and sore throats.
- **Liver Support:** Supports liver detoxification.
- **Immune Booster:** Rich in antioxidants and vitamin C.
- **Diuretic Effect:** Aids in eliminating excess fluids from the body.
- **Pain Relief:** Helps alleviate headaches and body aches.
- **Anti-Inflammatory:** Beneficial for arthritis.
- **Skin Health:** Soothes rashes, eczema, and wounds.
- **Digestive Aid:** Promotes digestion and relieves constipation.
- **Lymphatic Support:** Promotes detoxification and reduces swelling.
- **Mild Sedative:** Reduces stress and anxiety.

- **Dosage:** Standardized Extract: 200-400 mg daily.
- **Tincture:** 2-4 mL (40-80 drops), 2-3 times daily.
- **Tea:** 1-2 tsp of dried flowers or leaves per cup of water, 2-3 times daily.
- **Capsules:** 500-1,000 mg of dried herb, 1-2 times daily.

Safety:
- **Internal Use:** Safe in moderate amounts; excessive use may cause mild gastrointestinal upset.
- **Children:** Safe for children in small amounts, especially in teas or syrups for respiratory or skin conditions.

Preparation Methods:
- **Edible Flowers:** Violet flowers are edible and can be used in salads, desserts, or as a garnish.
- **Teas & Infusions:** Soothes respiratory issues, supports digestion, and promotes relaxation.
- **Decoctions:** Aids coughs, colds, and lymphatic congestion.
- **Tinctures:** Supports lymphatic drainage, inflammation, and skin health.
- **Syrups:** Soothes sore throats, coughs, and respiratory irritation.
- **Salves & Balms:** Soothes dry skin, rashes, minor burns, and eczema.
- **Poultices:** Reduces inflammation, soothes insect bites, and aids wound healing.
- **Topical Only:** Violet extracts or infused water can be used externally as a gentle skin wash or toner for acne, eczema, or other irritations.

WILD ROSE

Latin: Rosa species

Vital Parts: Fruit (Hips)
Harvest Season: Late Summer to Early Winter

Description: Wild rose is valued for its calming, mood-enhancing, and skin-nourishing properties. Rose petals are commonly used to reduce anxiety, promote relaxation, and support emotional well-being.

Native: Wild rose is native to Europe, Asia, and North America, with various species growing in temperate climates worldwide.

Cultivation: Wild rose thrives in well-drained, fertile soil and full sun. The petals and hips are harvested for use in herbal medicine, often prepared as teas, tinctures, and essential oils.

Ancient Usage: Rose, often called the "flower of love," has been cherished throughout history for its beauty, fragrance, and healing properties. Ancient civilizations, including the Greeks and Romans, used roses in perfumes, skincare, and rituals of love and protection. Rose petals were used in medicinal preparations to soothe inflammation and promote emotional balance. In folklore, roses were believed to offer protection against negative energy and symbolize purity, beauty, and love.

Wild rose is a woody, perennial shrub or climber with thorny stems and pinnate leaves made up of multiple oval, serrated leaflets. It produces large, fragrant flowers in a wide range of colors, including red, pink, white, and yellow. The flowers develop into round, red to orange fruits called rosehips.

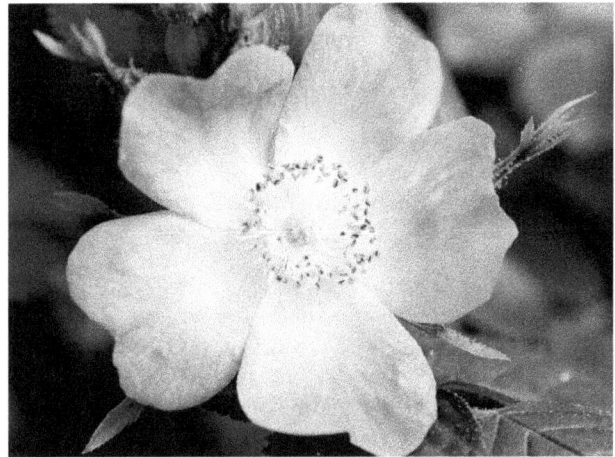

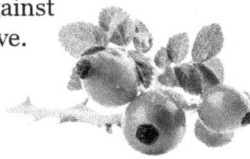

Medicinal Benefits:
- **Emotional & Stress Support:** Calms the nervous system, reduces anxiety, and uplifts mood.
- **Heart Health:** Improves circulation and blood pressure.
- **Digestive Aid:** Soothes indigestion and bloating.
- **Anti-Inflammatory:** Reduces joint pain and muscle soreness.
- **Skin & Wound Healing:** Promotes skin regeneration, hydrates, and soothes eczema and acne.
- **Hormonal Balance:** Helps ease menstrual discomfort, supports reproductive health, and alleviates PMS symptoms.
- **Immune Support:** Rich in antioxidants and vitamin C.

Dosage:
- **Standardized Extract:** 200-400 mg daily.
- **Tincture:** 2-4 mL (40-80 drops), 2-3 times daily.
- **Tea:** 1-2 tsp per cup of water, 2-3 times daily.
- **Capsules:** 500-1,000 mg, 1-2 times daily.

Safety:
- **Internal Use:** Excessive use may cause stomach upset.
- **Children:** Safe for soothing coughs or digestive issues.
- **Allergy Risk:** Individuals allergic to plants in the Rosaceae family (e.g., apples, strawberries) should use cautiously

Preparation Methods:
- **Edible Petals & Hips:** Rose petals and rose hips are edible.
- **Teas & Infusions:** Supports relaxation, uplifts mood, and promotes skin health.
- **Decoctions:** Aids digestion, boosts immunity, and soothes sore throats.
- **Tinctures:** Helps with emotional balance, supports heart health, and relieves stress.
- **Syrups:** Nourishes the skin, enhances immunity, and soothes coughs.
- **Salves & Balms:** Moisturizes skin, promotes healing, and reduces inflammation.
- **Poultices:** Soothes burns, relieves irritation, and helps with wound healing.

WILD YAM

Latin: Dioscorea villosa

Vital Parts: Roots, Rhizomes
Harvest Season: Late Summer to Early Autumn

Description: Wild yam is known for its hormone-supporting properties, traditionally used to alleviate symptoms of menopause, cramps, and other reproductive health concerns.

Native: Wild yam is native to North and Central America, particularly in moist woodlands, thickets, and along stream banks.

Cultivation: Wild yam thrives in well-drained, fertile soil with partial shade and moderate moisture. It is often cultivated in herbal gardens and can also be found growing wild in forested areas.

Ancient Usage: Wild yam, sometimes called the "balance root," has been used for centuries to support hormonal health and reduce inflammation. Native American tribes used it to relieve menstrual pain, promote fertility, and ease childbirth. Early herbalists in Europe and North America valued it for its antispasmodic properties, using it to treat muscle cramps and joint pain. Folklore associated wild yam with grounding and restoration, believed to enhance resilience and promote physical equilibrium.

Wild yam is a climbing, perennial vine with long, twisting stems and large, heart-shaped leaves with prominent veins. It produces small, yellowish-green flowers in clusters, with male and female flowers appearing on separate plants.

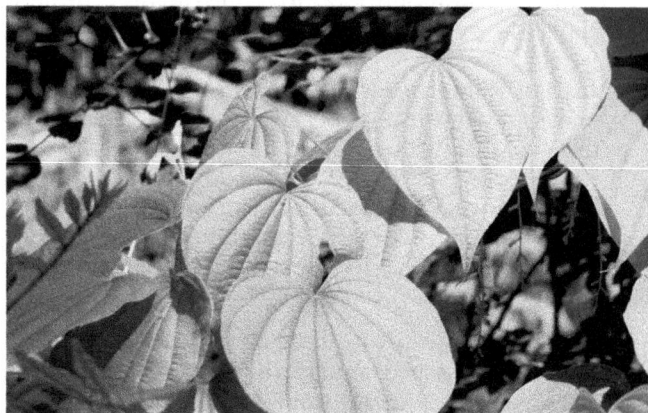

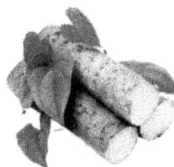

Medicinal Benefits:
- **Hormonal Balance:** Commonly used to ease menopausal symptoms, PMS, and menstrual cramps.
- **Anti-Inflammatory:** Beneficial for arthritis, joint pain, and muscle soreness.
- **Digestive Aid:** Soothes gastrointestinal discomfort, including cramps, gas, and bloating.
- **Muscle Relaxant:** Eases abdominal and uterine cramps.
- **Gallbladder Support:** Promotes bile flow, aiding in healthy gallbladder function.
- **Skin Health:** Improves skin elasticity and reduces dryness.

Dosage:
- **Standardized Extract:** 200-500 mg daily.
- **Tincture:** 2-4 mL (40-80 drops), 2-3 times daily.
- **Tea:** 1-2 tsp of dried root per cup of water, 1-2 times daily.
- **Capsules:** 500-1,000 mg, 1-2 times daily.

Safety:
- **Internal Use:** Excessive use may cause nausea.
- **Allergic Reactions:** Individuals sensitive to Wild Yam or related plants should avoid it.
- **Hormone-Sensitive Conditions:** Should be used cautiously in hormone-sensitive conditions (e.g., breast or uterine cancer).
- **Drug Interactions:** Use caution if taking medications for hormone therapy, blood pressure, or diabetes.

Preparation Methods:
- **Teas & Infusions:** Soothes menstrual cramps, supports digestive health, and alleviates inflammation.
- **Decoctions:** Aids arthritis pain, hormonal imbalances, and severe menstrual discomfort.
- **Tinctures:** Supports hormones, eases muscle spasms, and reduces joint inflammation.
- **Syrups:** Provides respiratory support and soothes menstrual and muscle pain.
- **Salves & Balms:** Relieves muscle aches, joint pain, and inflammation.
- **Poultices:** Aids sore muscles and inflamed joints; reduces pain and swelling.
- **Topical Only:** Provides hormonal balance.

WILLOW

Latin: Salix alba

Vital Parts: Bark
Harvest Season: Early Spring to Late Autumn

Description: Willow is known for its pain-relieving and anti-inflammatory properties, primarily due to the presence of salicin, a natural compound similar to aspirin.

Native: Willow is native to temperate regions across Europe, Asia, and North America, thriving in wetland areas such as riverbanks, marshes, and lakeshores.

Cultivation: Willow thrives in moist, well-drained soil and prefers full sun but can tolerate partial shade. It is commonly cultivated along waterways or in gardens.

Ancient Usage: Willow, often called the "tree of enchantment," has been used since ancient times for its pain-relieving properties. The ancient Greeks and Egyptians used willow bark to reduce fever and treat joint pain, inspiring the development of modern aspirin. Native American tribes valued it for relieving headaches and muscle soreness. In folklore, willow trees were seen as symbols of healing, intuition, and resilience, often associated with protection and emotional balance.

Medicinal Benefits:

- **Pain Relief:** Alleviates headaches, muscle aches, joint pain, and back pain.
- **Anti-Inflammatory:** Aids arthritis and tendinitis.
- **Fever Reduction:** Aids colds, flu, and infections.
- **Menstrual Cramp Relief:** Eases menstrual pain and discomfort.
- **Support for Rheumatic Conditions:** Helps reduce pain and stiffness in joints.
- **Mild Antiseptic:** Supports wound healing and infections.
- **Cardiovascular Support:** Supports circulation and heart health.
- **Digestive Health:** Soothes gastrointestinal discomfort.
- **Skin Health:** Treats acne.

Willow is a deciduous tree or shrub that can grow up to 25 meters (82 feet) tall, with long, flexible branches and narrow, lance-shaped leaves that are light green on top and silvery underneath. It produces small, catkin-like flowers.

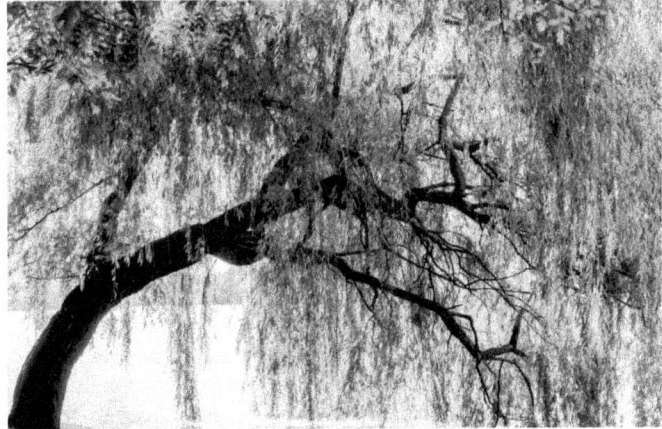

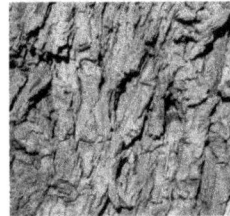

Dosage:
- **Standardized Extract:** 200-400 mg daily.
- **Tincture:** 2-4 mL (40-80 drops), 2-3 times daily.
- **Tea:** 1-2 tsp of dried bark per cup of water, 2-3 times daily.
- **Capsules:** 500-1,000 mg, 1-2 times daily.

Safety:
- **Internal Use:** Overuse can cause stomach upset.
- **Children:** Avoid use in children.
- **Drug Interactions:** May interact with blood-thinning medications, NSAIDs, and anticoagulants.
- **Allergy Risk:** Individuals allergic to aspirin, should avoid willow bark.

Preparation Methods:

- **Teas & Infusions:** Relieves pain, reduces inflammation, and soothes fevers.
- **Decoctions:** Aids severe pain relief and supports recovery during colds and flu.
- **Tinctures:** Provides relief for inflammation and pain.
- **Syrups:** Soothes sore throats and alleviates fever.
- **Salves & Balms:** Reduces joint pain, swelling, and inflammation.
- **Poultices:** Reduces swelling and promotes healing for sprains and bruises.
- **Oils & Infused Oils:** Targets localized pain and inflammation.
- **Vinegars & Oxymels:** Willow bark can be infused in vinegar or honey to create a potent remedy that provides internal relief for pain, fever, and inflammation.

WITCH HAZEL

Latin: *Hamamelis virginiana*

Vital Parts: Bark, Twigs, Leaves
Harvest Season: Early Spring or Late Autumn

Description: Witch hazel is known for its powerful astringent and anti-inflammatory properties, often used to soothe skin irritations, reduce swelling, and promote wound healing.

Native: Witch hazel is native to North America, particularly in woodland areas and along streambanks in the eastern United States and Canada.

Cultivation: Witch hazel thrives in temperate climates with moist, well-drained, slightly acidic soil and partial to full sunlight. It is often cultivated as an ornamental shrub in gardens and grows wild in forested regions.

Ancient Usage: Witch hazel, known as the "herb of clarity," has been used for centuries to soothe skin irritations, reduce swelling, and promote woun healing. Native American tribes used its bark and leaves to treat inflammation, bruises, and sore muscles. Early European settlers adopted witch hazel as a remedy for hemorrhoids, varicose veins, and other skin conditions. Folklore believed witch hazel could repel negative energies, with branches often used in rituals for purification and protection.

Medicinal Benefits:
- **Varicose Veins Support:** Reliefs swelling and discomfort.
- **Astringent:** Tightens and tones skin tissue, spores, and oiliness.
- **Anti-Inflammatory:** Calms rashes, eczema, psoriasis, and burns.
- **Wound Healing:** Heals cuts, scrapes, and bruises.
- **Hemorrhoid Relief:** Soothes itching, burning, and swelling.
- **Sunburn Relief:** Reduces irritation from sunburn.
- **Skin Irritation Soothing:** Relieves nsect bites, stings, and allergic reactions.
- **Sore Throat Relief:** Gargling reduces throat irritation.
- **Scalp Health:** Relieves dandruff and itching.
- **Anti-Microbial:** Prevents bacterial growth on skin.

Witch hazel is a deciduous shrub or small tree that can grow up to 6 meters (20 feet) tall, with smooth, gray bark and oval, toothed leaves. It produces unique, fragrant, yellow flowers with long, ribbon-like petals that bloom in late fall or winter.

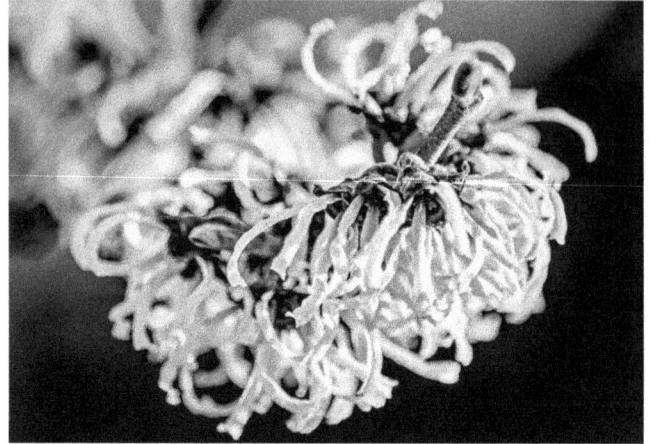

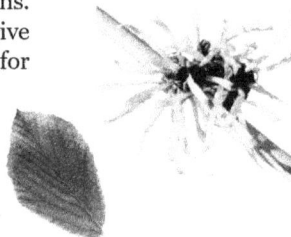

Dosage:
- **Tincture:** 2-4 mL (40-80 drops), up to 2 times daily for mild digestive support.
- **Infused Oil:** Apply externally to reduce skin irritation, inflammation, and bruising.

Safety:
- **Topical Use Only:** Safe for most skin types, though it may cause mild irritation for sensitive individuals.
- **Internal Use:** Use sparingly, as excessive consumption may cause stomach irritation.

Preparation Methods:
- **Teas & Infusions:** Soothes diarrhea and inflammation.
- **Decoctions:** Used for compresses and skin rinses.
- **Tinctures:** Aids wounds, bruises, and irritated skin.
- **Syrups:** Soothes sore throats, reduces inflammation, and supports digestive health.
- **Salves & Balms:** Soothes burns, hemorrhoids, and inflamed skin.
- **Poultices:** Aids bruises, swelling, and sprains to promote healing.
- **Topical:** Treats acne, varicose veins, and insect bites.

Planet: Venus

YARROW

Zodiac: ♎ Libra

Latin: *Achillea millefolium*

Vital Parts: Leaves, Flowers, Stems
Harvest Season: Late Spring to Early Autumn

Description: Yarrow is an herb known for its wound-healing, anti-inflammatory, and astringent properties, used to stop bleeding and reduce fever.

Native: Yarrow is native to temperate regions of Europe, Asia, and North America, where it is found in meadows, grasslands, and along roadsides.

Cultivation: Yarrow thrives in sunny locations with well-drained, sandy or loamy soil. It is drought-tolerant and commonly cultivated in herbal gardens.

Ancient Usage: Yarrow, often referred to as the "soldier's woundwort," has been used for centuries to stop bleeding, reduce inflammation, and promote healing. Ancient Greek warriors carried yyarrow to treat battlefield wounds. Native American tribes used yarrow to treat colds, flu, and pain. In folklore, yarrow was seen as a plant of protection and divination, believed to enhance psychic abilities and guard against harm.

Yarrow is a hardy, perennial herb that grows up to 90 cm (3 feet) tall, with finely divided, feathery green leaves. It produces clusters of small, white to pale pink flowers arranged in flat-topped umbels.

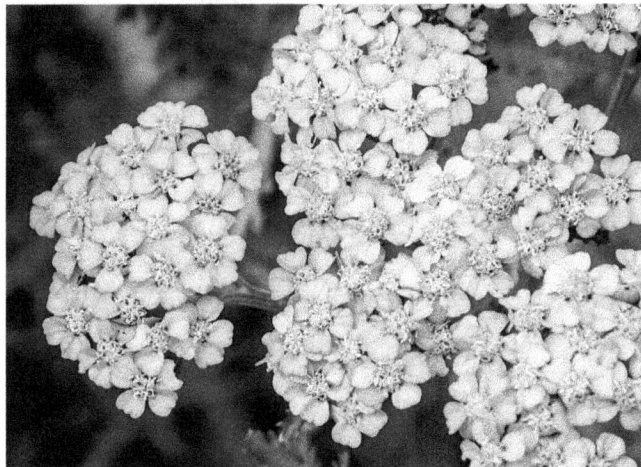

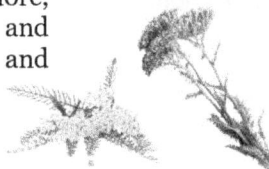

Medicinal Benefits:
- **Astringent:** Tightens and tones skin and reduced swelling.
- **Anti-Inflammatory:** Calms arthritis, digestive irritation, and skin rashes.
- **Wound Healing:** Heals cuts, scrapes, and bruises.
- **Fever Reduction:** Encourages sweating to help lower fever.
- **Menstrual Support:** Regulates menstrual cycles and alleviates cramps.
- **Digestive Aid:** Relieves bloating, cramping, and indigestion.
- **Blood Circulation:** Supports circulation and stops internal bleeding.
- **Urinary Health:** Aids in water retention and supporting urinary health.

Dosage:
- **Standardized Extract:** 200-400 mg daily.
- **Tincture:** 2-4 mL (40-80 drops), 2-3 times daily.
- **Tea:** 1-2 tsp of dried flowers or leaves per cup of water, 2-3 times daily.
- **Capsules:** 500-1,000 mg of dried herb, 1-2 times daily.

Safety:
- **Internal Use:** High doses can cause headaches.
- **Allergic Reactions:** Avoid if allergic to the Asteraceae family (e.g., ragweed, chamomile).
- **Photosensitivity:** May increase sensitivity to sunlight.
- **Blood Thinning:** Use cautiously if taking anticoagulants.

Preparation Methods:
- **Edible Flowers:** Adds a mild, herbal flavor to dishes.
- **Teas & Infusions:** Supports digestion, reduces fever, relieves menstrual discomfort, and boosts immunity.
- **Decoctions:** Addresses respiratory issues, fevers, and heavy menstrual bleeding.
- **Tinctures:** Manages fevers, improves circulation, and reduces inflammation.
- **Syrups:** Soothes sore throats, eases coughs, and supports respiratory health.
- **Salves & Balms:** Heals minor wounds, reduces bruising, and calms inflamed skin.
- **Poultices:** Stops bleeding, prevents infection, and relieves irritation.
- **Topical:** Treats skin conditions and alleviates muscle pain.

YELLOW DOCK

Latin: *Rumex crispus*

Vital Parts: Roots, Leaves
Harvest Season: Late Summer to Early Autumn

Description: Yellow dock is an herb known for its detoxifying and liver-supporting properties, often used to promote healthy digestion and alleviate constipation and skin disorders.

Native: Yellow dock is native to Europe and western Asia but has naturalized in North America, thriving in fields, roadsides, and disturbed soils.

Cultivation: Yellow dock thrives in a variety of climates and soil types, though it prefers well-drained, nutrient-rich soil and full to partial sunlight. It is commonly cultivated in herbal gardens and grows wild in many regions.

Ancient Usage: Yellow dock, sometimes known as the "blood purifier," has been used since ancient times to support liver health and promote detoxification. Native American tribes used the root to treat skin conditions, digestive issues, and inflammation. European herbalists valued it for its ability to cleanse the blood, improve digestion, and relieve constipation. Folklore associated yellow dock with renewal and vitality, symbolizing inner strength and purification.

Yellow dock is a perennial herb that can grow up to 1.5 meters (5 feet) tall, with slender, branching stems and large, lance-shaped, wavy-edged leaves. It produces clusters of small, greenish flowers that mature into reddish-brown seed pods.

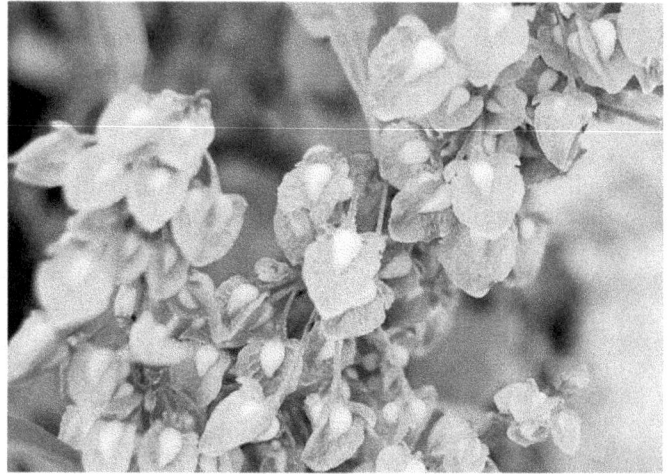

Medicinal Benefits:
- **Liver Detoxification:** Aids in the elimination of toxins.
- **Digestive Health:** Relieves constipation, stimulates digestion, and alleviates bloating.
- **Blood Purification:** Used to "cleanse the blood," aiding in eczema, acne, and psoriasis.
- **Iron Absorption:** Useful for addressing anemia.
- **Skin Health:** Helps soothe and heal skin irritations, rashes, and wounds.
- **Anti-Inflammatory:** Beneficial for joint and muscle discomfort.
- **Diuretic:** Supports kidney health and reduces water retention.

Dosage:
- **Standardized Extract:** 300-600 mg daily.
- **Tincture:** 2-4 mL (40-80 drops), 2-3 times daily.
- **Tea:** 1-2 tsp per cup of water, 2-3 times daily.
- **Capsules:** 500-1,000 mg, 1-2 times daily.

Safety:
- **Internal Use:** Excessive use may cause mild gastrointestinal discomfort.
- **Iron Overload:** Use cautiously if prone to hemochromatosis, as yellow dock can enhance iron absorption.

Preparation Methods:
- **Teas & Infusions:** Supports digestion, liver health, and mild detoxification.
- **Decoctions:** Aids in liver detox, constipation relief, and skin support.
- **Tinctures:** Aids in digestion, supports iron absorption, and promotes liver and kidney health.
- **Syrups:** Supports digestion and serves as a gentle laxative.
- **Salves & Balms:** Soothes skin conditions such as eczema, rashes, or psoriasis.
- **Poultices:** Reduces inflammation, soothes insect bites, and draws out toxins from wounds.

Chapter Five

HERBAL RECIPES FOR COMMON AILMENTS

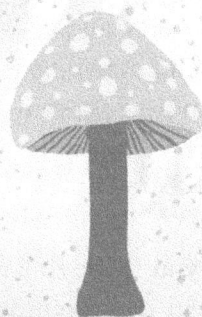

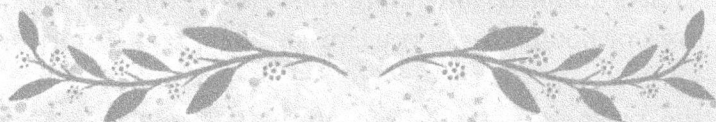

"Herbs are the medicines that heal not only the body, but also the spirit."
— Native American Proverb

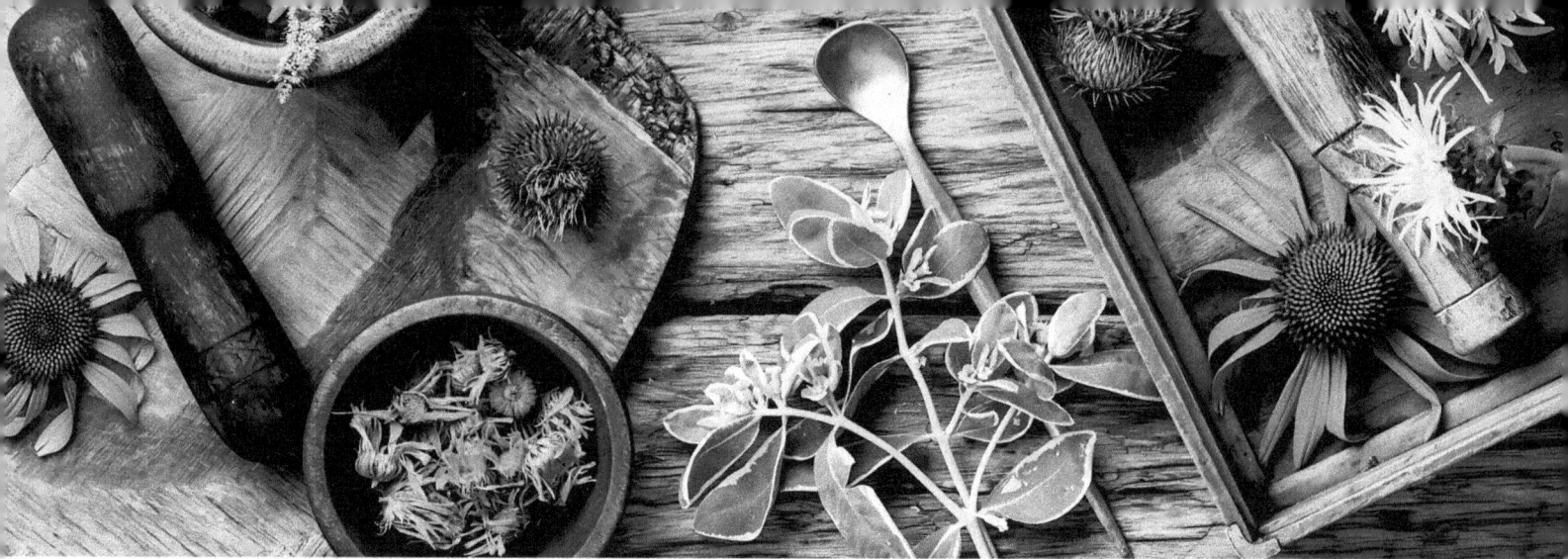

HERBAL REMEDIES

This chapter explores the vast and dynamic world of herbal remedies, offering practical insights into how different plants can support your health and well-being. Whether you're managing a common cold, digestive discomfort, anxiety, skin irritations, or chronic conditions, nature provides powerful solutions that work in harmony with your body's natural healing processes.

Herbs are diverse in their benefits and applications. Some, like ginger and peppermint, provide rapid relief for nausea and digestive issues. Others, such as chamomile and lavender, help soothe the nervous system and promote relaxation. Immune-strengthening herbs like echinacea and elderberry can be especially beneficial during cold and flu season, helping your body defend against illness.

The following pages will guide you through a comprehensive exploration of herbal remedies, beginning with their astrological correspondences, followed by solar and lunar influences, and finally moving into targeted herbal solutions for specific health concerns. Each remedy will be carefully outlined, including the best preparation methods—whether as teas, tinctures, salves, or poultices—so you can confidently integrate them into your daily routine.

However, true wellness extends beyond herbal remedies. A holistic approach includes healthy lifestyle choices such as regular exercise, maintaining a balanced weight, managing stress, and prioritizing quality sleep. Herbs can be a valuable tool, but they work best when combined with mindful habits that support overall well-being.

All remedies and recipes in this book are fully customizable. If you dislike an ingredient or have an allergy, feel free to omit it or substitute it with a similar alternative. Herbal healing is meant to be flexible, allowing you to create personalized solutions that align with your needs and preferences.

By embracing nature's wisdom and making intentional choices for your health, you can cultivate a balanced, vibrant, and resilient life. This chapter will equip you with the knowledge and confidence to harness the power of herbal medicine as part of your holistic wellness journey.

☀ Radiant Sun Vitality Tonic

Purpose: Boosts energy, enhances vitality, and awakens the body and mind with the power of the sun.

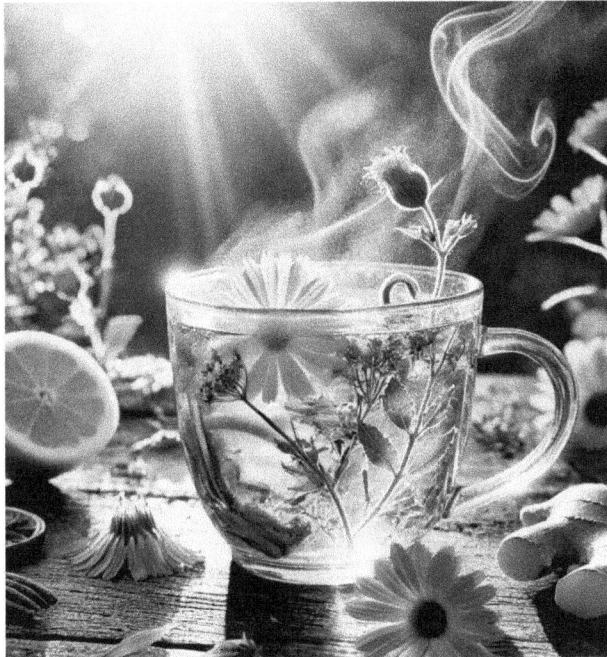

INGREDIENTS

- 1 tsp ashwagandha root (combats stress)
- 1 tsp lemon peel (supports mood and digestion)
- ½ tsp Ginger Root (stimulates circulation)
- ½ tsp Calendula Flowers (promotes immune support)
- 2 cups hot water

DIRECTIONS

1. Place all herbs into a large glass jar.
2. Pour room-temperature water over the herbs and stir gently.
3. Cover and place the jar in direct sunlight for 4–6 hours.
4. Strain the tea, and sweeten.
5. Serve over ice for a refreshing solar-infused drink.

Solar Bonus:

- Brew your tonic in direct sunlight to absorb its vibrant energy.
- Set an intention by whispering: "I embrace vitality, strength, and passion."
- Place a citrine or tiger's eye near your cup to amplify confidence and personal power.

☀ Sun-Kissed Energizing Tea

Purpose: Purpose: Refreshes the body, boosts focus, and uplifts mood.

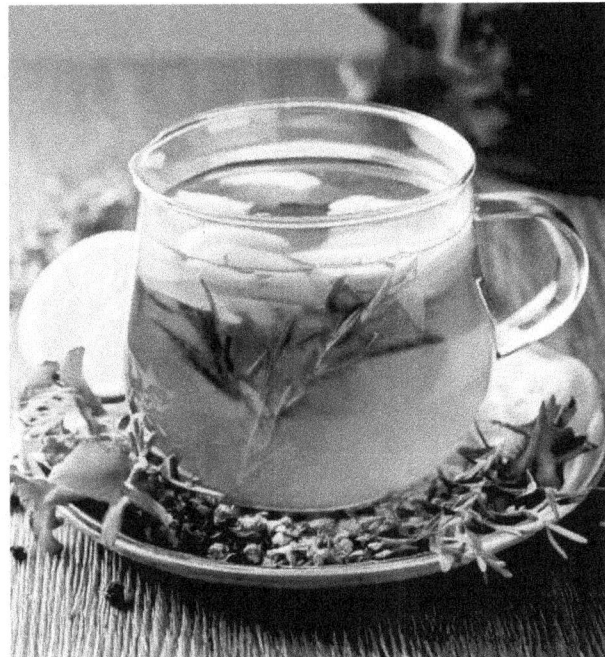

INGREDIENTS

- 2 tbsp dried rosemary (stimulating)
- 1 tbsp dried orange peel (brightening)
- 1 tbsp dried hibiscus flowers (cooling)
- 1 quart water
- 1 tbsp honey or agave (balancing)

DIRECTIONS

1. Place all herbs into a large glass jar.
2. Pour room-temperature water over the herbs and stir gently.
3. Cover and place the jar in direct sunlight for 4–6 hours.
4. Strain the tea, and sweeten.
5. Serve over ice for a refreshing solar-infused drink.

Solar Bonus:

- Brew your tonic in direct sunlight for 4-6 hours to absorb its vibrant energy.
- Set an intention by saying: "I welcome energy, clarity, and joy into my body and mind.
- Place a citrine or clear quartz near your jar to amplify focus, motivation, and vitality.

☀ Sunshine Healing Oil

Purpose: Soothes skin, speeds up wound healing, and reduces inflammation.

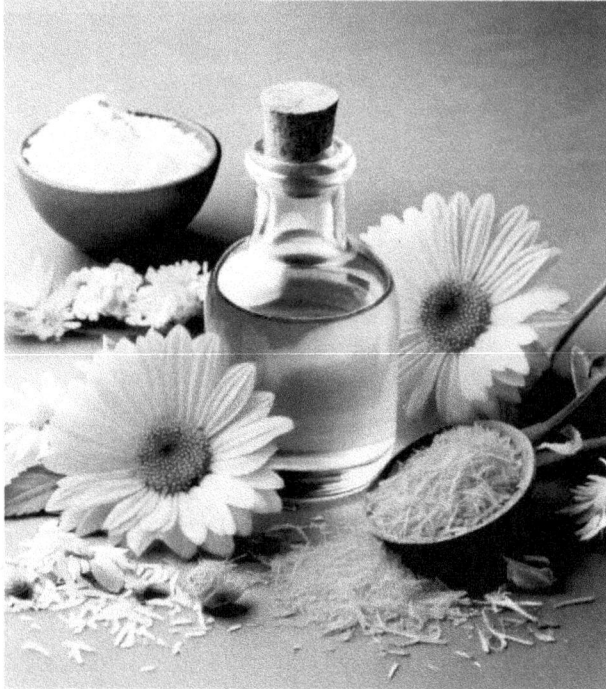

• •

INGREDIENTS

- ½ cup dried calendula flowers (healing)
- 1 cup coconut oil (anti-inflammatory)
- 1 tbsp dried chamomile (soothing)
- 1 clear glass jar

DIRECTIONS

1. Add calendula and chamomile to a glass jar.
2. Pour coconut oil over the herbs, ensuring they are fully covered.
3. Seal and place the jar in direct sunlight for 1–2 weeks, shaking gently every day.
4. Strain and store the golden-infused oil in a dark glass bottle.
5. Use as a moisturizer, massage oil, or after-sun skin soother.

Solar Bonus:
- Brew your tonic in direct sunlight to absorb its vibrant energy.
- Set an intention: by saying "I nourish and heal my skin with nature's golden warmth."
- Place a clear quartz near the jar to amplify the oil's restorative energy.

☀ Sun-Infused Herbal Elixir

Purpose: Supports immunity, soothes digestion, enhances mental clarity, and boosts mood.

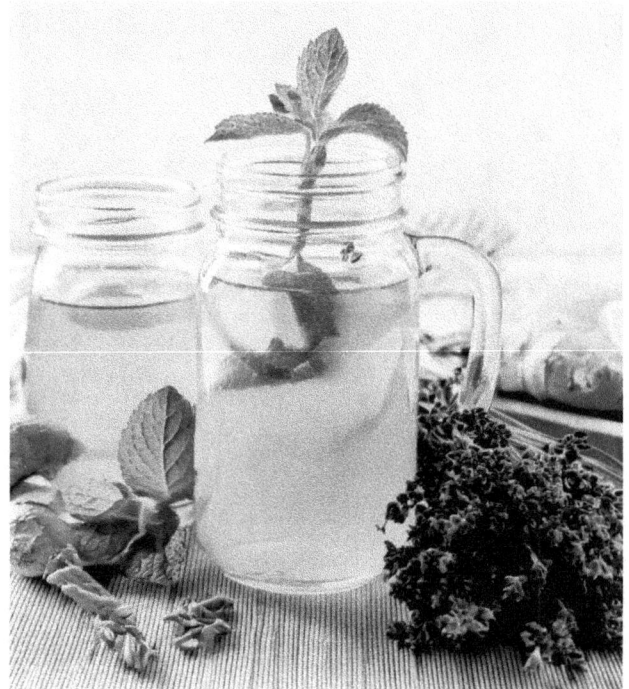

• •

INGREDIENTS

- ½ cup raw honey (antioxidant)
- 2 tbsp dried lemon balm (stress)
- 2 tbsp dried ginger slices (digestion)
- 1 tbsp dried lavender (relaxation)
- 1 small glass jar with lid

DIRECTIONS

1. Add all herbs to a clean glass jar.
2. Pour honey over the herbs until fully coated.
3. Seal the jar and place it in direct sunlight for 2–4 days, turning the jar occasionally.
4. Strain if desired, or leave the herbs in for extra potency.
5. Use 1 tsp daily in tea or on foods.

Solar Bonus:
- Brew your tonic in direct sunlight to absorb its vibrant energy.
- Whisper an intention: "I infuse my body with light, warmth, and healing."
- Place a tiger's eye or carnelian near your jar for strength and vitality.

Full Moon Dream Elixir

Purpose: Enhances intuition, promotes vivid dreams, and supports emotional release, aligning with the Full Moon's heightened energy for deep subconscious insight.

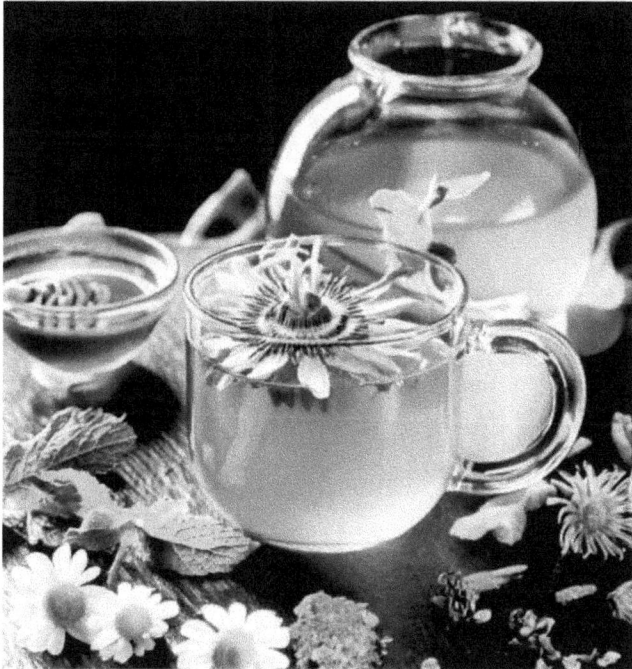

INGREDIENTS

- 1 tsp passionflower (calming)
- 1 tsp chamomile (sleep aid)
- ½ tsp lemon balm (stress)
- ½ tsp skullcap (anxiety)
- 1 tsp raw honey

DIRECTIONS

1. Steep herbs in hot water for 10-15 minutes while setting an intention for dream clarity.
2. Strain and add honey.
3. Drink before bed while gazing at the moon.
4. Keep a dream journal nearby for morning insights!

Lunar Bonus:
- Charge your tea under moonlight for extra dream-enhancing energy.
- Set an intention by whispering: "I welcome clarity and release the old."
- Place an amethyst or moonstone near your cup to amplify intuition.

New Moon Renewal Tonic

Purpose: Supports cleansing, intention-setting, and fresh beginnings, helping to release the old and welcome new opportunities with clarity and balance.

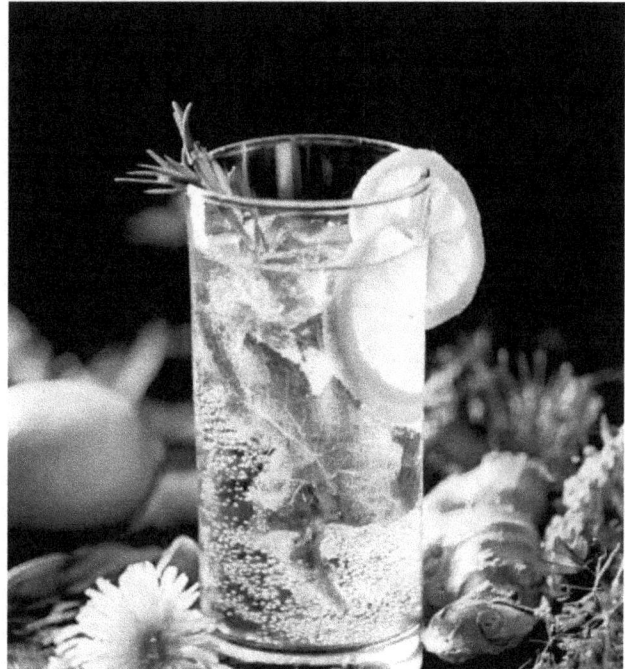

INGREDIENTS

- 1 tsp dandelion root (liver health and digestion)
- 1 tsp nettle (bone and joint health)
- ½ tsp lemon balm (anxiety and sleep)
- ½ tsp ginger (anti-inflammatory)
- 1 slice lemon

DIRECTIONS

1. Boil herbs in water for 15 minutes to extract full benefits.
2. Strain and squeeze in fresh lemon.
3. Drink while journaling new intentions.

Lunar Bonus:
- Charge your tonic under the New Moon to absorb fresh-start energy.
- Set an intention by whispering: "I welcome new beginnings and embrace change."
- Place a clear quartz or moonstone near your cup to enhance renewal.

145

Waxing Moon Energy Syrup

Purpose: Boosts motivation, vitality, and focus, aligning with the moon's growth phase to fuel ambition and manifest new goals.

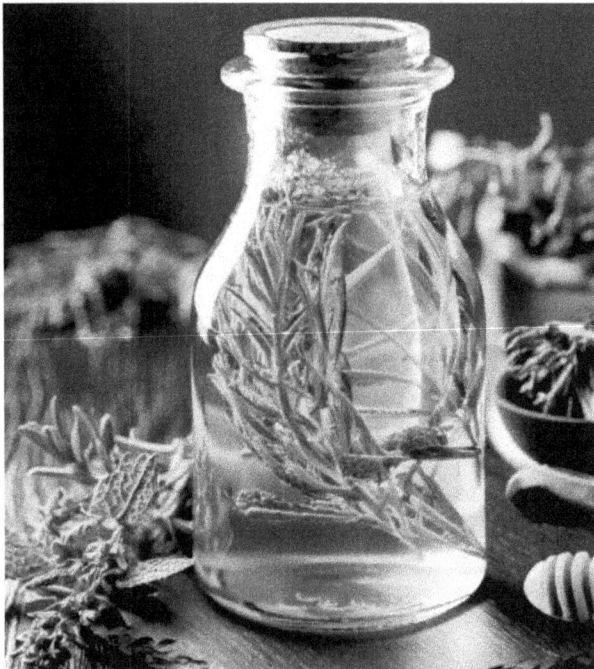

INGREDIENTS

- 1 cup fresh rosemary (memory)
- ½ cup fresh peppermint (digestion)
- ½ cup raw honey
- 2 cups water

DIRECTIONS

1. Simmer the herbs in water for 20 minutes until reduced.
2. Strain and mix with honey while warm.
3. Store in a jar and take 1 tsp daily for focus and energy.

Lunar Bonus:
- Charge your syrup under the Waxing Moon to amplify growth and momentum.
- Set an intention by whispering: "I embrace progress and build my dreams with strength."
- Place a citrine or carnelian near your cup to enhance motivation and confidence.

Waning Moon Release Tonic

Purpose: Promotes relaxation, letting go, and emotional cleansing, helping to release negativity and prepare for renewal.

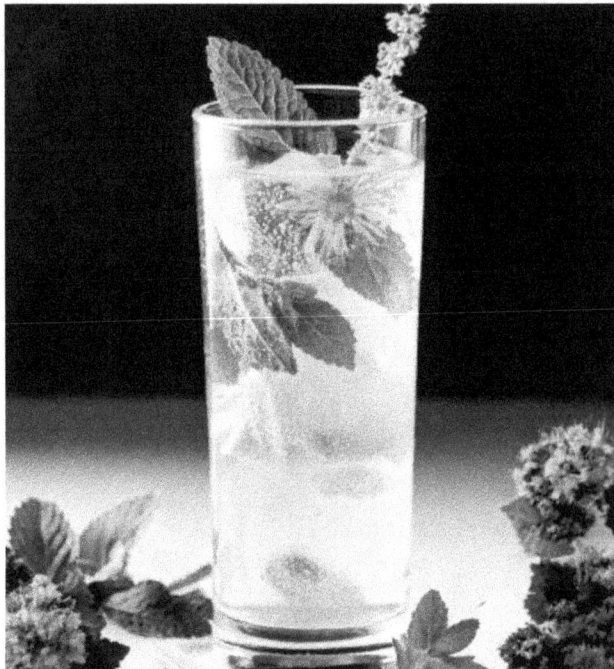

INGREDIENTS

- 1 tsp lemon balm (anxiety)
- 1 tsp passionflower (calmness)
- ½ tsp valerian root (relaxation and sleep)
- ½ tsp sage (memory)
- 1 tsp raw honey

DIRECTIONS

1. Steep the herbs in hot water for 10-15 minutes while focusing on what you wish to release.
2. Strain and stir in honey.
3. Sip slowly in a quiet, dimly lit space to reflect on what no longer serves you.

Lunar Bonus:
- Charge your tonic under the Waning Moon to enhance release and reflection.
- Set an intention by whispering: "I let go of what no longer serves me and welcome peace."
- Place an obsidian or amethyst near your cup to support cleansing and emotional healing.

♈ Aries (Fire): Courage and Vitality Tonic

Purpose: Boosts energy and supports adrenal health for Aries' dynamic nature.

INGREDIENTS

- 1 tsp cayenne pepper (stimulating)
- 1 tbsp fresh ginger (warming)
- 1 tsp rosemary (mental focus)
- 2 cups water
- Honey

DIRECTIONS

1. Steep ginger and rosemary in boiling water for 10 minutes.
2. Add cayenne and honey.
3. Drink to ignite passion and vitality.

Aries Courage Ritual
✦ Find a bold, energizing space, light a red or gold candle. Hold your cup as you envision confidence, courage, strength, and energy.
🔮 **Affirmation:** Say aloud, "I am strong, fearless, and full of vitality. I move forward with passion and purpose."
🔷 **Amplify the Energy:** Place a carnelian, garnet, or tiger's eye crystal near your tea to enhance motivation, courage, and fiery determination.

♉ Taurus (Earth): Grounding Serenity Infusion

Purpose: Brings relaxation and supports Taurus' love for comfort and beauty.

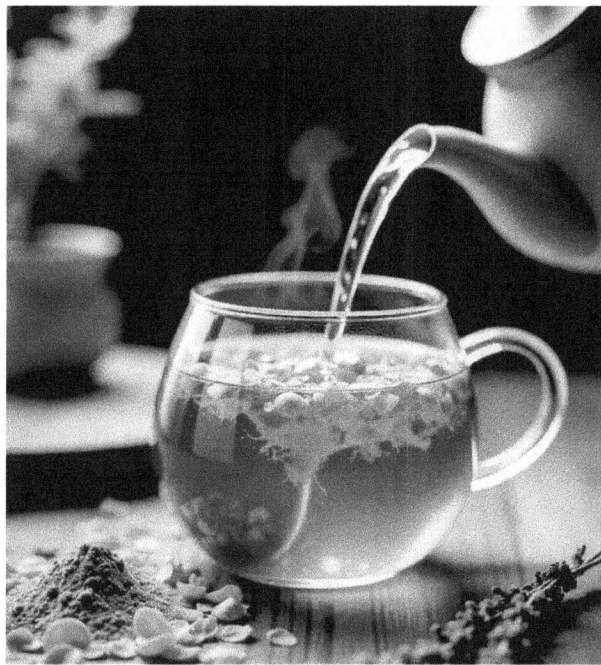

INGREDIENTS

- 1 tbsp rose petals (heart-soothing)
- 1 tsp lavender (calming)
- 1 tsp cinnamon (warming)
- 2 cups hot water

DIRECTIONS

1. Steep herbs in hot water for 10-15 minutes.
2. Strain. the rose petals.
3. Sip slowly while embracing serenity.

Taurus Serenity Ritual
✦ Find a calm, grounding space, light a green or brown candle. Hold your cup as you envision deep roots grounding you in strength and abundance.
🔮 **Affirmation:** Say aloud, "I am deeply rooted, calm, and secure. I welcome peace, stability, and abundance into my life."
🔷 **Amplify the Energy:** Place a green aventurine, moss agate, or smoky quartz crystal near your tea to enhance grounding, relaxation, and inner harmony.

♊ Gemini (Air): Mental Clarity Brew

Purpose: Enhances focus and communication for Gemini's active mind.

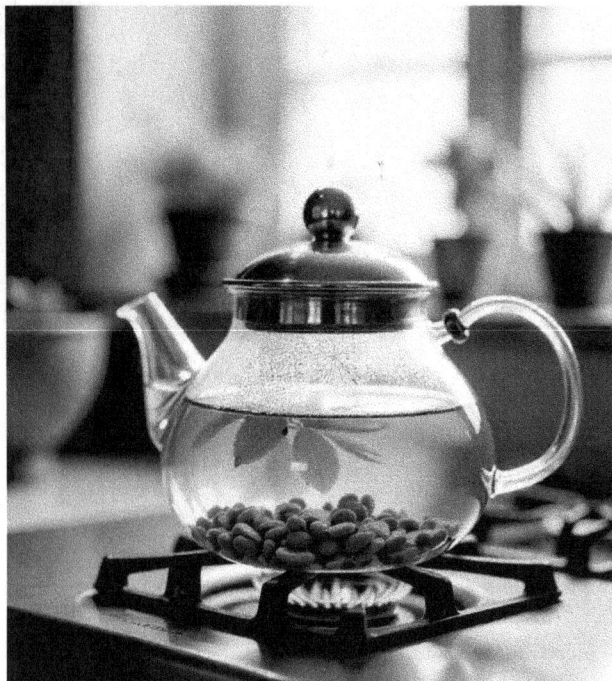

INGREDIENTS

- 1 tsp peppermint (clarity)
- 1 tsp fennel seeds (mental balance)
- 1/2 tsp gotu kola (cognitive support)
- 2 cups hot water

DIRECTIONS

1. Combine all ingredients in a teapot.
2. Steep herbs for 5-10 minutes.
3. Strain and enjoy during mentally demanding tasks.

Gemini Clarity Ritual

✦ Find a bright, airy space, light a yellow or light blue candle. Hold your cup as you visualize your thoughts becoming sharper, more focused, and free-flowing.

💀 **Affirmation:** Say aloud, "My mind is clear, sharp, and open to new insights. I communicate with ease and confidence."

🔮 **Amplify the Energy:** Place a blue lace agate, fluorite, or citrine crystal near your tea to enhance mental clarity, communication, and quick thinking.

♋ Cancer (Water): Comforting Tranquility Elixir

Purpose: Supports intuition, emotional balance and relaxation.

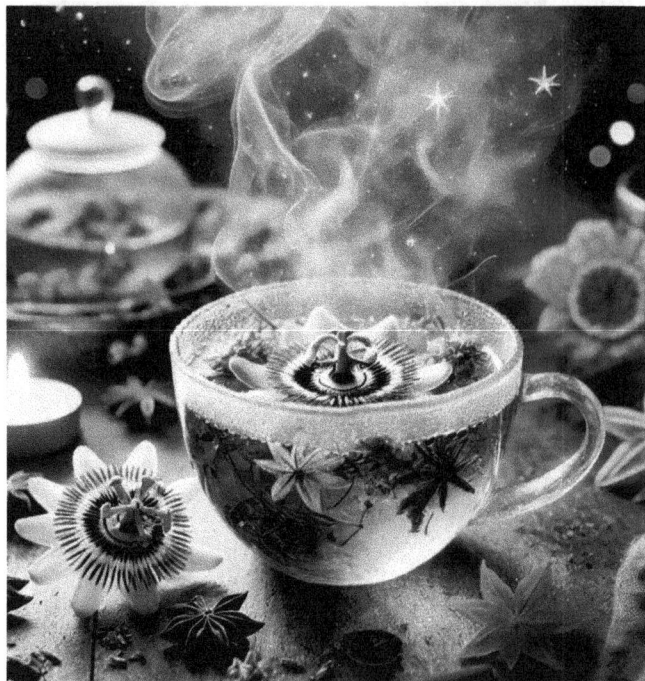

INGREDIENTS

- 1 tsp blue lotus (intuition and dream clarity)
- 1 tsp passionflower (calms emotions)
- ½ tsp anise seed (enhances dream recall and spiritual connection)
- 2 cups hot water

DIRECTIONS

1. Combine all ingredients in a cup.
2. Pour 2 cups of hot water over the herbs.
3. Cover and steep for 10–15 minutes, then strain.
4. Sip slowly to enhance emotional clarity, intuition, and dream connection.

Cancer Comforting Ritual

✦ Find a cozy, tranquil space, light a silver or white candle. Hold your cup as you breathe deeply, inviting emotional healing, comfort, and inner calm.

💀 **Affirmation:** Say aloud, "I am safe, loved, and deeply connected to my emotions. I embrace comfort, intuition, and inner peace."

🔮 **Amplify the Energy:** Place a moonstone, selenite, or rose quartz crystal near your tea to enhance emotional balance, self-love, and intuitive connection.

♌ Leo (Fire): Radiance Heart Tea

Purpose: Supports vitality and self-expression for Leo's confident energy.

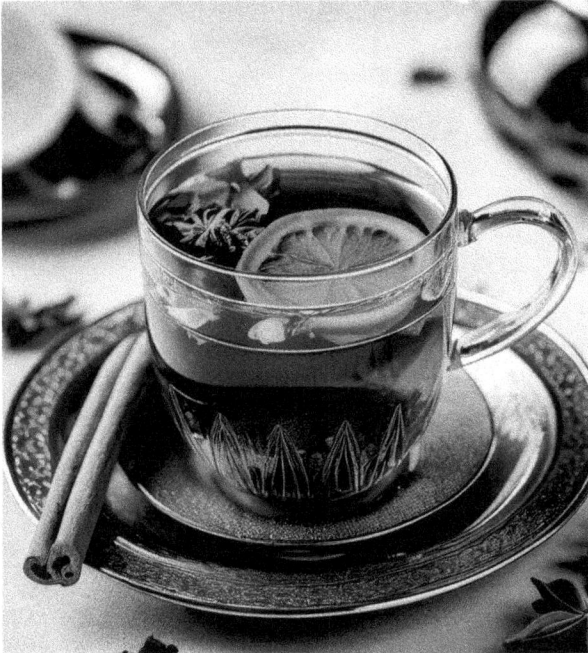

INGREDIENTS

- 1 tsp hibiscus (heart health)
- 1 tsp cinnamon (warming)
- 1 tsp orange zest (uplifting)
- 2 cups hot water

DIRECTIONS

1. Steep ingredients in hot water for 10 minutes.
2. Strain and drink with joyful intention.

Leo Radiance Confidenc Ritual

✦ Find a warm, inviting space, light a gold or orange candle. Hold your cup, and embrace the glow of self-love, confidence, and radiant energy.

🏮 **Affirmation:** Say aloud, "I shine with love, confidence, and passion. My heart is open, and my light inspires others."

🔮 **Amplify the Energy:** Place a sunstone, carnelian, or rose quartz crystal near your tea to enhance self-expression, courage, and joy.

♍ Virgo (Earth): Digestive Harmony Tonic

Purpose: Supports Virgo's sensitive digestion and promotes balance.

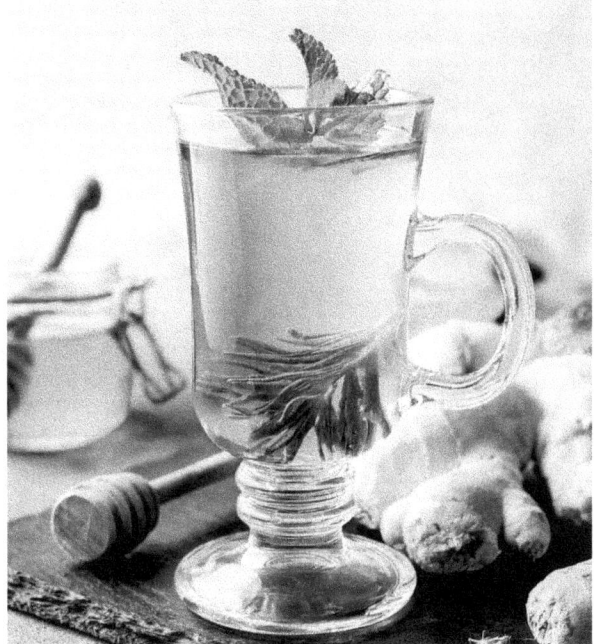

INGREDIENTS

- 1 tsp fennel seeds (digestive support)
- 1 tsp peppermint (soothing)
- 1/2 tsp ginger (warming)
- 1 tsp raw honey (antioxidant)
- 2 cups hot water

DIRECTIONS

1. Steep herbs for 10 minutes.
2. Strain and drink after meals for digestive harmony.

Virgo Harmony Ritual

✦ Find a clean, serene space, light a green or brown candle. Hold your cup as you set an intention for harmony, nourishment, and balance.

🏮 **Affirmation:** Say aloud, "I honor my body with care and balance. I welcome harmony, healing, and vitality."

🔮 **Amplify the Energy:** Place a green aventurine, jasper, or moss agate crystal near your tea to enhance grounding and digestive healing.

♎ Libra (Air): Love and Balance Infusion

Purpose: Promotes inner harmony and supports beauty and love.

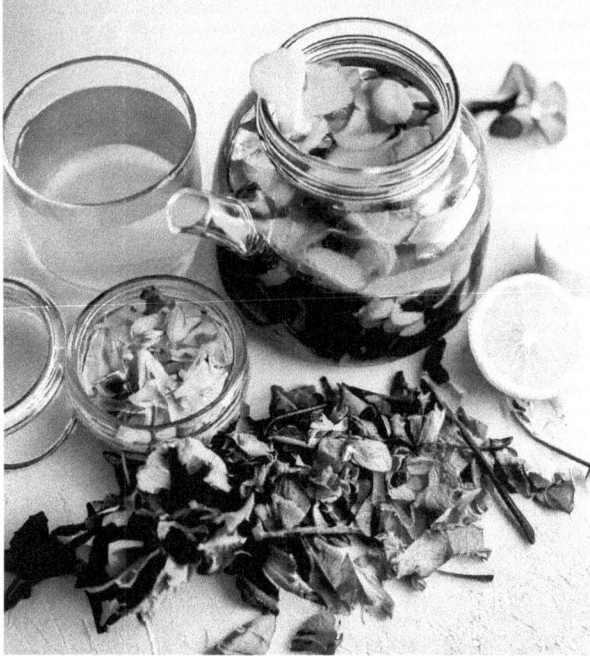

INGREDIENTS

- 1 tbsp rose petals (relaxation)
- 1 tbsp hibiscus flowers (antioxidants)
- 1 tsp dried chamomile (calming)
- 1 tsp lemon balm (reduces anxiety)
- 1 tsp vanilla bean
- 2 cups hot water

DIRECTIONS

1. Steep herbs for 10 minutes.
2. Strain and drink with an intention of love and balance.

Libra Love & Balance Ritual

✦ Find a quiet space and light a candle. Hold your cup focusing on its warmth and loving energy.

🕯 **Affirmation:** Say aloud, "I radiate love and harmony. My heart is open, my mind is at peace."

🔮 **Amplify the Energy:** Place a rose quartz or aventurine crystal near your tea to enhance love, balance, and emotional connection.

♏ Scorpio (Water): Transformative Detox Potion

Purpose: Supports emotional and physical detox for Scorpio's intense energy.

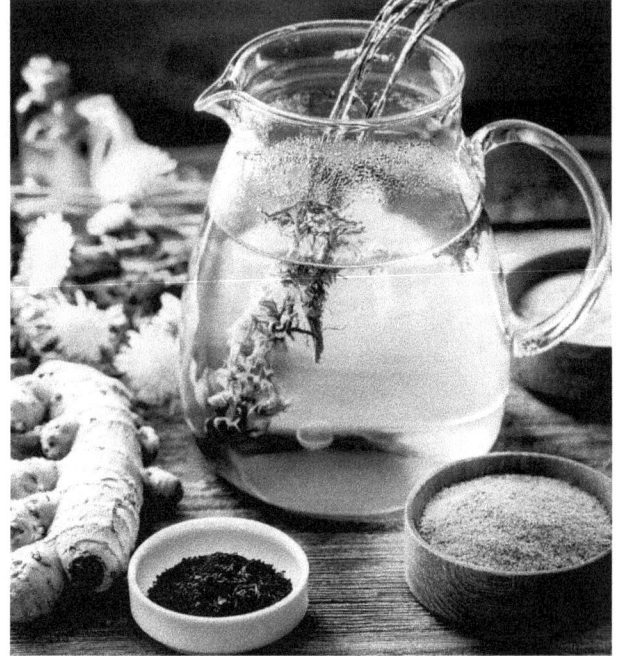

INGREDIENTS

- 1 tsp black cohosh (transformative energy)
- 1 tsp dandelion root (detox)
- 1/2 tsp ginger (warming)
- 2 cups water

DIRECTIONS

1. Simmer dandelion root and ginger for 15 minutes.
2. Add black cohosh and steep for 5 more minutes.
3. Strain and sip mindfully.

Scorpio Transformational Ritual

✦ Find a dark, quiet space, light a black candle. Hold your cup and focus on releasing negative energy.

🕯 **Affirmation:** Say aloud, "I release the old, embrace transformation, and step into my power."

🔮 **Amplify the Energy**: Place a black obsidian, malachite, or garnet crystal near your tea to enhance emotional detox, protection, and renewal.

♐ Sagittarius (Fire): Expansive Abundance Tea

Purpose: Promotes growth, optimism, and liver health.

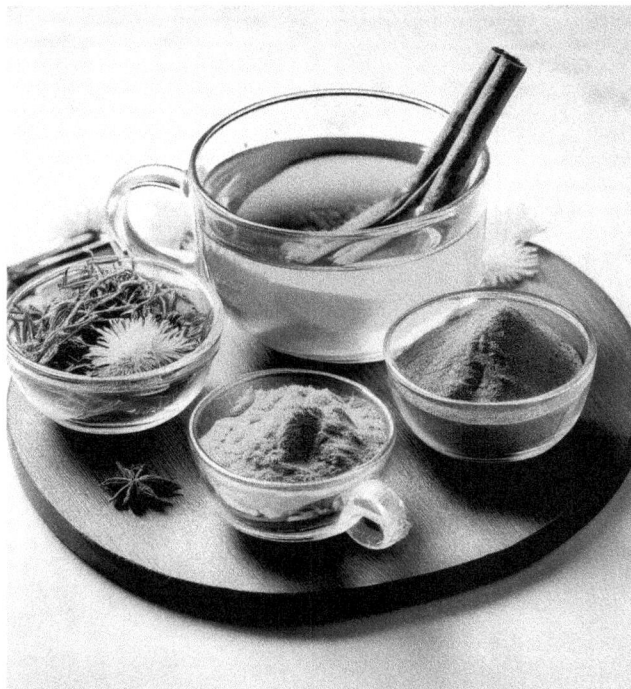

INGREDIENTS

- 1 tbsp dandelion root (liver support)
- 1 tsp turmeric (anti-inflammatory)
- 1 tsp cinnamon (uplifting)
- 2 cups water

DIRECTIONS

1. Simmer dandelion root and turmeric for 15 minutes.
2. Add cinnamon and steep for 5 more minutes.
3. Strain and drink to manifest abundance.

Sagittarius Abundance Ritual

✦ Find a bright, open space, light a gold or purple candle. Hold your cup and visualize limitless opportunities, inner fire, and passion.

🕯 **Affirmation:** Say aloud, "I welcome abundance, adventure, and limitless possibilities into my life."

🤍 **Amplify the Energy:** Place a citrine, amethyst, or tiger's eye crystal near your tea to enhance expansion, prosperity, and inspiration.

♑ Capricorn (Earth): Grounding and Strengthening Brew

Purpose: Strengthens bones and promotes stability for Capricorn's determined nature.

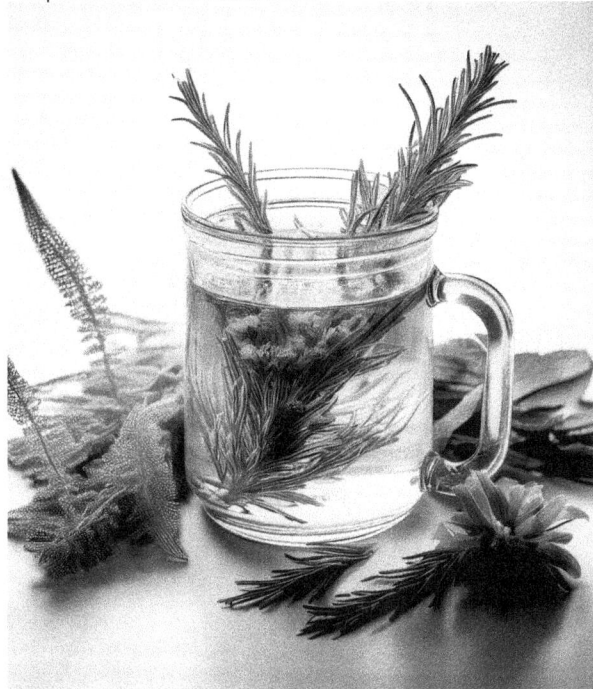

INGREDIENTS

- 1 tsp comfrey (bone support)
- 1 tsp horsetail (silica for strength)
- 1 tsp rosemary (mental resilience)
- 2 cups hot water

DIRECTIONS

1. Steep herbs in hot water for 10-12 minutes.
2. Strain and sip slowly to feel grounded.

Capricorn Grounding & Strength Ritual

✦ Find a quiet, earthy space, light a brown or green candle. Hold your cup and visualize roots growing from your feet and your inner strength.

🕯 **Affirmation:** Say aloud, "I am grounded, disciplined, and strong. I build my life with purpose and stability."

🤍 **Amplify the Energy:** Place a hematite, smoky quartz, or black tourmaline crystal near your tea to enhance grounding, resilience, and protection.

♒ Aquarius (Air): Innovative Inspiration Infusion

Purpose: Sparks creativity and supports the nervous system for Aquarius' visionary energy.

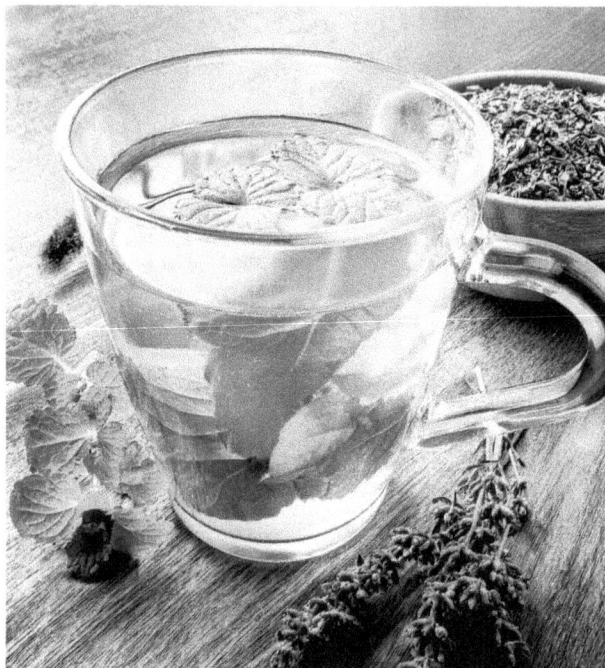

INGREDIENTS

- 1 tsp gotu kola (mental clarity)
- 1 tsp lemon balm (calming)
- 1/2 tsp lavender (soothing)
- 2 cups hot water

DIRECTIONS

1. Steep herbs in hot water for 10 minutes.
2. Strain and drink during creative endeavors.

Aquarius Innovation & Inspiration Ritual

✦ Find a peaceful space, light a blue or silver candle, and let go of distractions. Hold your cup, feeling its warmth and allowing new ideas to flow freely.

🕯 **Affirmation:** Say aloud, "I am open to inspiration and limitless creativity. My mind flows with new ideas and bold possibilities."

🪔 **Amplify the Energy:** Place an amethyst, lapis lazuli, or fluorite crystal near your tea to enhance intuition, mental expansion, and visionary thinking.

♓ Pisces (Water): Dreamy Intuition Elixir

Purpose: Enhances intuition and promotes vivid dreams.

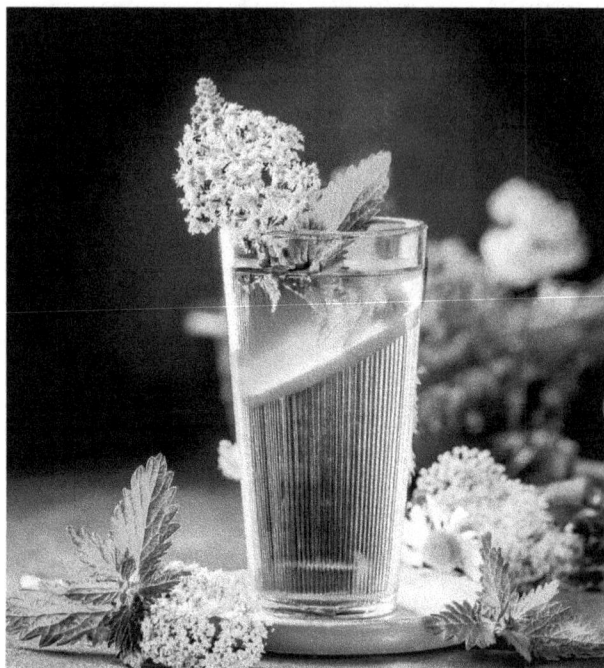

INGREDIENTS

- 1 tsp mugwort (dream enhancement)
- 1 tsp chamomile (relaxation)
- 1/2 tsp lemon balm (calming)
- 2 cups hot water

DIRECTIONS

1. Steep herbs in hot water for 10-15 minutes.
2. Strain and drink 30 minutes before bedtime.

Pisces Dreamy Intuition Ritual

✦ Find a quiet, tranquil space, dim the lights, and light a purple or blue candle. Hold your cup and open your mind to subtle insights and inner wisdom.

🕯 **Affirmation:** Say aloud, "I trust my intuition and embrace the flow of divine wisdom. My dreams guide me with clarity and purpose."

🪔 **Amplify the Energy:** Place an amethyst, moonstone, or labradorite crystal near your tea to deepen intuition, enhance dream recall.

Peppermint Allergy Relief Tea

Purpose: Reduces inflammation and relieves allergy symptoms.

INGREDIENTS
- 1 tsp dried nettle leaves
- 1 tsp dried peppermint leaves
- 1 cup boiling water

DIRECTIONS
1. Steep nettle and peppermint leaves in boiling water for 10 minutes.
2. Strain and drink warm.

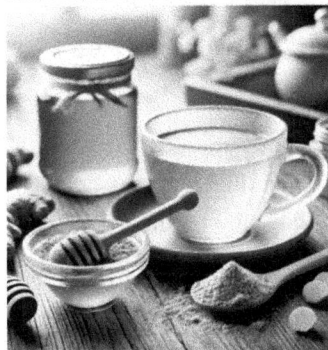

Turmeric & Honey Anti-Allergy Tonic

Purpose: Combats inflammation and boosts immunity.

INGREDIENTS
- 1 tsp turmeric powder
- 1 tsp raw honey
- 1 cup warm water

DIRECTIONS
1. Mix turmeric and honey into warm water.
2. Drink daily to manage allergy symptoms.

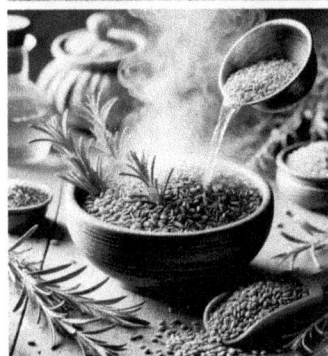

Rosemary & Fenugreek Steam Inhalation

Purpose: Clears nasal congestion and provides allergy relief.

INGREDIENTS
- 1 tablespoon dried rosemary
- 1 tablespoon fenugreek seeds
- 4 cups boiling water

DIRECTIONS
1. Place the rosemary and fenugreek seeds in a large bowl.
2. Pour the boiling water over the herbs.
3. Lean over the bowl with a towel over your head to create a tent.
4. Inhale the steam for 5-10 minutes.

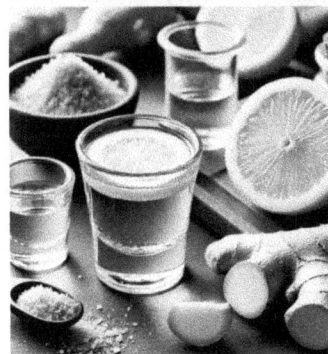

Ginger & Lemon Allergy Shot

Purpose: Reduces inflammation and soothes airways.

INGREDIENTS
- 1 tbsp grated ginger
- Juice of 1 lemon
- ½ cup water

DIRECTIONS
1. Blend all ingredients and strain.
2. Drink as a quick shot for symptom relief.

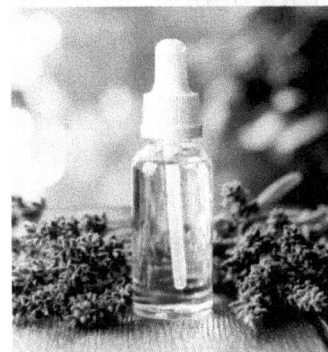

Lavender & Eucalyptus Nasal Spray

Purpose: Eases nasal congestion and promotes clear breathing.

INGREDIENTS
- 1 cup distilled water
- 5 drops lavender essential oil
- 5 drops eucalyptus essential oil

DIRECTIONS
1. Combine ingredients in a spray bottle.
2. Spray lightly into nostrils as needed.

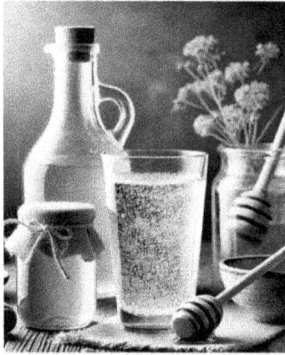

Apple Cider Vinegar Allergy Tonic

Purpose: Balances pH and reduces histamine response.

INGREDIENTS

- 1 tbsp apple cider vinegar
- 1 cup water
- 1 tsp honey

DIRECTIONS

1. Mix apple cider vinegar and honey into water.
2. Drink once daily during allergy season for cold prevention.

Calendula & Rose Petal Eye Compress

Purpose: Relieves itchy, irritated eyes.

INGREDIENTS

- 1 tbsp dried calendula flowers
- 1 tbsp dried rose petals
- 1 cup boiling water

DIRECTIONS

1. Steep calendula and rose petals in boiling water for 5 minutes.
2. Soak a clean cloth in the tea and wring out.
3. Place over closed eyes for 10 minutes.

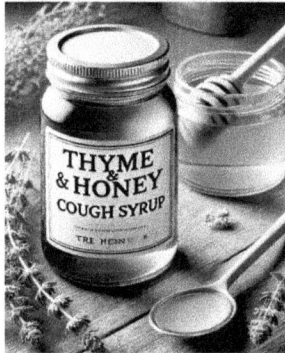

Thyme & Honey Cough Syrup

Purpose: Soothes allergy-related coughs and clears mucus.

INGREDIENTS

- Ingredients:
- 1 tbsp dried thyme
- 1 cup water
- 2 tbsp raw honey

DIRECTIONS

1. Simmer thyme in water for 10 minutes and strain.
2. Mix in honey and store in a jar.
3. Take 1 tsp as needed.

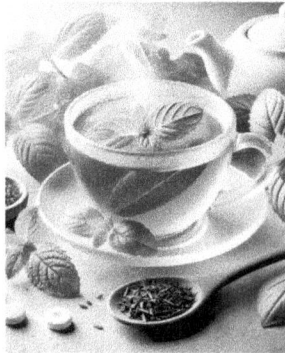

Peppermint & Basil Sinus Tea

Purpose: Relieves sinus pressure and clears nasal passages.

INGREDIENTS

- 1 tsp dried peppermint leaves
- 1 tsp dried basil leaves
- 1 cup boiling water

DIRECTIONS

1. Steep peppermint and basil leaves in boiling water for 10 minutes.
2. Strain and drink warm.

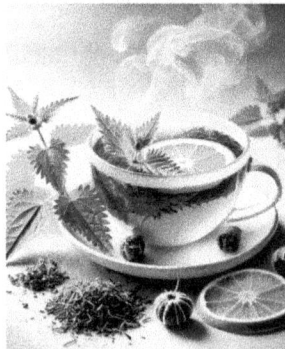

Nettle & Orange Tea

Purpose: Acts as a natural antihistamine to combat allergies.

INGREDIENTS

- 1 tsp dried nettle leaves
- Zest of 1 orange
- 1 cup boiling water

DIRECTIONS

1. Steep nettle and orange zest in boiling water for 10 minutes.
2. Strain and drink warm.

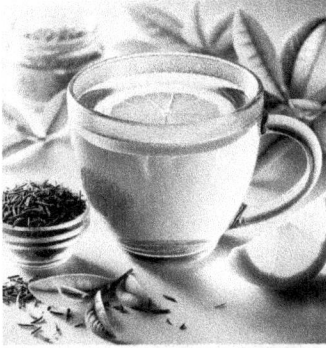

Green Tea & Lemon Antioxidant Tea

Purpose: Combats free radicals and promote youthful skin.

INGREDIENTS

- 1 tsp green tea leaves
- Juice of ½ lemon
- 1 cup boiling water

DIRECTIONS

1. Steep green tea leaves in boiling water for 5 minutes.
2. Add lemon juice, strain, and drink warm.

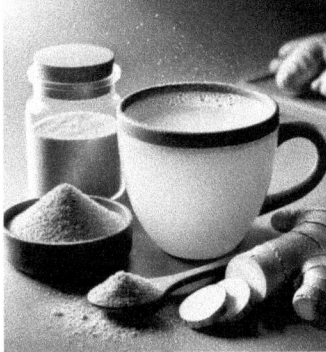

Turmeric Anti-Inflammatory Tonic

Purpose: Reduces inflammation and supports healthy aging.

INGREDIENTS

- ½ tsp turmeric powder
- ½ tsp grated ginger
- 1 cup warm water
- 1 tsp honey

DIRECTIONS

1. Mix turmeric and ginger into warm water.
2. Add honey and drink daily.

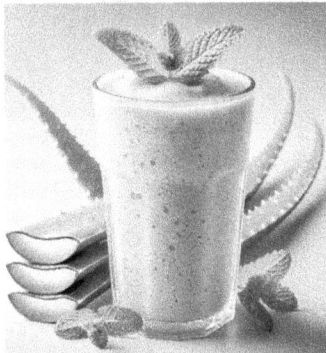

Aloe Mint Skin Hydration Smoothie

Purpose: Keeps skin hydrated and reduces signs of aging.

INGREDIENTS

- 2 tbsp fresh aloe vera gel
- 5 fresh mint leaves
- 1 cup coconut water
- ½ cucumber

DIRECTIONS

1. Blend all ingredients until smooth.
2. Drink for a refreshing hydration boost.

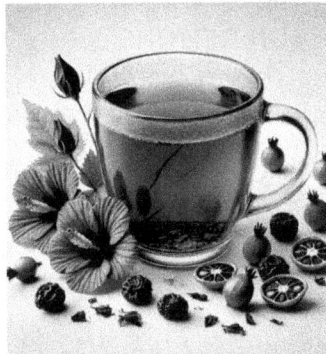

Hibiscus & Rosehip Anti-Aging Tea

Purpose: Reduces inflammation and soothes airways.

INGREDIENTS

- 1 tsp dried hibiscus flowers
- 1 tsp dried rosehips
- 1 cup boiling water

DIRECTIONS

1. Steep hibiscus flowers and rosehips in boiling water for 10 minutes.
2. Strain and enjoy warm or chilled.

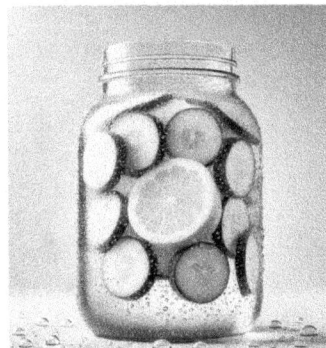

Cucumber & Lemon Detox Water

Purpose: Flushes toxins to promote healthy, glowing skin.

INGREDIENTS

- 1 cucumber, sliced
- Juice of ½ lemon
- 1 liter water

DIRECTIONS

1. Combine cucumber slices and lemon juice in water.
2. Let infuse for 2-3 hours and drink throughout the day.

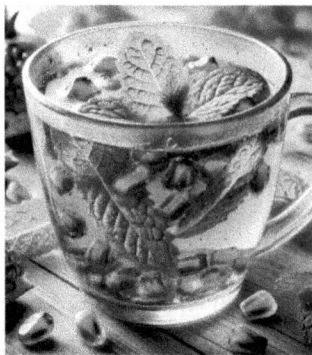

Pomegranate Youth-Boosting Tea

Purpose: Provides antioxidants to protect against aging.

INGREDIENTS

- ½ cup pomegranate seeds (lightly crushed)
- 5 fresh mint leaves
- 1 cup boiling water

DIRECTIONS

1. Steep pomegranate seeds and mint leaves in boiling water for 10 minutes.
2. Strain and enjoy warm.

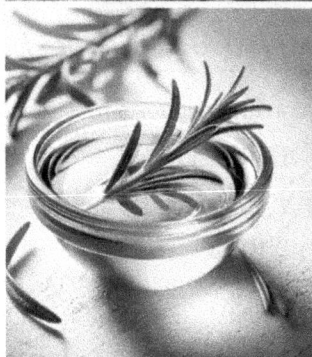

Rosemary Anti-Aging Massage Oil

Purpose: Improves circulation and skin elasticity.

INGREDIENTS

- 2 tbsp olive oil
- 5 drops rosemary essential oi

DIRECTIONS

1. Mix olive oil and rosemary essential oil.
2. Use as a massage oil on the face or body.

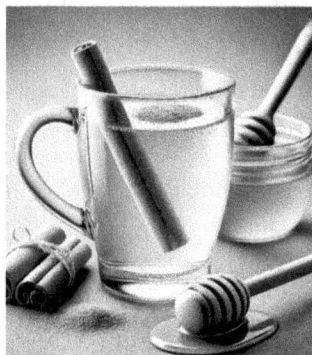

Cinnamon & Honey Longevity Drink

Purpose: Improves circulation and boosts overall vitality.

INGREDIENTS

- ½ tsp cinnamon powder
- 1 tsp raw honey
- 1 cup warm water

DIRECTIONS

1. Mix cinnamon and honey into warm water.
2. Drink daily to support healthy aging.

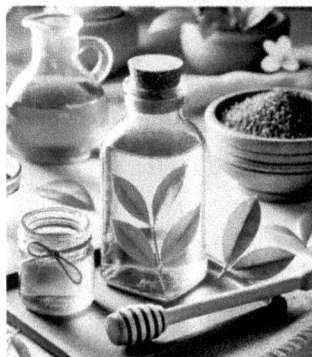

Aloe Vera Anti-Aging Facial Rinse

Purpose: Soothes and rejuvenates tired, aging skin.

INGREDIENTS

- 1 tsp green tea leaves (or 1 green tea bag)
- 2 tbsp fresh aloe vera gel
- 1 tsp raw honey

DIRECTIONS

1. Steep green tea leaves in a small amount of boiling water for 5 minutes, then let cool.
2. Mix cooled tea and honey with aloe vera gel to form a paste.
3. Apply to the face for 15 minutes, then rinse with cool water.

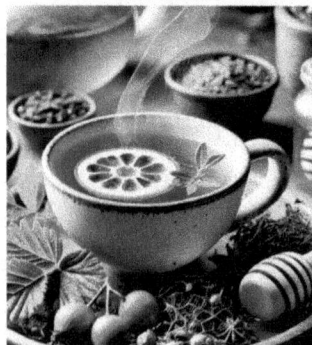

Youthful Rose Glow Infusion

Purpose: Supports skin elasticity, boosts collagen production, and fights stress.

INGREDIENTS

- 1 tbsp rosehip
- 1 tsp gotu kola
- 1 tsp ginseng
- 1 tsp horsetail
- 1 cup hot water
- 1 tsp honey

DIRECTIONS

1. Combine all herbs in a teapot.
2. Pour hot (not boiling) water over the herbs. Steep for 10-15 minutes.
3. Strain and add honey.
4. Drink daily for radiant skin.

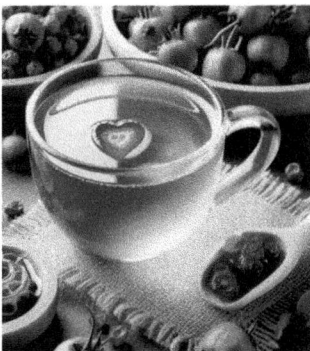

Hawthorn Berry Heart Tea

Purpose: Strengthens the heart and improves circulation.

INGREDIENTS
- 1 tsp dried hawthorn berries
- 1 tsp dried hibiscus petals
- 1 cup boiling water

DIRECTIONS
1. Steep hawthorn berries and hibiscus petals in boiling water for 10-15 minutes.
2. Strain and enjoy warm.

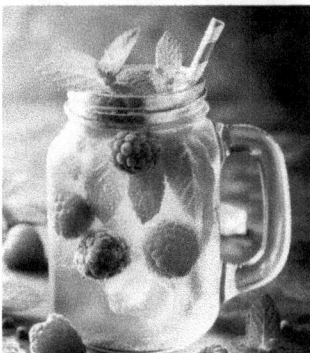

Raspberry & Mint Infused Water

Purpose: Supports arterial health and reduces oxidative stress.

INGREDIENTS
- ½ cup raspberries
- 5 fresh mint leaves
- 1 liter water

DIRECTIONS
1. Combine all ingredients in a pitcher.
2. Let infuse for at least 2 hours.
3. Drink throughout the day to relieve stress.

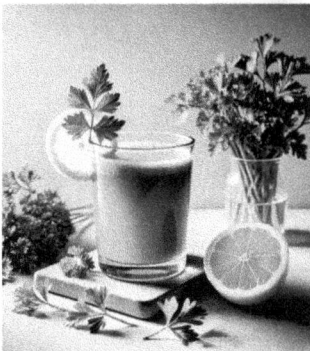

Parsley & Lemon Heart Cleansing Juice

Purpose: Flushes toxins and supports heart function.

INGREDIENTS
- 1 cup fresh parsley
- 1 small banana
- ½ avocado
- Juice of 1 lemon
- 1 cup water

DIRECTIONS
1. Chop the parsley, slice the banana, and peel the avocado.
2. Add all ingredients to a blender. Blend until smooth.
3. Add more water if needed for a thinner texture.

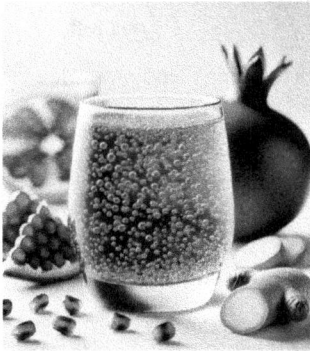

Pomegranate & Ginger Tonic

Purpose: Enhances blood flow and reduces oxidative stress.

INGREDIENTS
- ½ cup pomegranate juice
- 1 tsp grated ginger
- ½ cup sparkling water

DIRECTIONS
1. Mix pomegranate juice and fresh grated ginger.
2. Top with sparkling water.
3. Drink chilled.

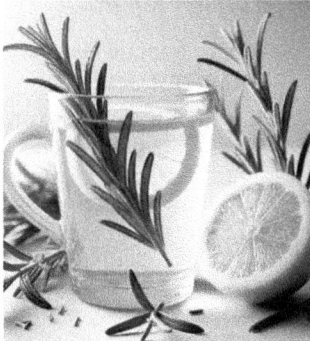

Rosemary & Lemon Circulatory Tea

Purpose: Enhances blood flow and supports vascular health.

INGREDIENTS
- 1 tsp dried rosemary
- ½ tsp dried ginger root
- ½ lemon juice
- 1 tsp raw honey
- 1 cup boiling water

DIRECTIONS
1. Steep rosemary and ginger root in boiling water for 10 minutes.
2. Stain and add lemon juice and honey.
3. Drink warm to increase blood flow.

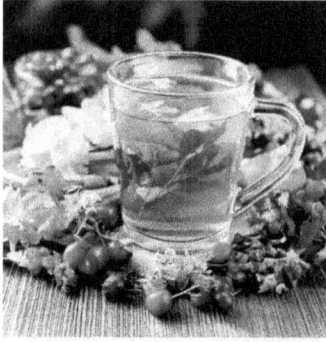

Heart-Strengthening Herbal Tonic

Purpose: Improves circulation and regulates blood pressure.

INGREDIENTS

- 1 tbsp hawthorn berries
- 1 tsp motherwort
- 1 tsp dried hibiscus flowers
- 1 tsp linden flowers
- ½ tsp cinnamon
- 1 quart filtered water
- 1 tbsp raw honey

DIRECTIONS

1. Add all herbs to a pot with 1 quart of water.
2. Bring to a gentle simmer and let steep for 20 minutes.
3. Strain, stir in honey.
4. Drink warm.

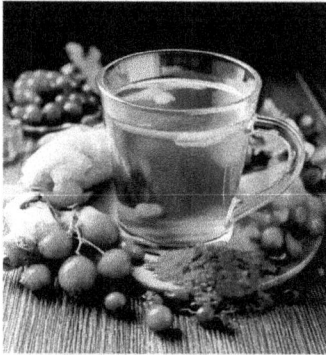

Circulation Herbal Heart Elixir

Purpose: Enhances blood flow, strengthens arteries, and prevents clotting.

INGREDIENTS

- 1 tbsp hawthorn berries
- 1 tsp ginger root
- 1 tsp ginkgo biloba
- ½ tsp cayenne pepper
- 1 tbsp beetroot powder
- 1 tbsp raw honey
- 1 cup warm water

DIRECTIONS

1. Add hawthorn, ginger, and ginkgo biloba to a cup of water.
2. Steep for 10 minutes, then strain.
3. Stir in beetroot powder, cayenne pepper, and honey.
4. Drink 1 cup daily.

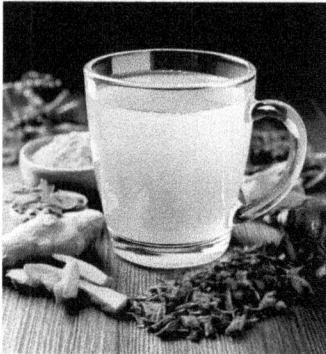

Golden Heart Vitality Infusion

Purpose: Supports circulation, enhances heart function, and reduces inflammation.

INGREDIENTS

- 1 tsp dried turmeric root
- ½ tsp dried ginger root
- ½ tsp cinnamon chips
- ½ tsp dried hibiscus flowers
- 1 cup hot filtered water
- 1 tsp raw honey

DIRECTIONS

1. Add ingredients to a cup or teapot.
2. Pour hot (not boiling) water over the herbs.
3. Cover and steep for 10–15 minutes.
4. Strain and stir in raw honey.
5. Enjoy warm.

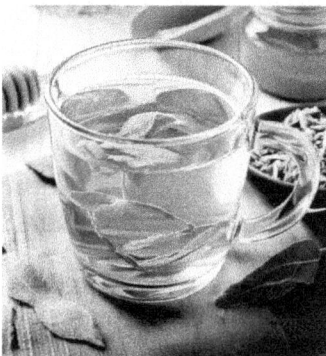

Sage & Lemon Balm Heart Tea

Purpose: Supports heart health, reduces stress, and promotes circulation.

INGREDIENTS

- 1 tsp dried sage leaves
- 1 tsp dried lemon balm
- ½ tsp dried rosemary
- 1 cup hot filtered water
- 1 tsp raw honey

DIRECTIONS

1. Add ingredients to a tea infuser or mug.
2. Pour hot water over the herbs and steep for 10–12 minutes.
3. Strain and stir in honey.
4. Drink warm.

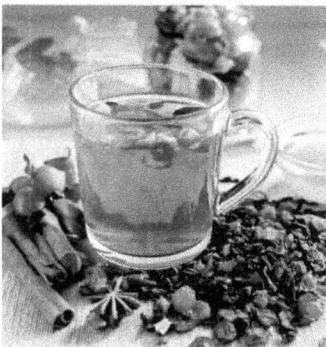

Berry Bliss Heart Tonic

Supports heart health, enhances circulation, and nourishes heart health.

INGREDIENTS

- 1/2 cup dried hawthorn berries
- 1/4 cup dried hibiscus flowers
- 1 tbsp rose petals
- 1 tsp cinnamon chips
- 1 tsp orange peel
- 4 cups filtered water
- 1 tbsp raw honey

DIRECTIONS

1. Add all ingredients (except honey) to a saucepan with 4 cups of water.
2. Bring to a gentle simmer and let steep for 20 minutes.
3. Strain and sweeten with honey.
4. Enjoy warm or chilled.

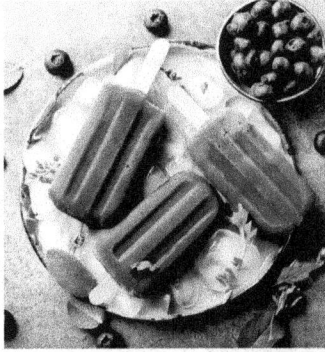

Blueberry Sage Popsicles

Purpose: Boosts brain health and supports memory.

INGREDIENTS
- 1 cup blueberries
- 1 tsp dried sage leaves
- 1/2 cup yogurt
- 1/2 cup water

DIRECTIONS
1. Blend all ingredients until smooth.
2. Pour into popsicle molds and freeze.
3. Enjoy these refreshing, brain-boosting treats.

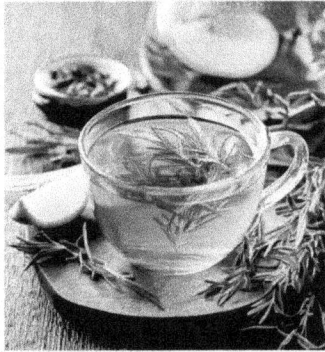

Rosemary & Gotu Kola Cognitive Tea

Purpose: Enhances memory, focus, and overall cognitive health.

INGREDIENTS
- 1 tablespoon dried rosemary
- 1 tablespoon dried gotu kola
- 1 teaspoon honey
- 1 cup boiling water

DIRECTIONS
1. Steep rosemary and gotu kola in boiling water for 10 minutes.
2. Strain and drink warm.

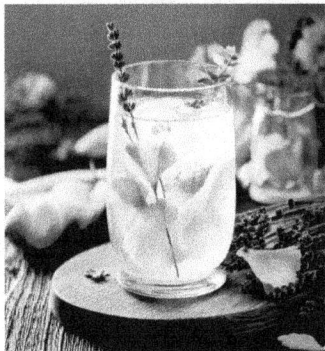

Gingko & Lavender Focus Tonic

Purpose: Supports mental clarity, focus, and reduces mental fatigue.

INGREDIENTS
- 1 tsp dried ginkgo biloba
- 1 tsp dried lavender
- 1 cup boiling water
- 1 tsp honey

DIRECTIONS
1. Steep ginkgo biloba and lavender in boiling water for 10–15 minutes.
2. Strain and sweeten with honey.

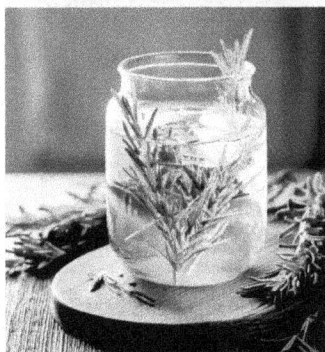

Rosemary & Sage Focus Infusion

Purpose: Stimulates the brain, enhances concentration, and improves memory.

INGREDIENTS
- 1 tsp dried rosemary
- 1 tsp dried sage
- 1 cup boiling water
- 1 tsp honey

DIRECTIONS
1. Steep rosemary and sage in boiling water for 10–15 minutes.
2. Strain and sweeten with honey.

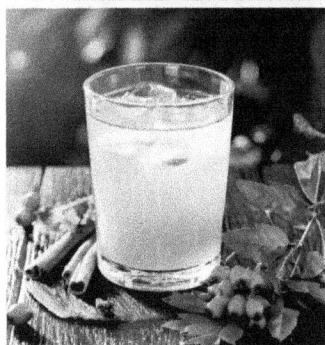

Ashwagandha Mind Calming Elixir

Purpose: Reduces stress, enhances cognitive function, and promotes relaxation.

INGREDIENTS
- 1 tsp dried ashwagandha
- 1 tsp dried hawthorn
- 1 cup boiling water
- 1 tsp honey

DIRECTIONS
1. Steep ashwagandha and hawthorn in boiling water for 10 minutes.
2. Strain and add honey.

Brain-Boosting Herbal Infusion

Purpose: Enhances mental clarity, memory, and cognitive function.

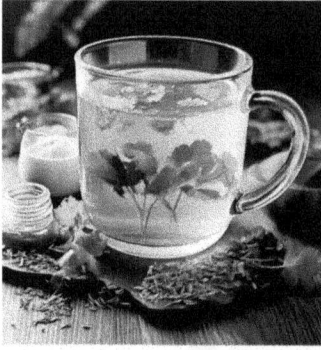

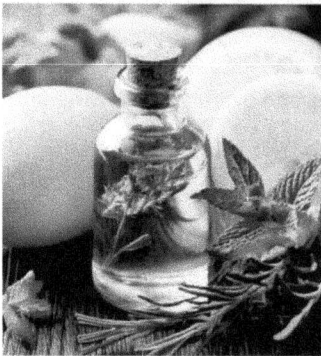

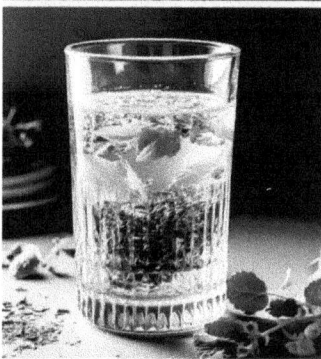

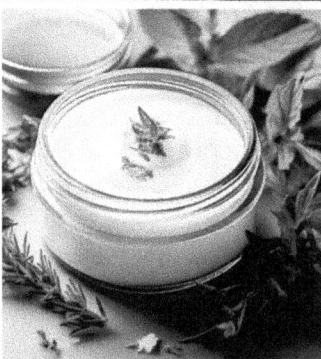

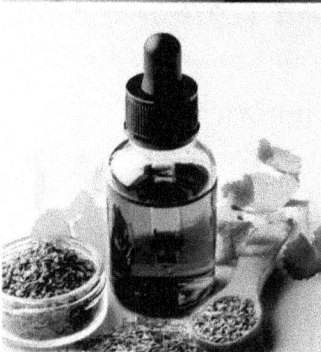

INGREDIENTS
- 1 tsp dried gotu kola
- 1 tsp dried ginkgo biloba
- ½ tsp dried rosemary
- ½ tsp dried peppermint
- 1 cup hot filtered water
- 1 tsp raw honey

DIRECTIONS
1. Add all herbs to a tea infuser or teapot.
2. Pour hot (not boiling) water over the herbs and steep for 10–15 minutes.
3. Strain and stir in raw honey, if desired.
4. Sip for a brain-boosting effect.

Focus-Enhancing Aromatherapy Oil

Purpose: Stimulates cognitive function, reduces brain fog, and sharpens focus.

INGREDIENTS
- 5 drops rosemary essential oil
- 5 drops peppermint essential oil
- 5 drops lemon essential oil
- 2 tbsp carrier oil (jojoba or coconut)

DIRECTIONS
1. Mix all oils in a small glass bottle.
2. Apply to wrists, temples, or inhale deeply before study sessions or work.
3. Diffuse to enhance focus.

Clarity & Focus Solar Infusion

Purpose: Boosts mental clarity, enhances focus, and supports cognitive longevity.

INGREDIENTS
- 1 tsp dried rosemary
- 1 tsp dried lemon balm
- ½ tsp dried gotu kola
- ½ tsp dried tulsi (holy basil)
- 1 quart filtered water

DIRECTIONS
1. Place all herbs in a clear glass jar.
2. Fill with room-temperature filtered water and stir gently.
3. Seal the jar and set it in direct sunlight for 4–6 hours to infuse.
4. Strain and drink for clarity.

Focus-Enhancing Herbal Salve

Purpose: Clears mental fog, refreshes the senses, and promotes alertness.

INGREDIENTS
- 2 tbsp coconut oil
- 1 tbsp beeswax
- 5 drops rosemary essential oil
- 5 drops peppermint essential oil
- 5 drops basil essential oil

DIRECTIONS
1. Melt coconut oil and beeswax in a double boiler over low heat.
2. Remove from heat and stir in essential oils.
3. Pour into a small glass jar or tin and let cool until solid.
4. Apply to temples, wrists, and back of the neck for clarity.

Cognitive Clarity Tincture

Purpose: Enhances memory, improves focus, and promotes mental agility.

INGREDIENTS
- 1 tbsp dried gotu kola
- 1 tbsp dried rosemary
- 1 tbsp dried tulsi (holy basil)
- ½ cup vodka or apple cider vinegar
- 1 glass jar with lid

DIRECTIONS
1. Add all herbs to a clean glass jar.
2. Pour vodka or apple cider vinegar over the herbs, until submerged.
3. Seal and store in a cool, dark place for 4–6 weeks, shaking occasionally.
4. Store in a dark glass dropper bottle.
5. Take ½ teaspoon diluted in water.

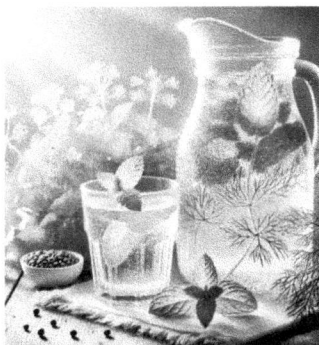

Peppermint and Dill Digestive Water

Purpose: Reduces bloating, enhances digestion, and provides gentle hydration.

INGREDIENTS

- 4-5 fresh peppermint leaves
- 1 tsp dried dill seeds
- 1-liter water

DIRECTIONS

1. Add peppermint leaves and dill seeds to a jug of water.
2. Infuse for at least 1 hour in the refrigerator.
3. Drink throughout the day to support reduce bloating.

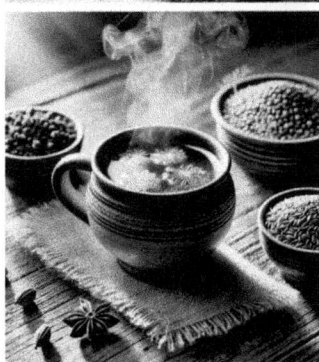

Cumin-Coriander-Dill Seed Decoction

Purpose: Improves digestion and stimulates enzyme production.

INGREDIENTS

- 1 tsp cumin seeds
- 1 tsp coriander seeds
- 1 tsp dill seeds
- 2 cups water

DIRECTIONS

1. Add all seeds to a small pot with water and bring to a boil.
2. Simmer for 10 minutes, then strain.
3. Drink warm, 1/2 cup at a time, before meals.

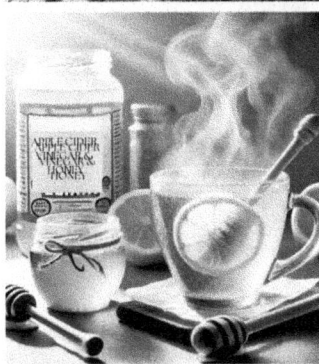

Apple Cider Vinegar and Honey Elixir

Purpose: Stimulates digestive enzymes, balances stomach acid, and alleviates gas.

INGREDIENTS

- 1 tbsp raw apple cider vinegar
- 1 tsp raw honey
- 1 cup warm water

DIRECTIONS

1. Mix apple cider vinegar and honey into a cup of warm water.
2. Stir well.
3. Drink 15-20 minutes before meals to prepare your digestive system for optimal function.

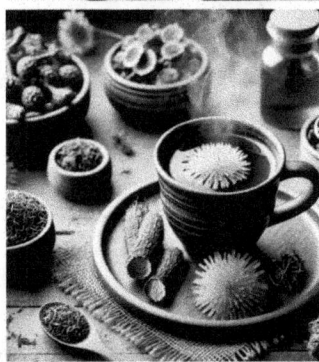

Dandelion & Burdock Root Detox Tea

Purpose: Supports liver function, promotes bile flow, and breaks down fats.

INGREDIENTS

- 1 teaspoon dried dandelion root
- 1 teaspoon dried burdock root
- 2 cups water

DIRECTIONS

1. Add dandelion root and burdock root to a pot with water.
2. Bring to a gentle boil, then reduce heat and simmer for 10-15 minutes.
3. Strain and enjoy warm before meals to stimulate digestion.

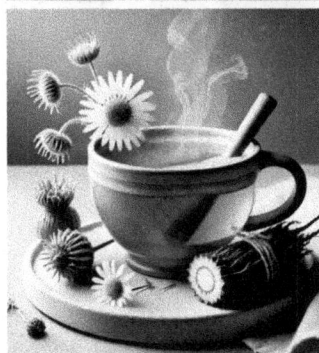

Burdock & Chamomile Digestive Tea

Purpose: Promotes liver health, aids digestion, and reduces inflammation.

INGREDIENTS

- 1 teaspoon dried burdock root
- 1 teaspoon dried chamomile flowers
- 2 cups water

DIRECTIONS

1. Simmer burdock root in 2 cups of water for 10 minutes.
2. Remove from heat, add chamomile, and steep for an additional 5 minutes.
3. Strain and drink warm for digestive support.

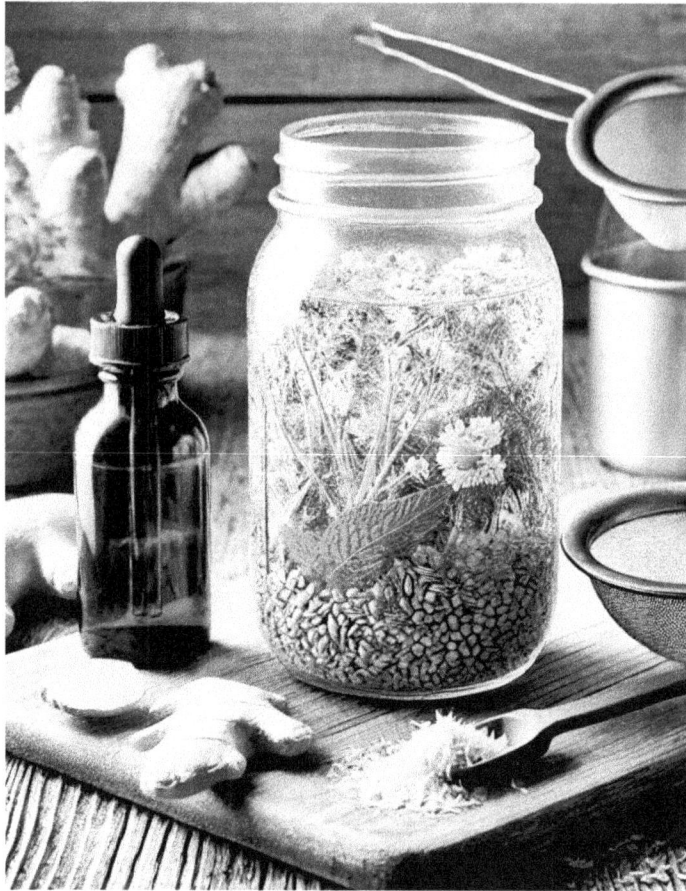

Digestive Tincture Recipe

Purpose: Supports gut health, relieves bloating, and soothes inflammation.

INGREDIENTS

- 1/4 cup dried fennel seeds
- 1/4 cup dried peppermint leaves
- 2 tbsp dried ginger root (or 1/4 cup fresh, chopped ginger)
- 1 tbsp dried chamomile flowers
- 1 tbsp dried dandelion root
- 1 cup high-proof vodka or food-grade alcohol (minimum 80 proof)

EQUIPMENT

- Glass jar with a tight-fitting lid (a mason jar)
- Fine mesh strainer or cheesecloth
- Dark glass tincture bottle with dropper (for storage)

DIRECTIONS

1. Add all the dried herbs to the glass jar. If using fresh ginger, chop it finely before adding it.
2. Pour the vodka or alcohol over the herbs until they are completely submerged, leaving about 1 inch of space at the top of the jar.
3. Seal the jar tightly and shake well to mix the ingredients.
4. Store the jar in a cool, dark place for 4-6 weeks. Shake the jar gently every day or at least a few times a week to ensure the herbs are evenly infused.
5. After the infusion period, strain the mixture through a fine mesh strainer or cheesecloth into a clean bowl, pressing the herbs to extract all liquid.
6. Pour the strained tincture into a dark glass tincture bottle with a dropper for easy use.

Dosage:
- Take 1-2 droppers (30-60 drops) diluted in a small glass of water or tea.
- Use 15-20 minutes before meals to stimulate digestion or after meals to ease bloating and discomfort.

Shelf Life:
- Store in a dark, cool place.
- This tincture lasts up to 1 year.

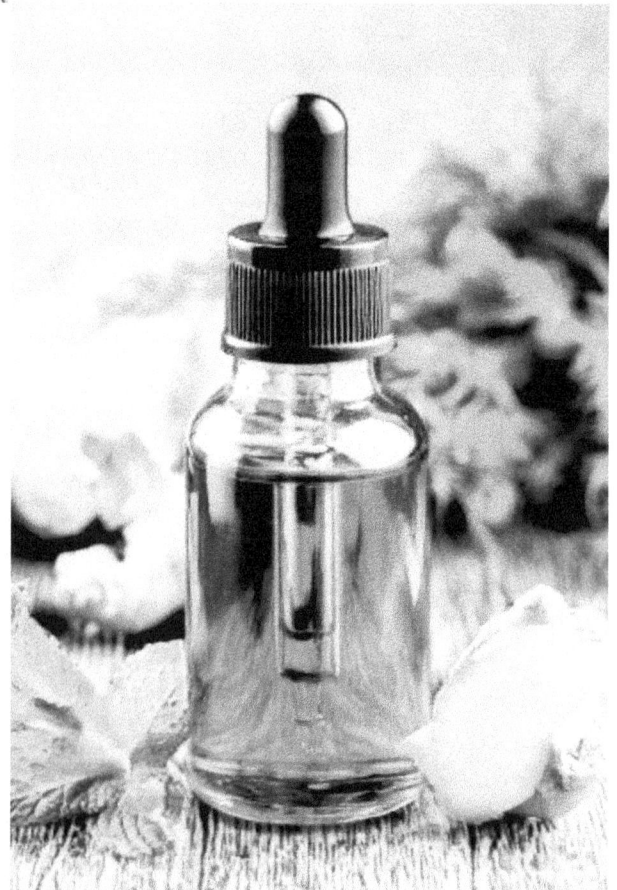

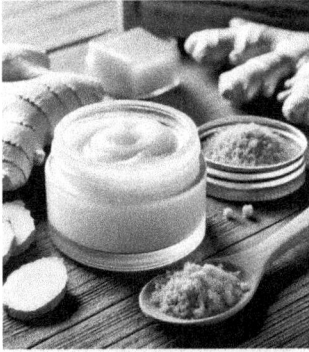

Ginger and Turmeric Gut Health Balm

Purpose: Contains antimicrobial benefits to support gut health topically.

INGREDIENTS

- 1/4 cup coconut oil
- 1 teaspoon grated fresh ginger
- 1 teaspoon ground turmeric
- 2 tablespoons beeswax

DIRECTIONS

1. Melt the coconut oil and beeswax together in a double boiler.
2. Stir in grated ginger and turmeric.
3. Pour the mixture into a sterilized jar and let cool.
4. Massage onto the abdomen in circular motions to promote gut health.

Artichoke Leaf Gut Tonic

Purpose: Stimulate bile production and enhance fat digestion.

INGREDIENTS

- 1 tablespoon dried artichoke leaf
- 1 teaspoon fresh lemon juice
- 1 cup boiling water
- Dash of cinnamon

DIRECTIONS

1. Steep the artichoke leaf in boiling water for 10 minutes.
2. Strain the infusion and stir in the lemon juice and cinnamon.
3. Drink before meals to prime digestion and support gut health.

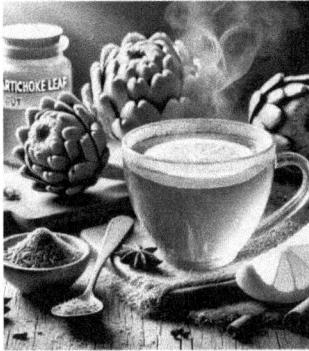

Aloe Vera, Lavender, & Fennel Poultice

Purpose: Soothes the stomach and supports a balanced gut microbiome.

INGREDIENTS

- 2 tablespoons fresh aloe vera gel
- 2 drops lavender essential oil
- 1 teaspoon fennel seeds
- A clean cloth or gauze

DIRECTIONS

1. Blend aloe vera gel, lavender oil, and fennel seeds into a smooth paste.
2. Spread the paste onto a clean cloth or gauze.
3. Apply the poultice to the abdomen for 20-30 minutes for gut health.

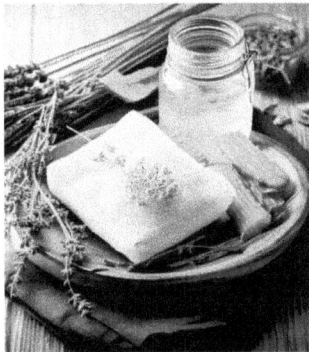

Slippery Elm and Licorice Decoction

Purpose: Soothes the gut lining and promotes the growth of beneficial bacteria.

INGREDIENTS

- 1 tablespoon slippery elm powder
- 1 tablespoon dried licorice root
- 3 cups water

DIRECTIONS

1. Combine ingredients in a saucepan with water.
2. Simmer gently for 15 minutes, then strain.
3. Drink 1 cup warm, up to twice daily, to support gut microbiome health.

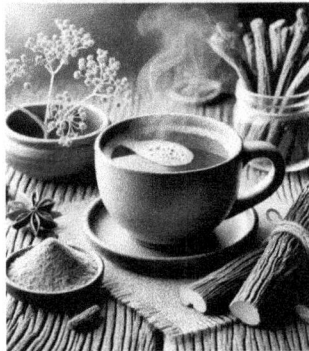

Peppermint and Caraway Infusion

Purpose: Relieves digestive discomfort and promotes microbial diversity.

INGREDIENTS

- 1 teaspoon dried peppermint leaves
- 1/2 teaspoon caraway seeds
- 1 cup hot water

DIRECTIONS

1. Combine peppermint leaves and caraway seeds in a teacup.
2. Pour hot water over the ingredients and cover. Steep for 10 minutes.
3. Strain and drink after meals to support digestion and the gut microbiome.

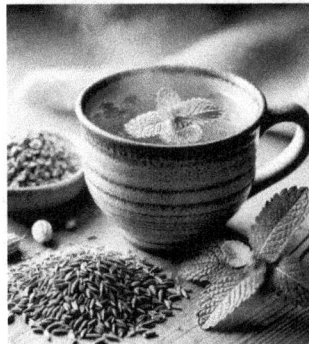

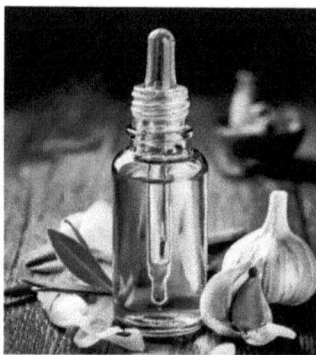

Garlic & Olive Oil Ear Drops

Purpose: Soothes ear pain, fights infection, and reduces inflammation.

INGREDIENTS

- 2 tbsp olive oil
- 1 clove fresh garlic (crushed)
- 2 drops tea tree essential oil

DIRECTIONS

1. Warm the olive oil slightly (not too hot).
2. Add crushed garlic; infuse for 15 minutes.
3. Strain the oil to remove garlic pieces and mix in tea tree essential oil.
4. Use 1–2 drops in the affected ear while laying on your side.
5. Let it sit for 5 minutes, then tilt to drain.

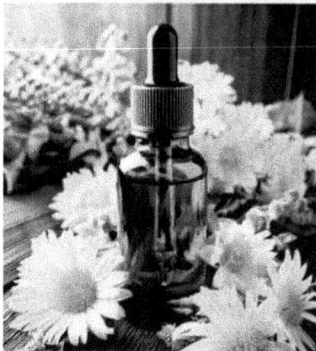

Mullein & Calendula Herbal Ear Oil

Purpose: Soothes inflammation, relieves pain, and supports natural healing.

INGREDIENTS

- 2 tbsp dried mullein flowers
- 1 tbsp dried calendula flowers
- ½ cup olive oil or almond oil

DIRECTIONS

1. Place mullein and calendula flowers in a small glass jar.
2. Pour warm oil over the herbs and let infuse for 4–6 hours.
3. Strain the oil into a clean dropper bottle.
4. Use 1–2 drops in the affected ear twice daily for soothing relief.

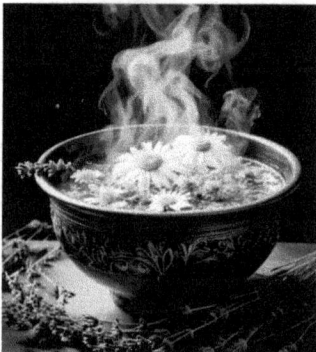

Chamomile & Lavender Steam Inhalation

Purpose: Clears congestion, reduces pressure, and eases ear pain.

INGREDIENTS

- 1 tbsp dried chamomile flowers
- 1 tbsp dried lavender flowers
- 4 cups hot water

DIRECTIONS

1. Add chamomile and lavender to a bowl of steaming hot water.
2. Lean over the bowl with a towel over your head, trapping the steam.
3. Inhale deeply for 10–15 minutes to help clear sinuses and ear pressure.
4. Repeat as needed to relieve ear pain.

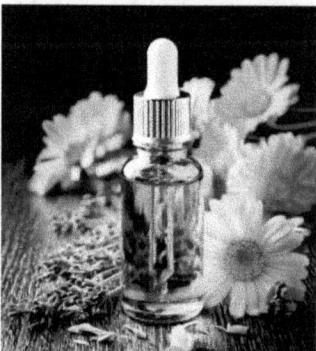

Calendula Ear Soothing Oil

Purpose: Calms irritation, reduces swelling, and promotes ear healing.

INGREDIENTS

- 2 tbsp almond oil or coconut oil
- 1 tbsp dried calendula flowers
- 1 tbsp dried lavender flowers

DIRECTIONS

1. Gently warm the oil and add the calendula and lavender.
2. Let it infuse over low heat for 10–15 minutes, then strain.
3. Store in a dropper bottle and use 1–2 drops in the affected ear for soothing relief.

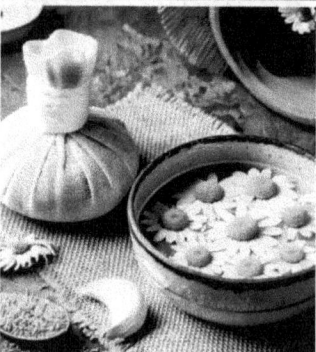

Warm Chamomile & Garlic Poultice

Purpose: Eases ear pain, reduces inflammation, and supports healing.

INGREDIENTS

- 2 tbsp dried chamomile flowers
- 1 clove fresh garlic (crushed)
- ½ cup warm water
- 1 clean cloth or cotton pad

DIRECTIONS

1. Soak chamomile flowers and garlic in warm water for 5 minutes.
2. Strain the herbs and dip a cloth or cotton pad into the warm infusion.
3. Place over the affected ear for 10–15 minutes to reduce pain.
4. Repeat 2–3 times daily as needed.

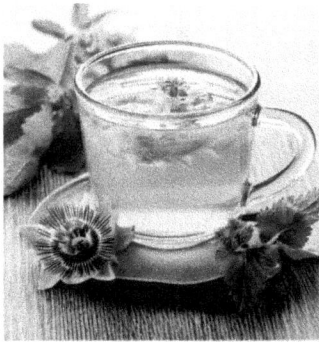

Serenity Soothing Tea

Purpose: Calms the nervous system, reduces stress, and eases anxiety.

INGREDIENTS

- 1 teaspoon dried lemon balm
- 1 teaspoon dried lavender
- 1 teaspoon dried passionflower
- 2 cups boiling water

DIRECTIONS

1. Combine all dried herbs in a teapot or heat-proof jar.
2. Pour boiling water over the herbs, cover, and steep for 10-15 minutes.
3. Strain and drink 1-2 cups daily to relax and unwind.
4. Store in the fridge for 24 hours.

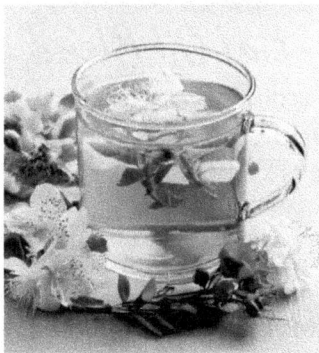

Mood-Lifting Herbal Infusion

Purpose: Uplifts mood, reduces depression, and restores emotional balance.

INGREDIENTS

- 1 teaspoon dried St. John's Wort
- 1 teaspoon dried rose
- 1 teaspoon dried holy basil
- 2 cups boiling water

DIRECTIONS

1. Add dried herbs to a teapot or heat-proof container.
2. Pour boiling water over the herbs; steep for 10-15 minutes.
3. Strain and drink to uplift mood.
4. Store in the fridge for 24 hours.

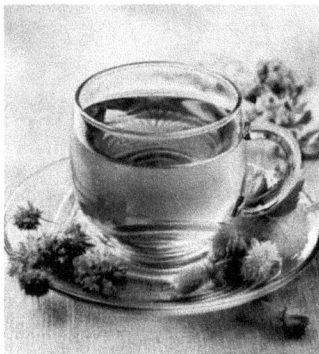

Anxiety & Overwhelm Relief Tea

Purpose: Reduces anxiety and restores emotional balance.

INGREDIENTS

- 1 teaspoon dried blue vervain
- 1 teaspoon dried motherwort
- 1 teaspoon dried hops
- 2 cups boiling water

DIRECTIONS

1. Add all dried herbs to a teapot or heat-proof container.
2. Pour boiling water over the herbs, cover, and steep for 10-15 minutes.
3. Strain and drink as needed to calm anxiety and restore balance.

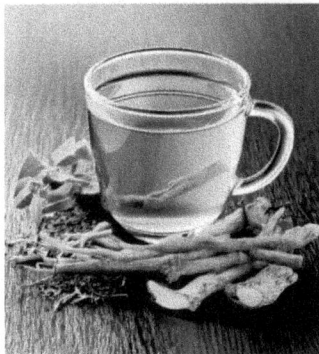

Adaptogenic Resilience Decoction

Purpose: Enhances resilience, boosts energy, and supports emotional strength.

INGREDIENTS

- 1 teaspoon dried ashwagandha
- 1 teaspoon dried licorice root
- 1 teaspoon dried ginseng
- 2 cups boiling water

DIRECTIONS

1. Add all dried herbs to a teapot or mug.
2. Pour boiling water over the herbs, cover, and steep for 15 minutes.
3. Strain and drink in the morning to boost emotional resilience.

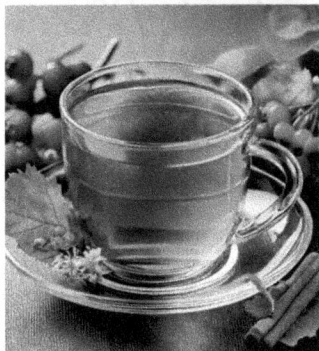

Heart-Centered Comfort Tea

Purpose: Supports emotional healing and provides emotional distress.

INGREDIENTS

- 1 teaspoon dried hawthorn berries
- 1 teaspoon dried linden
- 1 teaspoon dried cinnamon
- 2 cups boiling water

DIRECTIONS

1. Combine all dried herbs in a teapot or heat-proof jar.
2. Pour boiling water over the herbs, cover, and steep for 10-15 minutes.
3. Strain and drink when feeling emotionally heavy or in need of comfort.

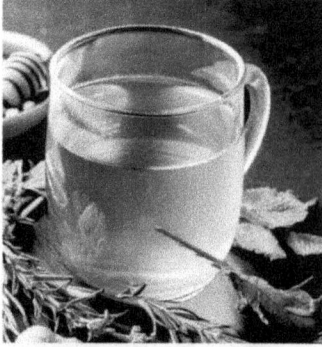

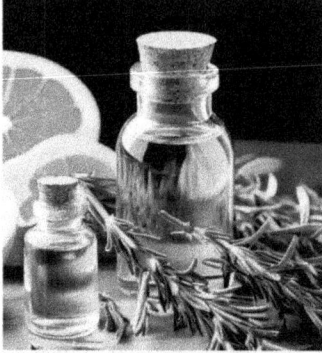

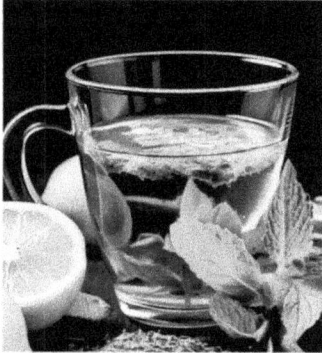

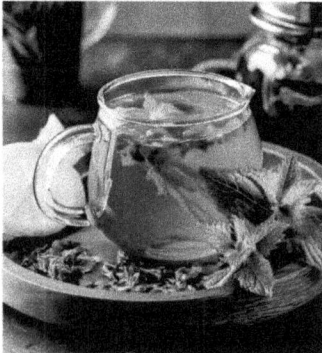

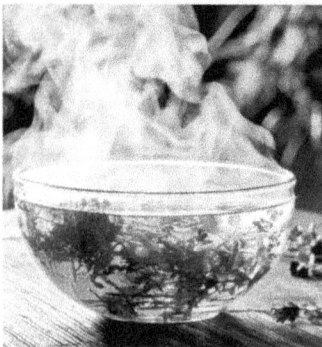

Energizing Herbal Infusion

Purpose: Boosts physical energy, mental clarity, and overall vitality.

INGREDIENTS

- 1 tsp dried ginseng root
- ½ tsp dried peppermint leaves
- ½ tsp dried rosemary
- 1 cup hot filtered water
- 1 tsp raw honey

DIRECTIONS

1. Add all herbs to an infuser.
2. Pour hot (not boiling) water over the herbs. Steep for 10–15 minutes.
3. Strain and stir in raw honey.
4. Sip in the morning or afternoon for a natural energy boost.

Invigorating Essential Oil Blend

Purpose: Clears brain fog, increases alertness, and fights fatigue.

INGREDIENTS

- 5 drops peppermint essential oil
- 5 drops rosemary essential oil
- 5 drops grapefruit essential oil
- 2 tbsp carrier oil (jojoba or coconut oil)

DIRECTIONS

1. Mix all oils in a glass bottle.
2. Apply to wrists, temples, or inhale deeply whenever you need an energy boost.
3. Diffuse in your workspace for enhanced focus and clarity.

Refresh & Focus Green Tea

Purpose: Sharpens focus, improves mental alertness, and keeps energy levels steady.

INGREDIENTS

- 1 tsp dried green tea leaves
- 1 tsp dried gotu kola
- ½ tsp dried rosemary
- ½ tsp dried spearmint leaves
- 1 cup hot filtered water
- 1 tsp fresh lemon

DIRECTIONS

1. Add all herbs to a tea infuser or teapot.
2. Pour hot (not boiling) water over the herbs and steep for 10–15 minutes.
3. Strain and stir in honey or agave.
4. Enjoy hot or iced for an energy boost!

Radiant Sun Energy Tea

Purpose: Enhances mood and vitality, providing a natural energy boost.

INGREDIENTS

- 1 tsp dried hibiscus flowers
- 1 tsp dried nettle leaves
- ½ tsp dried orange peel
- ½ tsp dried ginger root
- 1 cup hot filtered water
- 1 tsp raw honey or agave

DIRECTIONS

1. Combine ingredients in a saucepan with water.
2. Simmer gently for 15 minutes, then strain.
3. Drink 1 cup warm, up to twice daily, to support gut microbiome health.

Fatigue-Fighting Herbal Steam

Purpose: Clears brain fog, refreshes the senses, and awakens the mind.

INGREDIENTS

- 1 tbsp dried peppermint leaves
- 1 tbsp dried rosemary
- 1 tbsp dried eucalyptus leaves
- 4 cups boiling water

DIRECTIONS

1. Add herbs to a large bowl and pour boiling water over them.
2. Lean over the bowl, covering your head with a towel.
3. Inhale deeply for 5–10 minutes.
4. Allowing the steam to energize your body to boost alertness.

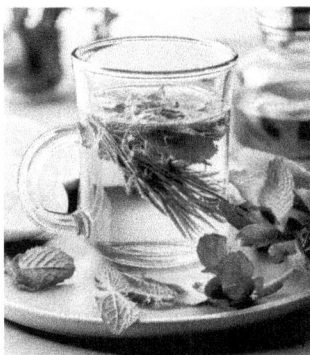

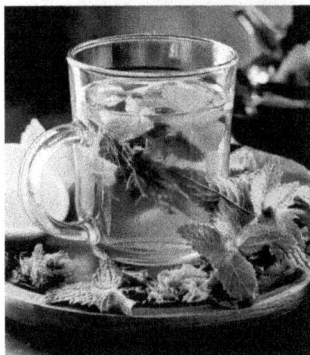

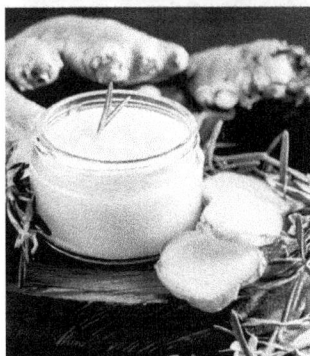

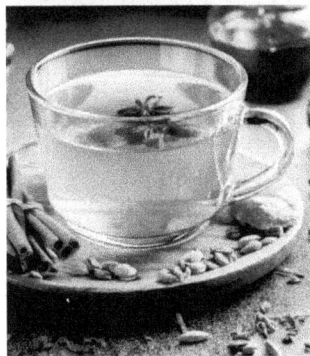

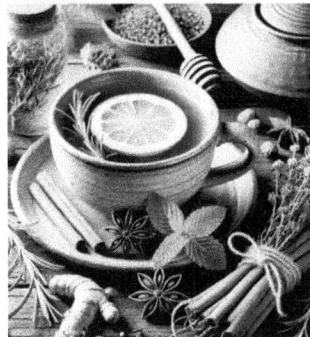

Revitalizing Green Energy Tea

Purpose: Enhances focus, mental clarity, and provides steady energy.

INGREDIENTS

- 1 tsp dried green tea leaves
- 1 tsp dried gotu kola
- ½ tsp dried peppermint leaves
- ½ tsp dried rosemary
- 1 cup hot filtered water
- 1 tsp fresh lemon juice

DIRECTIONS

1. Add all herbs to a tea infuser or teapot.
2. Pour hot (not boiling) water over the herbs; steep for 5–10 minutes.
3. Strain and stir in lemon juice.
4. Sip throughout the day.

Solar Vitality Infusion

Purpose: Invigorates the body, enhances endurance, sustains energy.

INGREDIENTS

- 1 tbsp dried nettle leaves
- 1 tbsp dried hibiscus flowers
- 1 tsp dried ginger root
- 1 tsp dried orange peel
- 1 quart filtered water

DIRECTIONS

1. Add herbs to a clear glass jar filled with room-temperature water.
2. Seal the jar and place in direct sunlight for 4–6 hours to infuse.
3. Strain and enjoy throughout the day for steady, natural energy.

Energizing Herbal Salve

Purpose: Boosts circulation, relieves fatigue, and refreshes the body.

INGREDIENTS

- 2 tbsp olive oil or coconut oil
- 1 tbsp beeswax
- 1 tbsp dried rosemary
- 1 tbsp dried ginger root
- 5 drops eucalyptus essential oil
- 5 drops black pepper essential oil

DIRECTIONS

1. Heat rosemary and ginger in olive or coconut oil for 30 minutes -low heat.
2. Strain out the herbs and return the oil to the double boiler.
3. Add beeswax and stir until melted.
4. Remove from heat and stir in oils.
5. Pour into a small glass jar or tin and allow to cool until firm.
6. Rub onto tired muscles or feet.

Spiced Honey Vitality Chai Tea

Purpose: Warms the body, supports metabolism, and provides energy.

INGREDIENTS

- 1 tsp dried cinnamon chips
- 1 tsp dried ginger root
- ½ tsp dried cardamom pods
- ½ tsp dried cloves
- 1 cup hot water or oat milk
- 1 tsp raw honey or coconut sugar

DIRECTIONS

1. Add all herbs to a small pan with water and simmer for 10 minutes.
2. Strain and pour into a cup.
3. Stir in honey or coconut sugar.
4. Enjoy warm.

Herbal Energy Booster Tea

Purpose: Enhances energy, improves focus, and combats fatigue.

INGREDIENTS

- 1 teaspoon ginseng root
- 1 teaspoon rosemary
- 1 teaspoon peppermint
- 1 teaspoon green tea
- ½ teaspoon cinnamon
- Honey and lemon

DIRECTIONS

1. In a teapot or heat-proof mug, add all the herbs.
2. Pour 1 cup of hot water (about 190°F, just before boiling) over the herbs.
3. Cover and let steep for 5-7 minutes.
4. Strain and add honey and lemon.
5. Drink warm.

Bay Leaf Headache Relief Compress

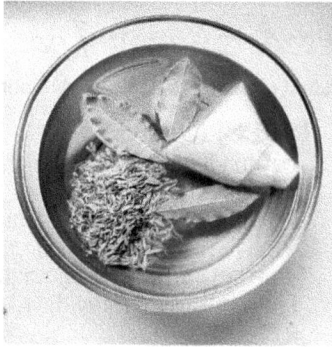

Purpose: Relieves tension headaches and soothes sinus-related discomfort.

INGREDIENTS

- 3-4 dried bay leaves
- 1 teaspoon fennel seeds
- 2 cups hot water
- A clean cloth or compress pad

DIRECTIONS

1. Place ingredients in a bowl and pour hot water over them.
2. Cover and steep for 10 minutes.
3. Soak the cloth in the herbal infusion, wring out excess liquid.
4. Apply to the forehead for 15-20 minutes.

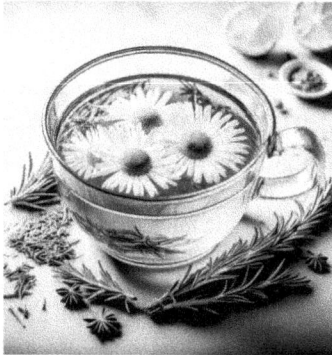

Chamomile & Rosemary Relaxing Tea

Purpose: Reduces stress and tension.

INGREDIENTS

- 1 tsp dried chamomile flowers
- 1 tsp dried rosemary
- 1 cup boiling water

DIRECTIONS

1. Steep chamomile and rosemary in boiling water for 10 minutes.
2. Strain and drink warm.

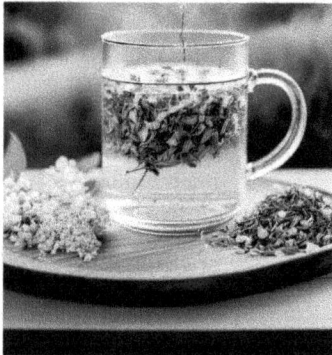

Wood Betony & Meadowsweet Soothing Tea

Purpose: Reduces stress and alleviates headache discomfort naturally.

INGREDIENTS

- 1 teaspoon dried wood betony leaves
- 1 teaspoon dried meadowsweet leaves
- 1 cup hot water
- 1 teaspoon raw honey

DIRECTIONS

1. Combine wood betony and meadowsweet in a teapot or mug.
2. Pour hot water over the herbs and steep for 8-10 minutes.
3. Strain, sweeten with honey if desired, and sip slowly.

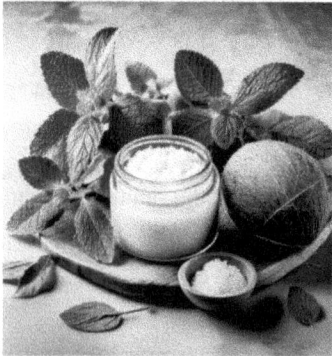

Eucalyptus & Mint Chest Rub

Purpose: Opens airways and relieves headache pressure.

INGREDIENTS

- 2 tbsp coconut oil
- 5 drops eucalyptus oil
- 3 drops peppermint essential oil

DIRECTIONS

1. Mix coconut oil with essential oils.
2. Massage onto the chest and temples for relief.

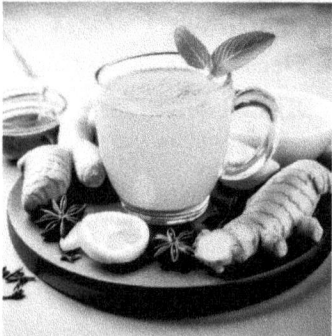

Turmeric & Ginger Anti-Inflammatory Tea

Purpose: Combats inflammation that contributes to headaches.

INGREDIENTS

- ½ tsp turmeric powder
- ½ tsp grated ginger
- 1 cup boiling water
- 1 tsp honey

DIRECTIONS

1. Steep turmeric and ginger in boiling water for 10 minutes.
2. Add honey and drink warm.

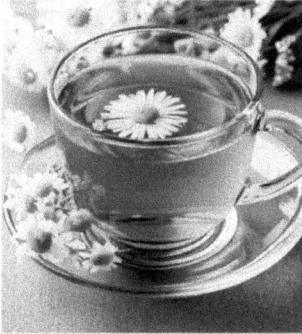

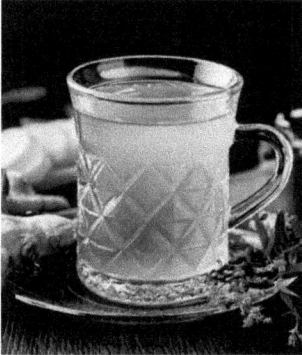

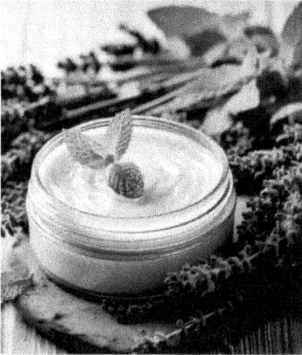

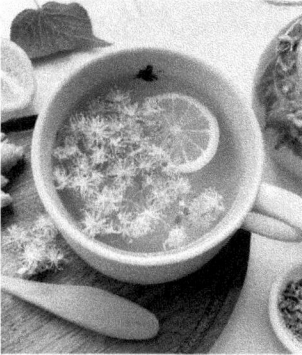

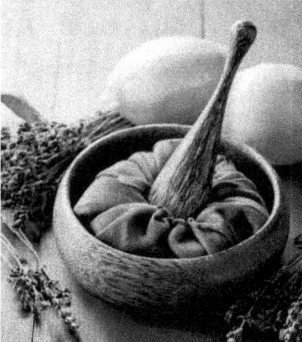

Feverfew & Chamomile Herbal Infusion

Purpose: Prevents and eases migraines by reducing inflammation.

INGREDIENTS

- 1 tsp dried feverfew leaves
- 1 tsp dried chamomile flowers
- 1 cup hot water
- ½ tsp lemon juice

DIRECTIONS

1. Place feverfew and chamomile in a mug or teapot.
2. Pour hot water over the herbs and let steep for 10 minutes.
3. Strain, add lemon juice if desired, and drink slowly.

Ginger & Willow Bark Pain-Relief Tea

Purpose: Alleviates migraines and inflammatory headaches by reducing pain.

INGREDIENTS

- 1 tsp dried willow bark
- 1 tsp fresh or dried ginger root
- 2 cups hot water
- 1 tsp honey

DIRECTIONS

1. Add ingredients to a teapot.
2. Pour hot water over the herbs and steep for 10–15 minutes.
3. Strain, add honey, and drink warm

Peppermint & Lavender Cooling Balm

Purpose: Relieves tension headaches by relaxing muscles and promoting circulation.

INGREDIENTS

- 2 tbsp coconut oil (or shea butter)
- 5 drops peppermint essential oil
- 5 drops lavender essential oil

DIRECTIONS

1. Melt the coconut oil in a bowl.
2. Add peppermint and lavender essential oils, then mix well.
3. Pour into a small container and allow it to solidify.
4. Apply a small amount to the temples, forehead, or neck.

Linden & Angelica Calming Infusion

Purpose: Reduces stress and headaches.

INGREDIENTS

- 1 teaspoon dried linden flowers
- 1/2 teaspoon dried angelica root
- 1 slice of fresh lemon
- 1 cup hot water

DIRECTIONS

1. Add linden flowers and angelica root to a teapot.
2. Pour hot water over the herbs and steep for 10–12 minutes.
3. Strain, add a slice of lemon for flavor, and enjoy warm.

Lavender & Lemon Cold Compress

Purpose: Relieves throbbing headaches and promotes relaxation.

INGREDIENTS

- 5 drops lavender oil
- Juice of ½ lemon
- A bowl of cold water
- A clean cloth or towel

DIRECTIONS

1. Mix water with 5 drops of lavender oil and of ½ lemon juice.
2. Soak a clean cloth, wring out excess water, and apply to the forehead, temples, or neck.
3. Relax for 10–15 minutes and reapply as needed.

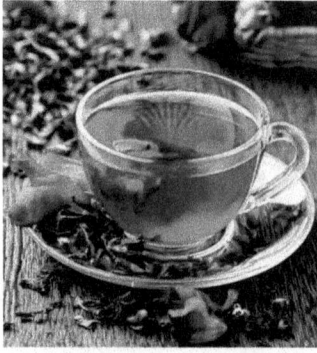

Rose Hormone Support Tea

Purpose: Balances hormones and soothes menstrual symptoms.

INGREDIENTS

- 1 tsp dried hibiscus flowers
- 1 tsp dried rose petals
- 1 cup boiling water

DIRECTIONS

1. Steep hibiscus flowers and rose petals in boiling water for 10 minutes.
2. Strain and enjoy warm or chilled.

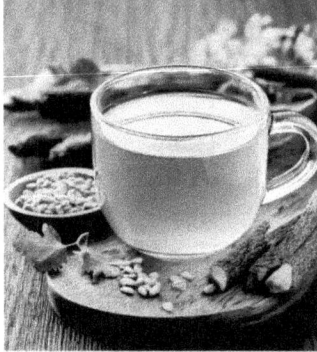

Fenugreek Hormone Decoction

Purpose: Promotes hormonal regulation and boosts reproductive health.

INGREDIENTS

- 1 teaspoon fenugreek seeds
- 1 teaspoon dried licorice root
- 2 cups water

DIRECTIONS

1. Simmer fenugreek seeds and licorice root in water for 15 minutes.
2. Strain and drink warm.

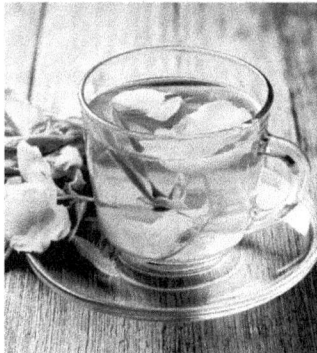

Evening Primrose & Sage Hormone Infusion

Purpose: Reduces symptoms of hormonal imbalances like hot flashes and mood swings.

INGREDIENTS

- 1 teaspoon dried evening primrose leaves
- 1 teaspoon dried sage leaves
- 1 cup boiling water

DIRECTIONS

1. Combine evening primrose and sage in a teapot or mug.
2. Pour boiling water over the herbs and steep for 10 minutes.

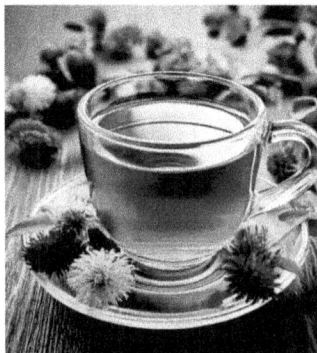

Black Cohosh Hormonal Balance Tea

Purpose: Eases menopausal symptoms and supports reproductive health.

INGREDIENTS

- 1 teaspoon dried black cohosh root
- 1 teaspoon dried red clover flowers
- 1 cup boiling water

DIRECTIONS

1. Combine black cohosh and red clover in a mug.
2. Pour boiling water over the herbs and steep for 10 minutes.
3. Strain and sip warm.

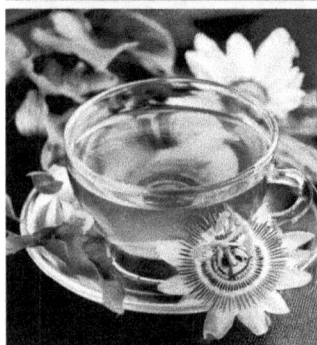

Motherwort Hormonal Balance Tea

Purpose: Supports menstrual regulation and reduces PMS.

INGREDIENTS

- 1 teaspoon dried motherwort leaves
- 1 teaspoon dried passionflower leaves
- 1 cup boiling water

DIRECTIONS

1. Combine motherwort and passionflower in a mug.
2. Pour boiling water over the herbs and steep for 10 minutes.
3. Strain and drink warm.

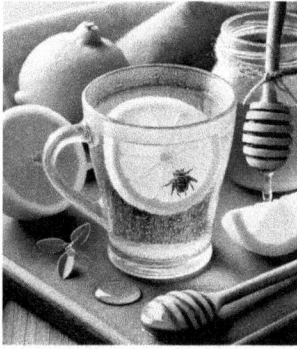

Local Honey & Lemon Tonic

Purpose: Fights colds and strengthens the body's natural defenses.

INGREDIENTS

- 1 tsp local raw honey
- Juice of ½ lemon
- 1 cup warm water

DIRECTIONS

1. Heat 1 cup of water until warm.
2. Stir in 1 tsp local raw honey.
3. Add the juice of ½ lemon and mix.
4. Drink warm for a refreshing boost.

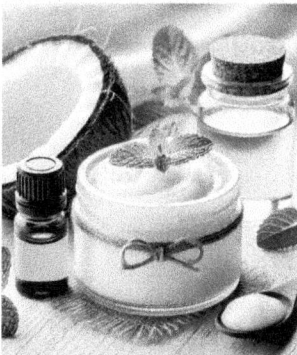

Peppermint & Eucalyptus Vapor Rub

Purpose: Supports the body's defense against colds, flu, and respiratory infections.

INGREDIENTS

- 2 tbsp coconut oil
- 5 drops peppermint essential oil
- 5 drops eucalyptus essential oil

DIRECTIONS

1. Melt 2 tbsp coconut oil until soft.
2. Add 5 drops peppermint oil and 5 drops eucalyptus essential oil.
3. Stir well. Store in a small jar and apply to the chest as needed.

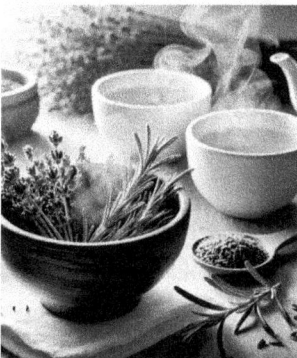

Rosemary & Lavender Sinus Steam

Purpose: Reduces nasal inflammation and boosts immunity.

INGREDIENTS

- 1 tbsp dried rosemary
- 1 tbsp dried lavender
- 4 cups boiling water

DIRECTIONS

1. Add 1 tbsp dried rosemary and 1 tbsp dried lavender to a bowl.
2. Pour 4 cups of boiling water over the herbs.
3. Lean over the bowl, cover your head with a towel, and inhale the steam for 5–10 minutes.
4. Enjoy the clearing benefits.

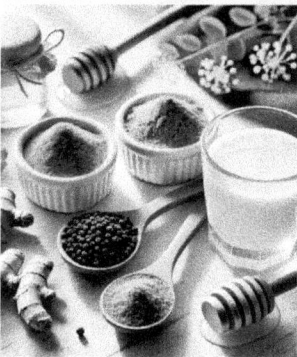

Turmeric Anti-Allergy Shot

Purpose: Reduces inflammation and boosts immunity.

INGREDIENTS

- ½ tsp turmeric powder
- Pinch of black pepper
- 1 cup warm water
- 1 tsp honey

DIRECTIONS

1. Heat 1 cup of water until warm.
2. Stir in ½ tsp turmeric powder.
3. Add a pinch of black pepper.
4. Mix in 1 tsp honey for sweetness.
5. Stir well and drink warm.

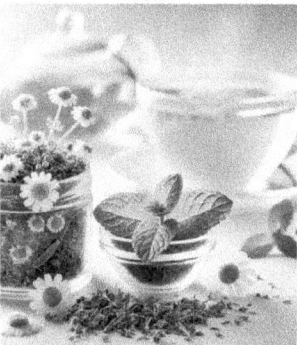

Chamomile & Mint Eye Rinse

Purpose: Soothes eyes and supports immune defense against eye infections.

INGREDIENTS

- 1 tsp dried chamomile
- 1 tsp dried mint
- 1 cup boiling water

DIRECTIONS

1. Steep chamomile and mint in boiling water for 10 minutes.
2. Strain, let cool, and use as an eye rinse with a clean cloth or dropper.

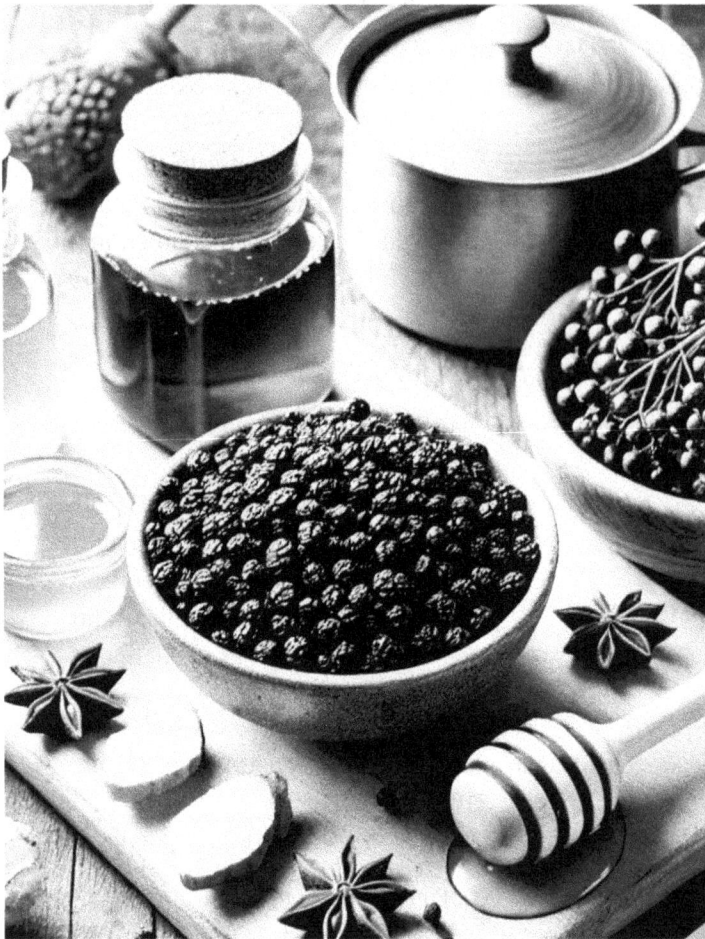

Elderberry Immunity Syrup

Purpose: Promotes restful sleep and calms anxiety.

INGREDIENTS

- 1 cup dried elderberries
- 4 cups water
- 1 cinnamon stick
- 3-4 whole cloves
- 1 tablespoon fresh grated ginger (or 1 teaspoon dried ginger)
- 1/2 cup raw honey

DIRECTIONS

1. Combine elderberries, water, cinnamon, cloves, and ginger in a medium saucepan. Bring the mixture to a boil, then reduce the heat to a simmer. Cook for 30-45 minutes, stirring occasionally, until the liquid reduces by half.
2. Remove from heat and allow to cool slightly. Strain the liquid through a fine mesh strainer or cheesecloth, pressing the berries to extract all the juice. Discard the solids.
3. Stir in the raw honey while the liquid is warm (not hot) to preserve its beneficial properties. Mix thoroughly.
4. Transfer the syrup into a sterilized glass jar or bottle. Seal tightly and refrigerate. The syrup will remain fresh for up to 3 months.
5. Take 1 teaspoon daily for immune support or 1 tablespoon every few hours when feeling unwell.

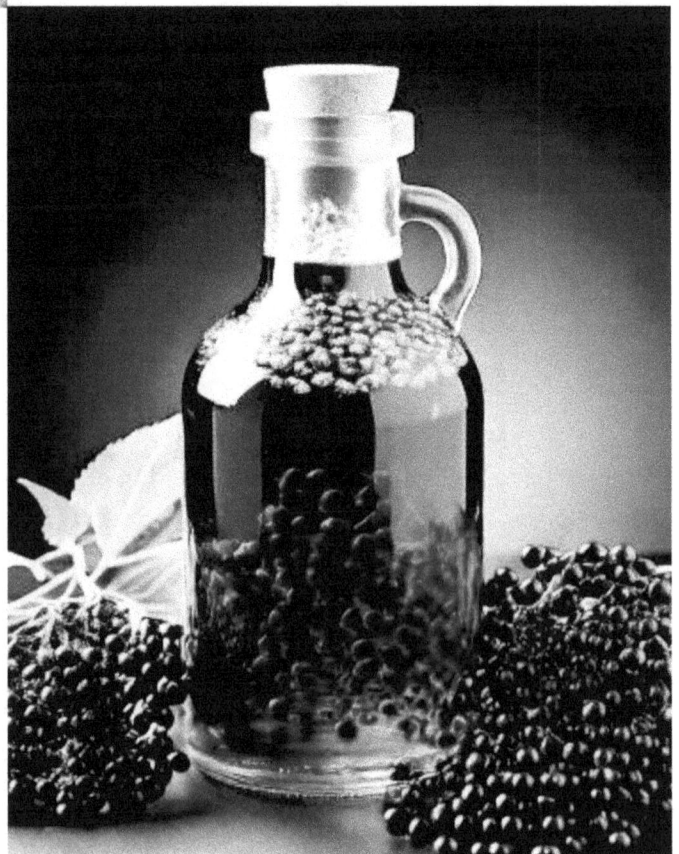

IMMUNE SUPPORT

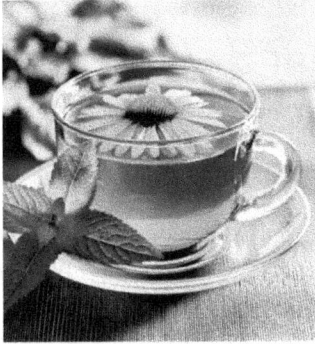

Echinacea and Peppermint Tea

Purpose: Stimulates the immune system and provides antiviral support.

INGREDIENTS
- 1 tbsp dried echinacea leaves or root
- 1 tsp dried peppermint leaves
- 1 cup boiling water

DIRECTIONS
1. Steep echinacea and peppermint in boiling water for 10 minutes.
2. Strain and enjoy warm.

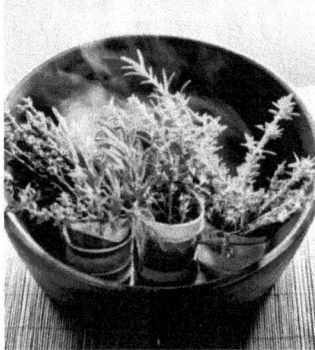

Immune-Boosting Herbal Steam

Purpose: Clears sinuses and supports respiratory health.

INGREDIENTS
- 1 tbsp dried rosemary
- 1 tbsp dried thyme
- 1 tbsp dried oregano
- Bowl of boiling water

DIRECTIONS
1. Add herbs to a bowl of boiling water.
2. Place a towel over your head and lean over the bowl.
3. Inhale the steam for 5-10 minutes.

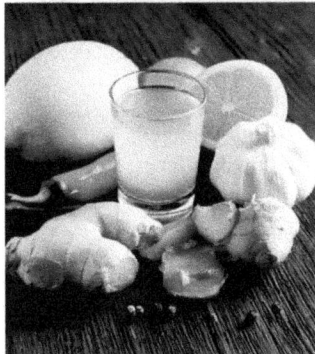

Ginger-Garlic Immune Shot

Purpose: Strengthens the immune system.

INGREDIENTS
- 1-inch piece of fresh ginger (grated)
- 1 clove garlic (minced)
- Juice of 1 lemon
- 1/4 tsp cayenne pepper
- 1/4 cup warm water

DIRECTIONS
1. Mix all ingredients in a small glass.
2. Strain and drink immediately.
3. Drink once daily when you feel the onset of a cold.

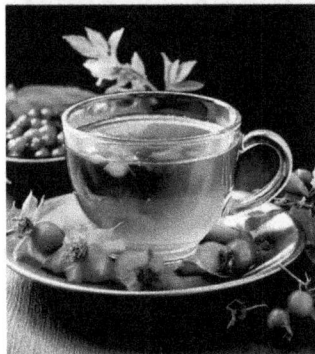

Rosehip and Hibiscus Vitamin C Tea

Purpose: Supports immune health and fights free radicals.

INGREDIENTS
- 1 tbsp dried rosehips
- 1 tsp dried hibiscus petals
- 1 cup boiling water

DIRECTIONS
1. Add rosehips and hibiscus to a teapot or mug.
2. Pour boiling water over the herbs and steep for 10 minutes.
3. Strain and drink warm or chilled.

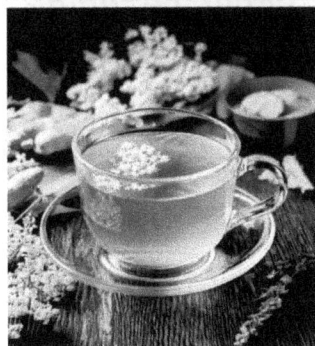

Elderflower Immune-Boosting Tea

Purpose: Supports respiratory health and helps ward off colds and flu.

INGREDIENTS
- 1 teaspoon dried astragalus root
- 1 teaspoon dried elderflower
- 1 slice fresh ginger
- 2 cups water

DIRECTIONS
1. Combine astragalus and elderflower in a pot with water.
2. Bring to a boil, then reduce heat and simmer for 10 minutes.
3. Strain into a cup and sip warm.

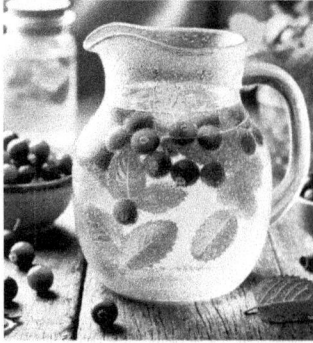

Cranberry & Mint Infused Water

Purpose: Prevents bacterial adhesion and promotes urinary tract health.

INGREDIENTS

- 1 cup fresh cranberries (slightly crushed)
- 5 fresh mint leaves
- 1 liter water

DIRECTIONS

1. Combine cranberries and mint leaves in a pitcher of water.
2. Let infuse for 2-3 hours in the refrigerator and drink.

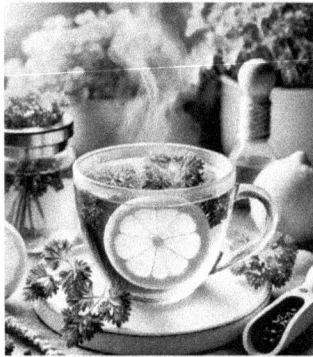

Parsley & Lemon Diuretic Drink

Purpose: Flushes bacteria and toxins from the urinary tract.

INGREDIENTS

- 1 handful fresh parsley leaves
- 1 slice of lemon
- 1 cup boiling water

DIRECTIONS

1. Add parsley and lemon to a cup.
2. Pour boiling water over the ingredients and cover.
3. Steep for 10 minutes and strain.
4. Drink warm 1-2 times daily.

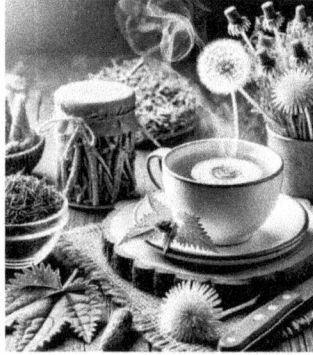

Dandelion & Nettle Detox Tea

Purpose: Promotes kidney function and supports urinary tract detoxification.

INGREDIENTS

- 1 teaspoon dried dandelion root
- 1 teaspoon dried nettle leaves
- 2 cups water

DIRECTIONS

1. Add dandelion root and nettle leaves to a pot of water.
2. Bring to a boil, then reduce heat and simmer for 10 minutes.
3. Strain and drink warm, ideally in the morning for detox benefits.

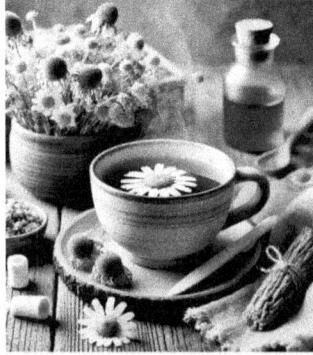

Chamomile & Marshmallow Root Tea

Purpose: Reduces inflammation and soothes urinary tract discomfort.

INGREDIENTS

- 1 tablespoon dried chamomile flowers
- 1 tablespoon dried marshmallow root
- 2 cups boiling water

DIRECTIONS

1. Add ingredients to a heatproof bowl.
2. Pour boiling water over the herbs and cover.
3. Let the mixture steep for 10-15 minutes, then strain.
4. Drink warm 2-3 times daily for soothing relief.

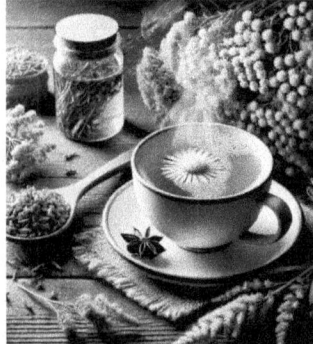

Goldenrod & Yarrow Infusion

Purpose: Reduces inflammation and prevents bacterial adhesion.

INGREDIENTS

- 1 tablespoon dried goldenrod flowers
- 1 tablespoon dried yarrow flowers
- 2 cups boiling water
- 1 teaspoon honey (for taste)

DIRECTIONS

1. Steep goldenrod and yarrow in boiling water for 10-15 minutes.
2. Strain and remove herbs.
3. Drink warm, optionally adding honey; enjoy 2-3 times daily.

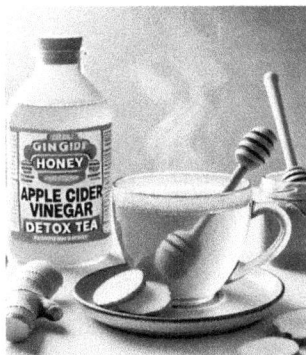

Apple Cider Vinegar Detox Tea

Purpose: Reduces mucus and clears sinus congestion.

INGREDIENTS

- 1 tsp grated ginger
- 1 tbsp apple cider vinegar
- 1 cup boiling water

DIRECTIONS

1. Steep ginger in boiling water for 5 minutes.
2. Add apple cider vinegar and drink warm.

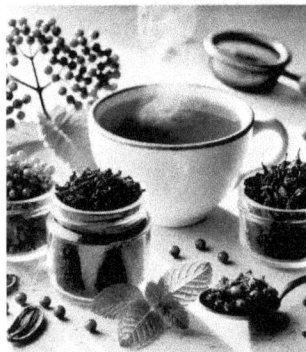

Elderberry Immune Support Tea

Purpose: supports immune function, digestion, and detoxification.

INGREDIENTS

- 1 tsp dried elderberries
- 1 tsp dried peppermint leaves
- 1 cup boiling water

DIRECTIONS

1. Steep elderberries and peppermint in boiling water for 10 minutes.
2. Strain and enjoy warm.

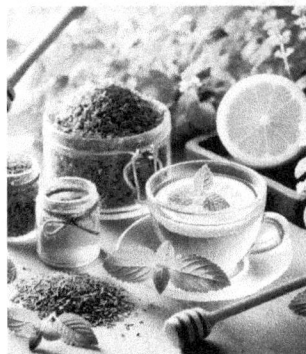

Tulsi & Lemon Anti-Allergy Detox Elixir

Purpose: Helps the body eliminate allergens, toxins, and inflammatory compounds.

INGREDIENTS

- 1 teaspoon dried tulsi (holy basil)
- 1 teaspoon dried lemon balm
- 1 teaspoon raw honey
- 1/4 teaspoon fresh lemon juice
- 1 cup hot water

DIRECTIONS

1. Steep tulsi and lemon balm in hot water for 8-10 minutes.
2. Strain and stir in raw honey and lemon juice.
3. Sip slowly for allergy relief and a calming effect on the body.

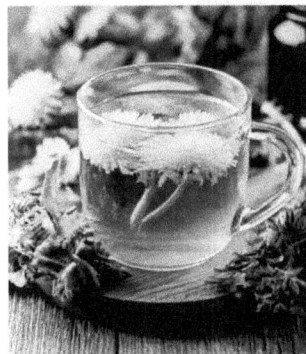

Dandelion & Burdock Liver Detox Tea

Purpose: Supports liver function, aids digestion, and flushes toxins.

INGREDIENTS

- 1 tsp dried dandelion root
- 1 tsp dried burdock root
- ½ tsp fresh grated ginger
- 2 cups water
- 1 tsp raw honey

DIRECTIONS

1. Add dandelion and burdock root to boiling water.
2. Simmer for 10–15 minutes.
3. Add ginger and steep for 5 more minutes.
4. Strain, add honey and drink warm.

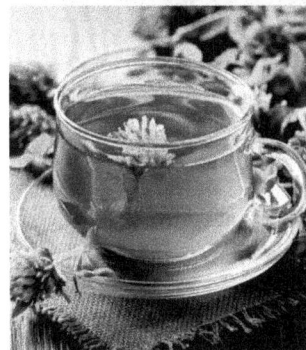

Cleavers & Red Clover Detox Tea

Purpose: Reduces lymphatic congestion, inflammation, and flushes toxins.

INGREDIENTS

- 1 tsp dried cleavers
- 1 tsp dried red clover
- ½ tsp fresh grated ginger
- 1 cup hot water

DIRECTIONS

1. Add cleavers and red clover to a teapot or mug.
2. Pour hot water over the herbs and steep for 10–15 minutes.
3. Strain and add ginger.
4. Drink warm for toxin removal.

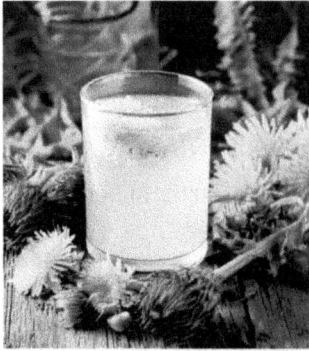

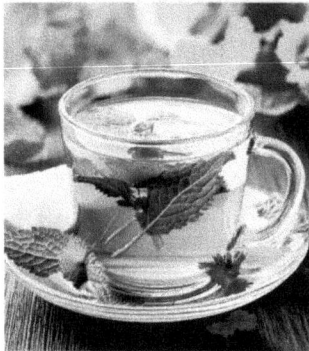

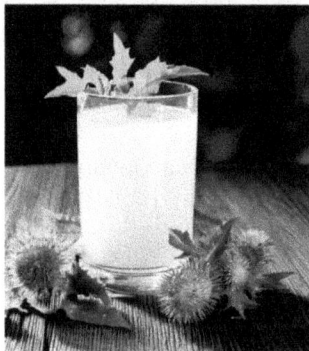

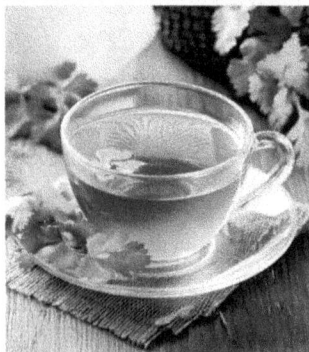

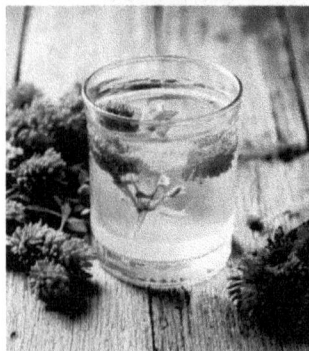

Dandelion & Burdock Detox Tonic

Purpose: Supports liver function, cleanses the blood, and promotes detox.

INGREDIENTS

- 1 tsp dried dandelion root
- 1 tsp dried burdock root
- 1 cup boiling water
- 1 tsp honey

DIRECTIONS

1. Steep dandelion root and burdock root in boiling water for 10–12 minutes.
2. Strain and add honey.
3. Drink warm and enjoy.

Nettle & Lemon Balm Detox Tea

Purpose: Supports detoxification, reduces stress, and promotes overall wellness.

INGREDIENTS

- 1 tsp dried nettle
- 1 tsp dried lemon balm
- 1 cup boiling water
- 1 tsp honey

DIRECTIONS

1. Steep nettle and lemon balm in boiling water for 10–12 minutes.
2. Strain and add honey.
3. Drink warm and enjoy.

Cleavers & Milk Thistle Detox Infusion

Purpose: Cleanses the lymphatic system, supports liver detoxification.

INGREDIENTS

- 1 tsp dried Cleavers
- 1 tsp dried Milk Thistle
- 1 cup boiling water
- 1 tsp honey

DIRECTIONS

1. Steep cleavers and milk thistle in boiling water for 10–12 minutes.
2. Strain and add honey.
3. Drink warm,

Parsley & Cilantro Detox Tea

Purpose: Helps remove toxins, supports kidney function, and aids in digestion.

INGREDIENTS

- 1 tsp dried parsley
- 1 tsp dried cilantro leaves
- 1 cup boiling water
- 1 tsp honey

DIRECTIONS

1. Steep parsley and cilantro leaves in boiling water for 10 minutes.
2. Strain and add honey.
3. Drink Warm.

Red Clover & Yellow Dock Detox Elixir

Purpose: Detoxifies the lymphatic system and cleanses the blood.

INGREDIENTS

- 1 tsp dried red clover
- 1 tsp dried yellow dock root
- 1 cup boiling water
- 1 tsp lemon juice

DIRECTIONS

1. Steep red clover and yellow dock root in boiling water for 10–15 minutes.
2. Strain and add lemon juice.
3. Drink warm.

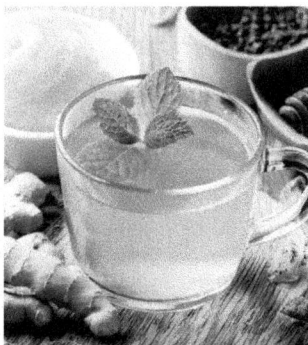

Revitalizing Tea for Men's Health

Purpose: Boosts energy, supports testosterone levels, and enhances overall vitality.

INGREDIENTS
- 1 tbsp dried ashwagandha root
- 1 tbsp dried ginseng root
- 1 tsp dried nettle leaf
- 1 tsp dried peppermint
- 2 cups hot water
- 1 tsp honey and lemon

DIRECTIONS
1. Place ingredients in a teapot.
2. Pour hot water over the herbs and let steep for 10-15 minutes.
3. Strain; add honey and lemon.
4. Drink 1-2 cups daily.

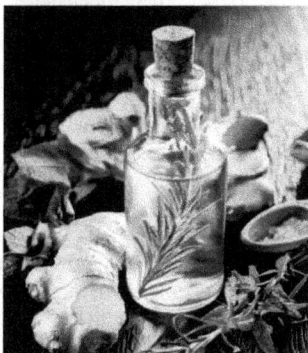

Invigorating Ginger Hair Growth Oil

Purpose: Stimulates hair follicles, strengthens roots, and promotes scalp health.

INGREDIENTS
- ½ cup jojoba oil or coconut oil
- 2 tbsp dried rosemary leaves
- 1 tbsp grated fresh ginger
- 10 drops peppermint essential oil

DIRECTIONS
1. Add rosemary and ginger to a glass jar.
2. Pour oil over the herbs and stir well.
3. Let the mixture infuse in a warm, sunny spot for 2 weeks, shaking occasionally.
4. Strain the herbs and add peppermint oil.
5. Massage into the scalp 2–3 times per week.

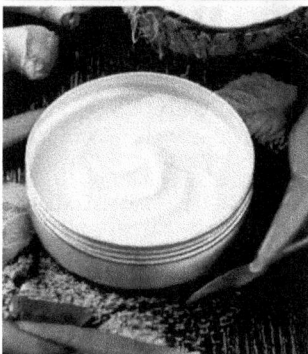

Circulation-Enhancing Muscle Rub Balm

Purpose: Improves blood flow, relieves sore muscles, and reduces stiffness.

INGREDIENTS
- ½ cup coconut oil
- 1 tbsp cayenne pepper powder
- 1 tbsp ginger powder
- 10 drops peppermint essential oil
- 10 drops eucalyptus essential oil

DIRECTIONS
1. Gently heat coconut oil and stir in cayenne and ginger powder.
2. Remove from heat and let sit for 15 minutes to infuse.
3. Strain out solids and stir in oils.
4. Store in a small jar and massage onto sore muscles and joints.

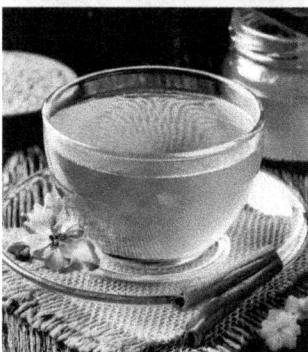

Testosterone-Boosting Fenugreek Tonic

Purpose: Supports testosterone levels, boosts stamina, and enhances metabolism.

INGREDIENTS
- 1 tbsp fenugreek seeds
- 1 cup hot water
- 1 tsp honey
- ½ tsp cinnamon powder

DIRECTIONS
1. Steep fenugreek seeds in hot water for 10–15 minutes.
2. Strain, then stir in honey and cinnamon.
3. Drink daily in the morning.

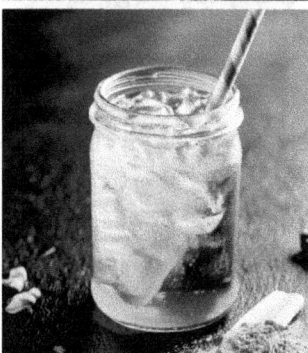

Energy-Boosting Ginseng Iced Tea

Purpose: Improves stamina, mental clarity, and supports endurance.

INGREDIENTS
- 1 tbsp dried ginseng root
- 1 tbsp dried green tea leaves
- 2 cups hot water
- Juice of ½ a lemon
- 1 tsp honey

DIRECTIONS
1. Steep ginseng and green tea in hot water for 10–15 minutes.
2. Strain, then stir in lemon juice and honey.
3. Chill in the refrigerator and serve over ice for a refreshing energy boost.

MEN'S HEALTH

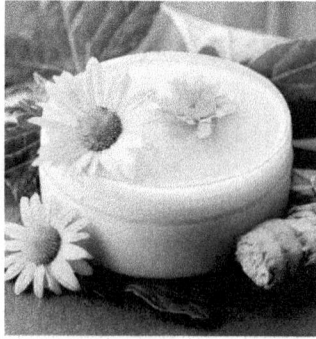

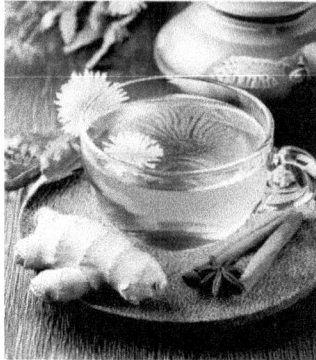

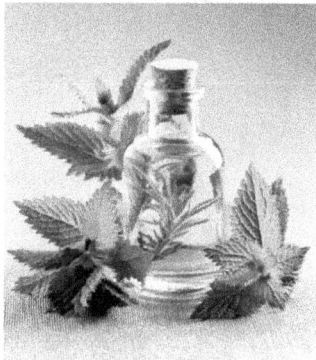

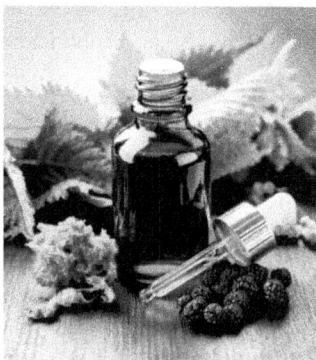

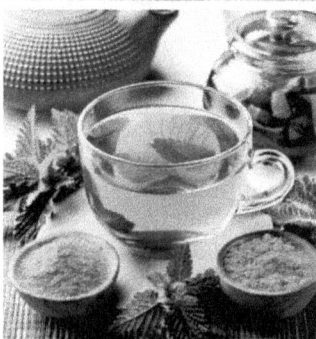

Muscle Recovery Herbal Salve

Purpose: Relieves sore muscles, inflammation, and promotes recovery.

INGREDIENTS

- ½ cup olive oil or coconut oil
- 2 tablespoons dried arnica flowers
- 2 tablespoons dried comfrey leaf
- 1 tablespoon dried ginger root
- 2 tablespoons beeswax

DIRECTIONS

1. Heat the oil in a double boiler and add the dried herbs.
2. Let the herbs infuse in the oil for 1 hour on low heat.
3. Strain the oil and return it to the double boiler, adding beeswax.
4. Stir until melted, pour into a small container. Allow to harden before use.

Metabolism-Boosting Herbal Tea

Purpose: Supports healthy metabolism, digestion, and weight management.

INGREDIENTS

- 1 teaspoon dried green tea leaves
- 1 teaspoon dried ginger root
- 1 teaspoon dried cinnamon
- 1 teaspoon dried dandelion root
- 2 cups boiling water

DIRECTIONS

1. Combine all dried herbs in a teapot or heat-proof container.
2. Pour boiling water over the herbs, cover, and steep for 10-15 minutes.
3. Strain and drink 1-2 cups daily to support digestion and metabolism.
4. Store extra in the fridge.

Hair & Beard Growth Herbal Oil

Purpose: Stimulates hair and beard growth while nourishing the scalp and skin.

INGREDIENTS

- ½ cup jojoba oil or coconut oil
- 2 tablespoons dried rosemary
- 2 tablespoons dried nettles
- 1 tablespoon dried peppermint
- 10 drops cedarwood essential oil

DIRECTIONS

1. Add dried herbs to a glass jar and cover with carrier oil.
2. Seal and let infuse in a warm, sunny spot for 4-6 weeks, shaking occasionally.
3. Strain the herbs and store the infused oil in a glass bottle.
4. Massage into the scalp or beard 2-3 times per week to promote growth.

Prostate Function Tincture

Purpose: Supports healthy prostate function and reduces frequent urination.

INGREDIENTS

- 1 tablespoon dried saw palmetto berries
- 1 tablespoon dried nettles root
- 1 tablespoon dried willow bark
- 1 cup vodka or brandy

DIRECTIONS

1. Place all dried herbs in a glass jar and cover with alcohol.
2. Seal and store in a cool, dark place for 4-6 weeks, shaking occasionally.
3. Strain the liquid and transfer to a dropper bottle.
4. Take 1-2 dropperfuls daily.

Anti-Inflammatory Prostate Tea

Purpose: Helps reduce prostate swelling and improves urinary function.

INGREDIENTS

- 1 teaspoon dried nettles root
- 1 teaspoon dried turmeric root
- 1 teaspoon dried ginger root
- 1 teaspoon dried green tea leaves
- 2 cups boiling water

DIRECTIONS

1. Combine all dried herbs in a teapot or heat-proof container.
2. Pour boiling water over the herbs, and steep for 15 minutes.
3. Strain and drink 1-2 cups daily to support prostate health.

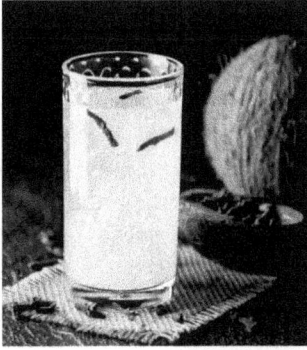

Clove & Coconut Oil Fresh Breath Rinse

Purpose: Removes bacteria, freshens breath, and supports gum health.

INGREDIENTS

- 1 tbsp coconut oil
- 2 drops clove essential oil
- 2 drops peppermint essential oil

DIRECTIONS

1. Place the coconut, clove, and peppermint oils in your mouth.
2. Swish for 10–15 minutes, making sure not to swallow.
3. Spit into a trash can (not the sink, to avoid clogging pipes) and rinse with warm water.

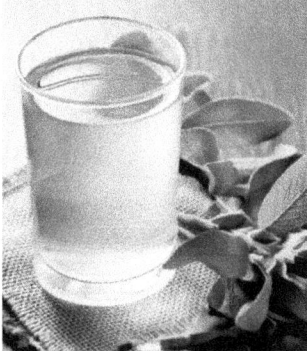

Sage Gum-Healing Mouth Rinse

Purpose: Soothes inflamed gums, reduces bacteria, and strengthens oral tissues.

INGREDIENTS

- 1 tbsp dried sage leaves
- 1 tsp sea salt
- 1 cup hot green tea
- ½ tsp apple cider vinegar

DIRECTIONS

1. Steep sage leaves in hot green tea for 15 minutes.
2. Strain and dissolve sea salt and apple cider vinegar to the infusion.
3. Let cool, then swish around the mouth for 30 seconds before spitting.
4. Use twice daily for gum health.

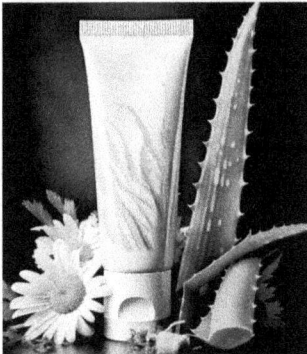

Aloe Vera Gum-Soothing Paste

Purpose: Heals sore gums, reduces irritation, and promotes oral healing.

INGREDIENTS

- 1 tbsp myrrh powder
- 1 tbsp dried chamomile flowers
- 1 tsp honey
- ½ tsp coconut oil
- ½ tsp aloe vera gel

DIRECTIONS

1. Grind chamomile flowers into a fine powder.
2. Mix with myrrh powder, honey, coconut oil, and aloe vera to form a paste.
3. Apply directly to sore gums; let sit for 5 minutes before rinsing.

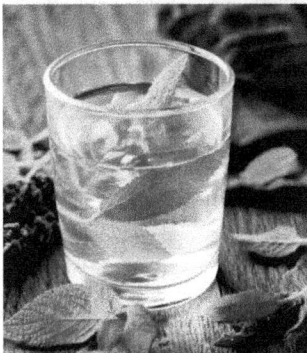

Sage Gum-Healing Mouth Rinse

Purpose: Soothes irritated gums, neutralizes bacteria, and freshens breath.

INGREDIENTS

- 1 tbsp dried sage leaves
- 1 tsp sea salt
- 1 cup hot water
- ½ tsp dried peppermint leaves

DIRECTIONS

1. Steep sage and peppermint in hot water for 15 minutes.
2. Strain and stir in sea salt.
3. Let cool, then swish in the mouth for 30 seconds before spitting. Use twice daily.

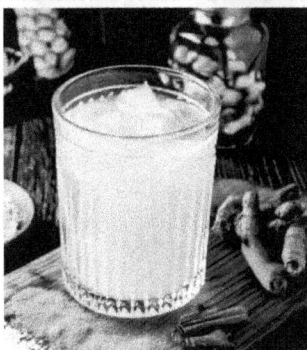

Turmeric & Sea Salt Mouth Rinse

Purpose: Freshens breath, reduces bacteria, and supports gum health.

INGREDIENTS

- 1 cup warm water
- 1 tsp sea salt
- ½ tsp ground cinnamon
- ½ tsp ground turmeric

DIRECTIONS

1. Heat the water and stir in all ingredients until dissolved.
2. Let the mixture cool before use.
3. Swish in the mouth for 30 seconds, then spit out.
4. Use twice daily for fresh breath.

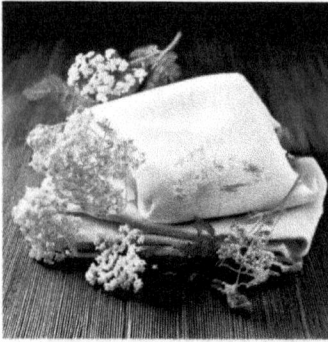

Meadowsweet Pain-Relief Compress

Purpose: Eases localized pain, reduces swelling, and promotes healing.

INGREDIENTS

- 1 tablespoon dried yarrow
- 1 tablespoon dried meadowsweet
- 2 cups boiling water
- A clean cloth or compress pad

DIRECTIONS

1. Steep yarrow and meadowsweet in boiling water for 15 minutes.
2. Strain and soak a clean cloth in the infusion.
3. Apply the cloth to the affected area for 20-30 minutes.

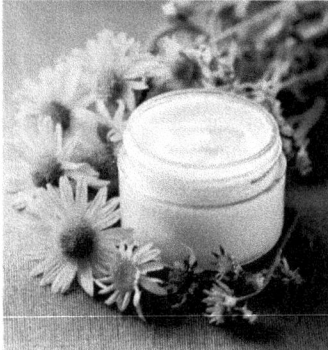

Arnica Pain-Soothing Salve

Purpose: Alleviates muscle soreness, joint pain, and minor bruising.

INGREDIENTS

- 1/4 cup dried arnica flowers
- 1/4 cup dried St. John's Wort flowers
- 1/2 cup olive oil
- 2 tablespoons beeswax pellets
- 5 drops lavender essential oil

DIRECTIONS

1. Infuse the olive oil with arnica and St. John's Wort for 1-2 hours on low heat.
2. Strain the infused oil into a double boiler, add the beeswax, and heat until melted.
3. Stir in lavender oil, pour into a small jar or tin. Cool before use.

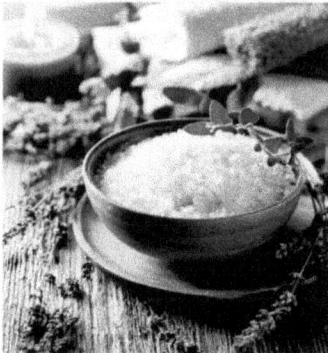

Eucalyptus and Lavender Bath Soak

Purpose: Relaxes sore muscles and reduces joint pain while promoting overall relaxation.

INGREDIENTS

- 1 cup Epsom salts
- 5 drops eucalyptus essential oil
- 5 drops lavender essential oil

DIRECTIONS

1. Mix the essential oils with the Epsom salts in a bowl.
2. Add the mixture to a warm bath, stirring to dissolve the salts.
3. Soak for 20 minutes to relieve pain and relax your body.

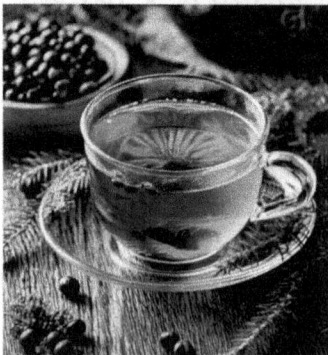

Juniper Berry & Willow Bark Pain Tea

Purpose: Alleviates headaches, joint pain, and muscle soreness.

INGREDIENTS

- 1 teaspoon dried juniper berries
- 1 teaspoon dried willow bark
- 1 cup boiling water
- 1 slice fresh lemon

DIRECTIONS

1. Add juniper berries and white willow bark to a teapot or mug.
2. Pour boiling water over the herbs and steep for 10 minutes.
3. Strain, add a slice of lemon if desired, and drink warm for relief.

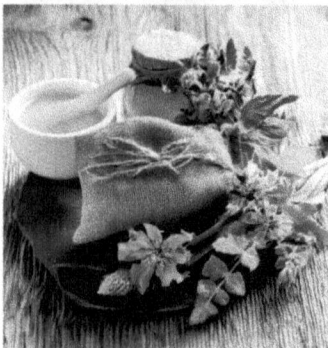

Borage & Plantain Poultice

Purpose: Alleviates pain in injured areas.

INGREDIENTS

- 1 tablespoon fresh or dried borage leaves
- 1 tablespoon fresh or dried plantain leaves
- Warm water to make a paste
- A clean cloth or gauze

DIRECTIONS

1. Crush the borage and plantain leaves (if fresh) or rehydrate with warm water if dried.
2. Mix to form a thick paste.
3. Spread the paste onto a clean cloth or gauze and apply to the affected area for 20-30 minutes.

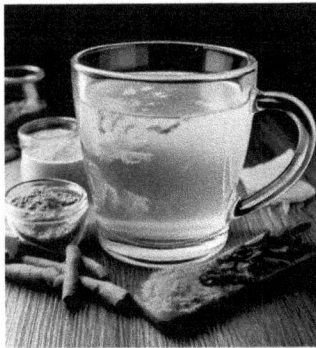

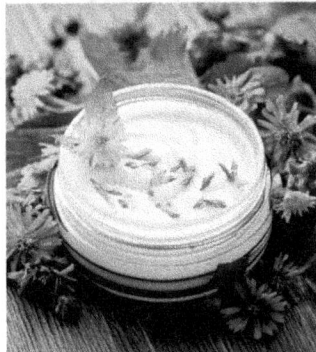

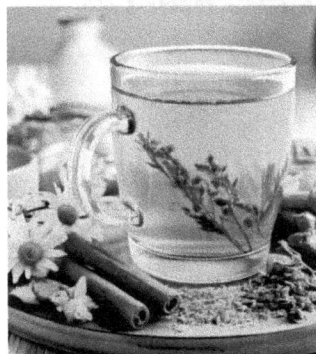

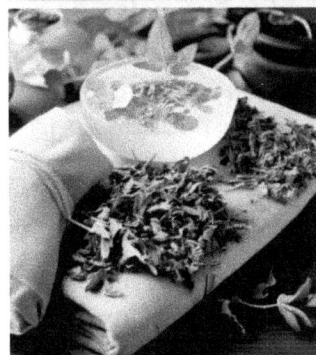

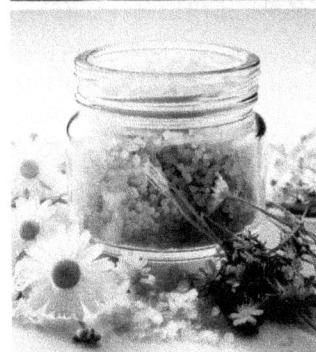

Soothing Herbal Pain-Relief Decoction

Purpose: Relieves joint pain, muscle aches, and inflammation.

INGREDIENTS

- 1 tbsp dried turmeric root
- 1 tsp dried ginger root
- 1 tsp dried willow bark
- ½ tsp cinnamon chips
- 3 cups filtered water
- 1 tsp raw honey

DIRECTIONS

1. Add all herbs to a small saucepan with water.
2. Bring to a gentle simmer, and steep for 20 minutes.
3. Strain and drink 1 cup as needed for pain relief.

Herbal Pain-Relief Salve

Purpose: Eases sore muscles, joint pain, and tension headaches.

INGREDIENTS

- 2 tbsp coconut oil
- 1 tbsp beeswax
- 1 tbsp dried arnica flowers
- 1 tbsp dried comfrey leaves
- 5 drops peppermint essential oil
- 5 drops eucalyptus essential oil

DIRECTIONS

1. Melt coconut oil and beeswax in a double boiler.
2. Stir in arnica and comfrey and let infuse for 15 minutes.
3. Strain herbs and stir in oils.
4. Pour into a small glass jar or tin and let cool until solid.
5. Apply to sore muscles and joints.

Soothing Herbal Pain-Relief Tea

Purpose: Eases inflammation, relaxes muscles, and relieves pain naturally.

INGREDIENTS

- 1 tsp dried white willow bark
- 1 tsp dried turmeric root
- ½ tsp dried ginger root
- ½ tsp dried chamomile flowers
- ½ tsp dried cinnamon chips
- 1 cup hot filtered water
- 1 tsp raw honey

DIRECTIONS

1. Add all herbs to a tea infuser or teapot.
2. Pour hot (not boiling) water over the herbs and let steep for 10–15 minutes.
3. Strain and stir in raw honey, if desired.
4. Sip slowly to relieve pain.

Eucalyptus Pain-Relief Compress

Purpose: Soothes headaches, relieves tension, and calms inflammation.

INGREDIENTS

- 1 tbsp dried peppermint leaves
- 1 tbsp dried eucalyptus leaves
- 1 tsp dried lavender flowers
- 2 cups hot or cold filtered water
- 1 clean cloth or towel

DIRECTIONS

1. Add herbs to a bowl of hot or cold water and let steep for 10 minutes.
2. Soak a clean cloth in the infusion, wring out excess liquid, and apply to the painful area.
3. Leave on for 15–20 minutes,

Herbal Pain-Relief Bath Soak

Purpose: Eases sore muscles, reduces inflammation, and soothes joint pain.

INGREDIENTS

- 1 cup Epsom salt
- ½ cup dried chamomile flowers
- ½ cup dried comfrey leaves
- ¼ cup dried yarrow
- 5 drops eucalyptus essential oil

DIRECTIONS

1. Mix all dried herbs and Epsom salt in a bowl.
2. Add 5 drops of eucalyptus oil and stir well.
3. Store in a glass jar.
4. Add ½ cup to a warm bath and soak for 20–30 minutes.

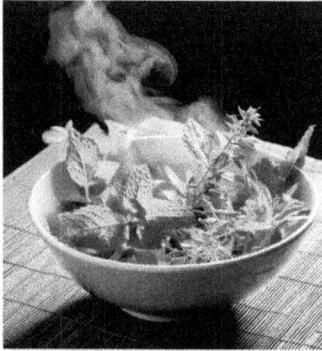

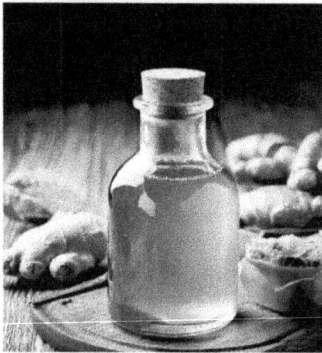

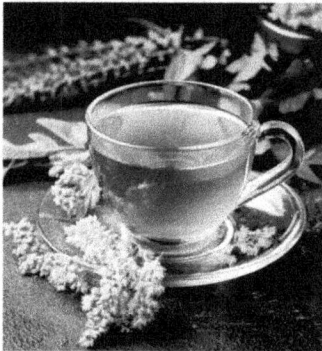

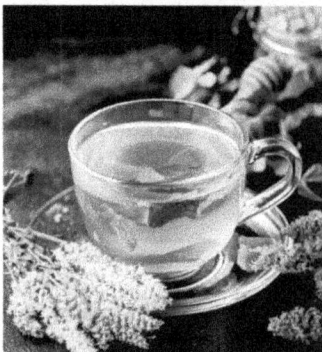

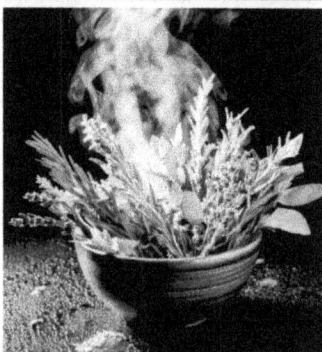

Steam Inhalation for Congestion Relief

Purpose: Clears nasal passages, soothes airways, and supports lung health.

INGREDIENTS

- 4 cups hot water
- 1 tbsp dried eucalyptus leaves (or 5 drops eucalyptus essential oil)
- 1 tbsp dried thyme leaves
- 1 tbsp dried peppermint leaves,

DIRECTIONS

1. Pour hot water into a large bowl.
2. Add eucalyptus, thyme, and peppermint.
3. Lean over the bowl, cover your head with a towel, and inhale the steam for 10 minutes.
4. Repeat as needed to clear congestion and open airways.

Soothing Ginger & Honey Cough Syrup

Purpose: Eases coughs, reduces throat irritation, and aids respiratory health.

INGREDIENTS

- 1 cup water
- 1 tbsp grated fresh ginger
- 1 tbsp raw honey
- ½ tsp cinnamon powder
- Juice of ½ a lemon

DIRECTIONS

1. Boil water and add grated ginger. Let simmer for 10 minutes.
2. Strain and stir in honey, cinnamon, and lemon juice.
3. Take 1 tbsp every few hours to soothe coughs and sore throats.

Lung-Cleansing Herbal Tea

Purpose: Supports lung function, reduces mucus, and eases breathing.

INGREDIENTS

- 1 tbsp dried mullein leaves
- 1 tsp dried licorice root
- 1 tsp dried marshmallow root
- 1 cup hot water

DIRECTIONS

1. Place herbs in a teapot or strainer.
2. Pour hot water over the herbs and steep for 10–15 minutes.
3. Strain and drink warm, 1–2 times daily for lung support and mucus relief.

Lung Support Infusion

Purpose: Clears mucus, soothes the throat, and supports lung function.

INGREDIENTS

- 1 tsp Mullein
- 1 tsp Thyme
- 1 tsp Peppermint
- 1 cup boiling water
- Honey for sweetness

DIRECTIONS

1. Place the herbs in a teacup or tea infuser.
2. Pour boiling water over the herbs.
3. Cover and steep for 10-15 minutes.
4. Strain and drink 2-3 times daily.

Decongestant Steam Inhalation

Purpose: Clears nasal congestion, soothes airways, and helps with breathing.

INGREDIENTS

- 2 tbsp Eucalyptus leaves
- 1 tbsp Rosemary
- 1 tbsp Lavender
- 4 cups boiling water

DIRECTIONS

1. Pour boiling water over the herbs in a heatproof bowl.
2. Lean over the bowl, cover the head with a towel, and inhale deeply for 5-10 minutes.
3. Repeat as needed for congestion relief.

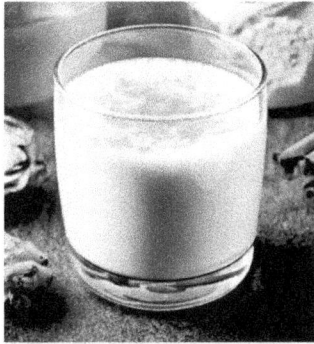

Libido-Boosting Maca Love Elixir

Purpose: Enhances libido, increases stamina, and supports overall sexual health.

INGREDIENTS

- 1 cup warm almond or oat milk
- 1 tsp maca root powder
- 1 tsp cacao powder
- ½ tsp cinnamon powder
- 1 tsp honey or maple syrup

DIRECTIONS

1. Warm the milk over low heat.
2. Stir in ingredients until blended.
3. Sweeten with honey or maple syrup if desired.
4. Drink 30 minutes before intimacy to boost desire.

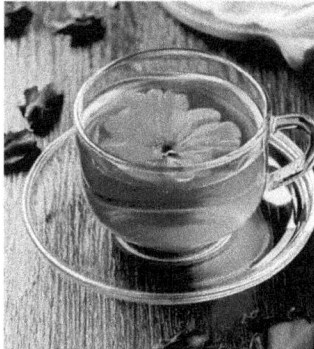

Sensual Rose & Damiana Love Tea

Purpose: Increases circulation, reduces stress, and enhances intimacy.

INGREDIENTS

- 1 tbsp dried damiana leaves
- 1 tbsp dried rose petals
- 1 tsp dried hibiscus flowers
- 2 cups hot water
- 1 tsp honey or lemon

DIRECTIONS

1. Add all herbs to a teapot or strainer.
2. Pour hot water over them and steep for 10-15 minutes.
3. Strain and sweeten with honey or lemon if desired.
4. Enjoy as a heart-opening tea.

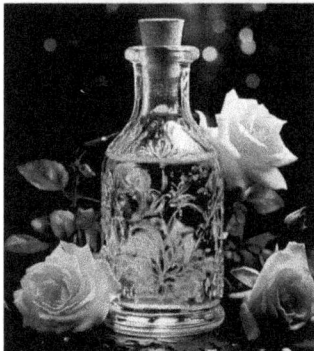

Passionate Rose Massage Oil

Purpose: Relaxes muscles and enhances sensual touch.

INGREDIENTS

- ½ cup sweet almond oil or coconut oil
- 10 drops ylang-ylang oil
- 5 drops rose essential oil
- 5 drops sandalwood essential oil

DIRECTIONS

1. Combine all ingredients in a small glass bottle.
2. Shake well before each use.
3. Warm a few drops in your hands and massage onto the skin to enhance intimacy.

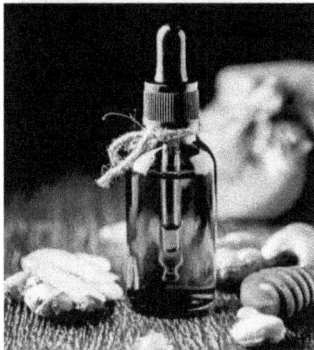

Honey & Ginseng Libido Tincture

Purpose: Boosts libido, enhances endurance, and improves sexual vitality.

INGREDIENTS

- ½ cup dried ginseng root
- ½ cup raw honey
- 1 cup brandy or 100-proof vodka
- 1 mason jar with lid

DIRECTIONS

1. Add ginseng root to a clean mason jar.
2. Pour honey and alcohol over the ginseng until submerged.
3. Seal and store in a cool, dark place for 4-6 weeks, shaking occasionally.
4. Strain into a dropper bottle and take 1-2 dropperfuls daily.

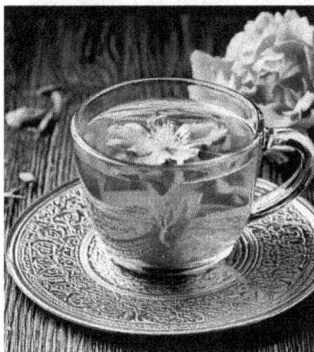

Sensual Saffron & Rose Herbal Tea

Purpose: Increases blood flow and naturally enhances mood and attraction.

INGREDIENTS

- 3 saffron threads
- 1 tbsp dried rose petals
- 1 tsp dried cardamom pods (lightly crushed)
- 2 cups hot water
- 1 tsp honey

DIRECTIONS

1. Add saffron, rose petals, and crushed cardamom pods to a teapot or cup.
2. Pour hot water over the herbs and steep for 10 minutes.
3. Strain and sweeten with honey.
4. Enjoy to enhance sensuality.

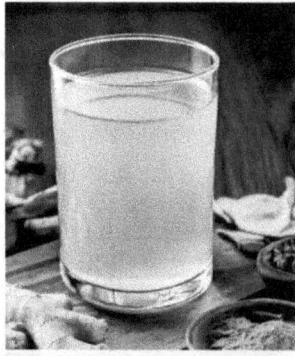

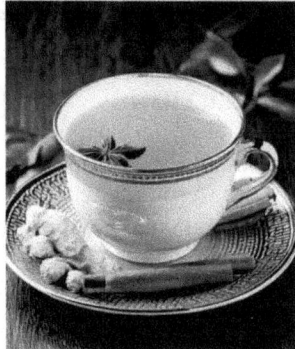

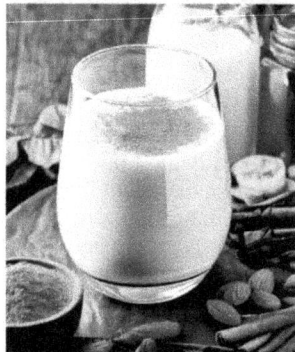

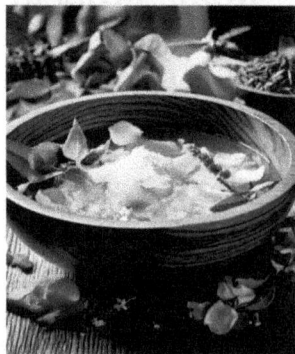

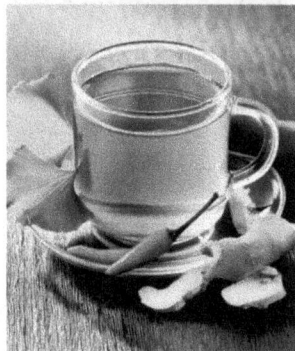

Circulation-Boosting Aphrodisiac Elixir

Purpose: Improves blood flow, enhances sensitivity, and supports arousal.

INGREDIENTS

- 1 tablespoon dried ginseng root
- 1 tablespoon dried ginger root
- 1 teaspoon dried cayenne pepper
- 1 teaspoon dried cinnamon
- 1 cup honey

DIRECTIONS

1. Mix all herbs with honey in a glass jar.
2. Let the mixture infuse for 24 hours, stirring occasionally.
3. Take 1 teaspoon daily.
4. Store in a cool, dark place for up to two weeks.

Endurance & Stamina Herbal Tea

Purpose: Boosts physical stamina, energy levels, and sexual performance.

INGREDIENTS

- 1 teaspoon dried ginseng root
- 1 teaspoon dried maca root
- 1 teaspoon dried cacao nibs
- 1 teaspoon dried cinnamon
- 2 cups boiling water

DIRECTIONS

1. Add all dried herbs to a teapot or heat-proof jar.
2. Pour boiling water over the herbs and steep for 15-20 minutes.
3. Strain and drink 1 cup daily to enhance stamina and endurance.
4. Store in the fridge for 24 hours.

Aphrodisiac Chocolate Love Potion

Purpose: Enhances mood, increases circulation, and stimulates desire.

INGREDIENTS

- 1 cup almond milk
- 1 tablespoon raw cacao powder
- 1 teaspoon dried maca root powder
- 1 teaspoon dried damiana leaf
- 1 teaspoon raw honey
- ½ teaspoon dried cinnamon

DIRECTIONS

1. Heat almond milk in a saucepan until warm (do not boil).
2. Stir in cacao, maca, damiana, cinnamon, and honey.
3. Whisk until smooth and let steep for 5 minutes.
4. Strain (if using whole herbs) and drink warm to enhance passion.

Sensuality Herbal Bath Soak

Purpose: Relaxes the body, enhances circulation, and promotes sensuality.

INGREDIENTS

- ½ cup dried rose petals
- ½ cup dried damiana leaves
- ½ cup dried lavender flowers
- ¼ cup Epsom salts
- 10 drops sandalwood essential oil

DIRECTIONS

1. Mix all dried herbs and place in a muslin bag or cheesecloth.
2. Fill the bathtub with warm water and add the herb bag.
3. Let the herbs steep for 10 minutes before getting in.
4. Soak for at least 20 minutes to relax and stimulate the senses.

Blood Flow & Erectile Support Tea

Purpose: Improves circulation, blood flow, and supports erectile function.

INGREDIENTS

- 1 teaspoon dried ginkgo biloba
- 1 teaspoon dried horny goat weed
- 1 teaspoon dried cayenne pepper
- 1 teaspoon dried ginger root
- 2 cups boiling water

DIRECTIONS

1. Combine all dried herbs in a teapot or heat-proof container.
2. Pour boiling water over the herbs; steep for 15-20 minutes.
3. Strain and drink 1 cup daily.
4. Store any extra in the fridge for up to 24 hours.

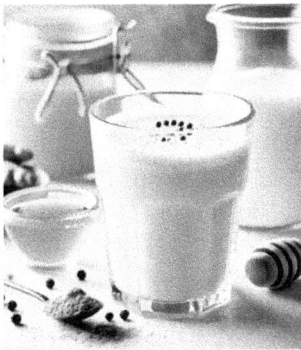

Turmeric & Black Pepper Golden Elixir

Purpose: Combats inflammation and promotes radiant skin.

INGREDIENTS
- ½ tsp turmeric powder
- A pinch of black pepper
- 1 cup warm almond milk
- 1 tsp honey

DIRECTIONS
1. Mix turmeric and black pepper into almond milk.
2. Add honey and drink in the evening

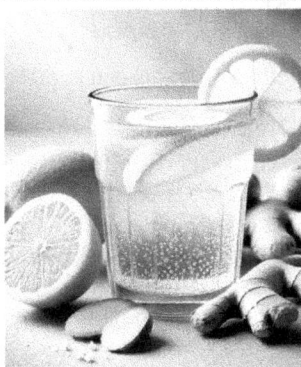

Ginger & Lemon Youth Tonic

Purpose: Detoxifies and promotes healthy, glowing skin.

INGREDIENTS
- 1 tsp grated ginger
- Juice of 1 lemon
- 1 cup warm water

DIRECTIONS
1. Combine ginger and lemon juice with warm water.
2. Drink in the morning for a daily detox boost.

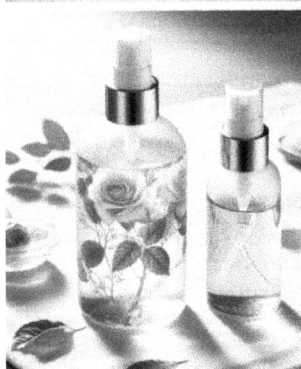

Rosewater & Green Tea Toner

Purpose: Rejuvenates and tightens the skin.

INGREDIENTS
- ½ cup rosewater
- ½ cup brewed green tea (cooled)

DIRECTIONS
1. Mix rosewater and green tea in a spray bottle.
2. Spritz onto the face after cleansing.

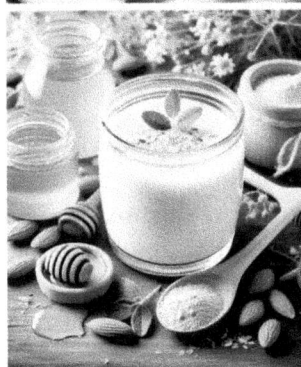

Ashwagandha Skin Glow Tonic

Purpose: Reduces stress and promotes youthful skin tone.

INGREDIENTS
- 1 tsp ashwagandha powder
- 1 tsp raw honey
- 1 cup warm almond milk

DIRECTIONS
1. Mix ingredients into warm almond milk.
2. Drink in the evening to reduce stress.

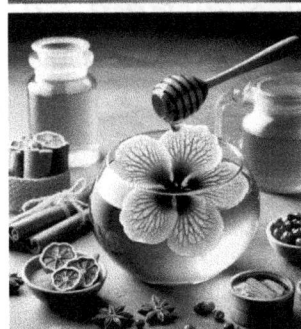

Reishi & Hibiscus Youthful Elixir

Purpose: Fights oxidative stress to promote healthy, youthful skin.

INGREDIENTS
- 1 teaspoon dried reishi mushroom powder
- 1 teaspoon dried hibiscus petals
- 1/2 teaspoon cinnamon powder
- 1 cup hot water
- 1 teaspoon raw honey or maple syrup

DIRECTIONS
1. Steep reishi mushroom powder and hibiscus petals in hot water for 8-10 minutes.
2. Strain and stir in cinnamon and honey or maple syrup.
3. Sip warm to enhance skin health and vitality.

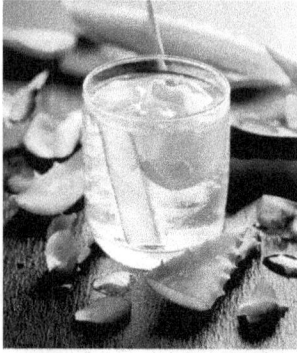

Aloe Vera & Rose Skin-Glow Tonic

Purpose: Hydrates and balances skin from the inside for glowing skin.

INGREDIENTS

- 1 tablespoon rose water
- ¼ cup aloe vera juice
- 1 cup chamomile tea

DIRECTIONS

1. Brew a cup of chamomile tea and let it cool.
2. Mix in 1 tablespoon of rose water.
3. Add ¼ cup of aloe vera juice.
4. Drink this tonic daily.

Comfrey & Violet Skin Repair Mask

Purpose: Promotes skin regeneration, soothes irritation, and hydrates skin.

INGREDIENTS

- 1 teaspoon dried comfrey leaves
- 1 teaspoon dried violet leaves
- 1 tablespoon plain yogurt or aloe vera gel

DIRECTIONS

1. Grind leaves into a fine powder.
2. Mix with yogurt or aloe vera gel to create a paste.
3. Apply to clean skin and leave on for 15-20 minutes.
4. Rinse with warm water.

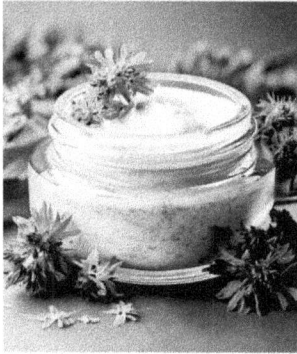

Nettle & Horsetail Mineral Face Steam

Purpose: Opens pores, detoxifies skin, and provides minerals for a healthy glow.

INGREDIENTS

- 1 tablespoon dried nettle leaves
- 1 tablespoon dried horsetail leaves
- 4 cups boiling water

DIRECTIONS

1. Add nettle and horsetail to a large bowl.
2. Pour boiling water over the herbs and cover your head with a towel to trap steam.
3. Lean over the bowl and steam your face for 5-10 minutes.

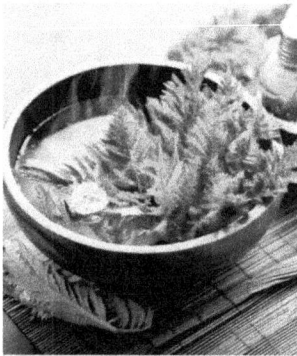

Rosemary & Aloe Vera Scalp Serum

Purpose: Stimulates hair growth and soothes the scalp for healthier, stronger hair.

INGREDIENTS

- ½ cup fresh aloe vera gel
- 10 drops rosemary essential oil
- 1 tbsp castor oil
- ½ cup distilled water

DIRECTIONS

1. Blend the aloe vera gel until smooth.
2. Mix in the rosemary oil and castor oil and add distilled water.
3. Store in a small bottle and apply to the scalp 2-3 times per week.

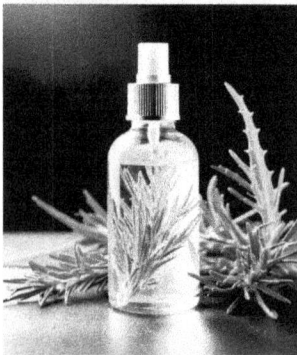

Burdock & Calendula Soothing Salve

Purpose: Reduces redness, soothes eczema, and promotes skin healing.

INGREDIENTS

- 1 teaspoon dried burdock root
- 1 teaspoon dried calendula flowers
- 1/2 cup coconut oil
- 2 tablespoons beeswax pellets

DIRECTIONS

1. Infuse the ingredients by heating gently for 1-2 hours.
2. Strain the oil and mix with melted beeswax in a double boiler.
3. Pour into a container and let cool before applying to irritated skin.

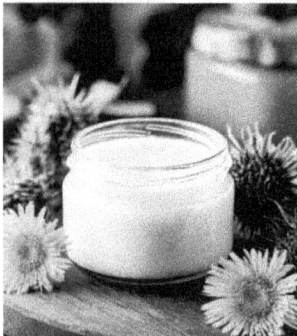

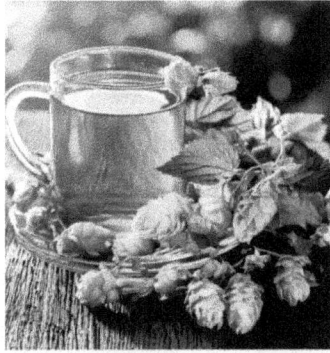

Hops & Valerian Restful Sleep Tea

Purpose: Helps ease stress, reduce anxiety, and promote restful sleep.

INGREDIENTS

- 1 teaspoon dried hops flowers
- 1 teaspoon dried valerian root
- 1 cup boiling water
- 1 teaspoon raw honey

DIRECTIONS

1. Add hops and valerian root to a teapot or mug.
2. Pour boiling water over the herbs and steep for 10 minutes.
3. Strain and sweeten with honey.
4. Drink warm.

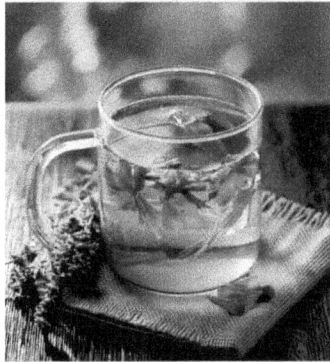

Skullcap & Hyssop Insomnia Infusion

Purpose: Promotes relaxation and improve sleep quality helping with insomnia.

INGREDIENTS

- 1 teaspoon dried skullcap leaves
- 1 teaspoon dried hyssop leaves
- 2 cups boiling water

DIRECTIONS

1. Add skullcap and hyssop to a teapot or mug.
2. Pour boiling water over the herbs and cover. Let steep for 15 minutes.
3. Strain and drink warm.

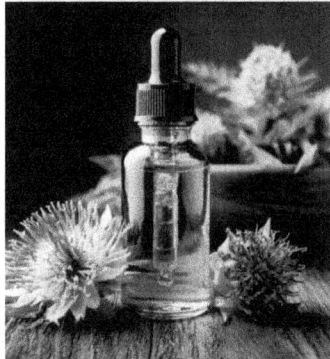

Valerian Root Deep Sleep Tincture

Purpose: Eases stress and encourages deep sleep.

INGREDIENTS

- 1/4 cup dried valerian root
- 1/4 cup dried passionflower
- 1 cup vodka or food-grade alcohol
- Honey

DIRECTIONS

1. Add ingredients to a clean glass jar and cover with vodka.
2. Seal the jar tightly and store in a cool, dark place for 4-6 weeks, shaking occasionally.
3. Strain the mixture into a dark glass bottle with a dropper.
4. Take 1-2 droppers (30-60 drops) diluted in water before bedtime.

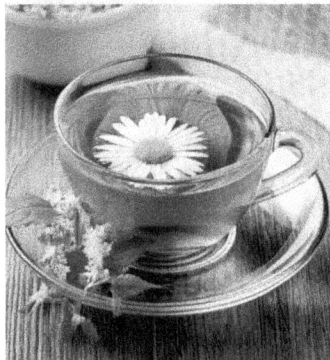

Chamomile and Holy Basil Sleep Tea

Purpose: Calms the mind and promotes restful sleep.

INGREDIENTS

- 1 tbsp dried chamomile flowers
- 1 tsp dried holy basil
- 1 cup boiling water
- Honey

DIRECTIONS

1. Combine ingredients in a mug.
2. Pour boiling water over the herbs and steep for 10 minutes.
3. Strain and sweeten with honey..
4. Drink warm before bed.

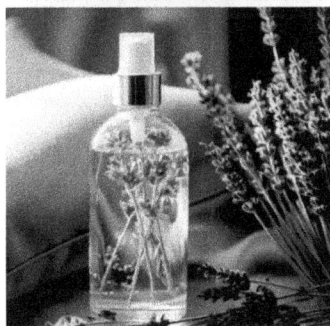

Lavender Aromatherapy Pillow Spray

Purpose: Calms the mind and enhances sleep quality with soothing scents.

INGREDIENTS

- 1/2 cup distilled water
- 1 tbsp witch hazel
- 5 drops lavender essential oil
- 3 drops rose essential oil

DIRECTIONS

1. Mix all ingredients in a small spray bottle.
2. Shake well before each use.
3. Lightly mist your pillow and bedding before bedtime.

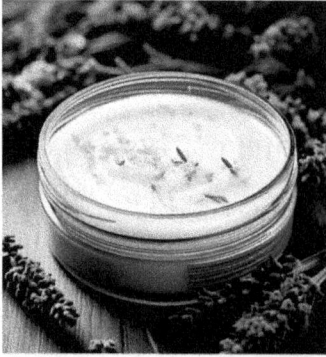

Restful Nights Sleep Balm

Purpose: Soothes the senses, relaxes the body, and encourages restful sleep.

INGREDIENTS

- 2 tbsp coconut oil or shea butter
- 1 tbsp beeswax
- 5 drops lavender essential oil
- 5 drops cedarwood essential oil
- 5 drops roman chamomile essential oil

DIRECTIONS

1. Melt coconut oil and beeswax together in a double boiler.
2. Remove from heat and stir in the essential oils.
3. Pour into a small container and let cool until solid.
4. Rub onto wrists, temples, and the soles of your feet before bed.

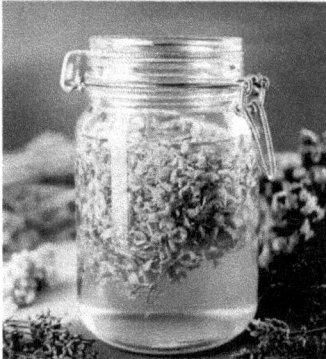

Tranquil Night Syrup

Purpose: Encourages relaxation, relieves stress, and supports deep sleep.

INGREDIENTS

- 1 tbsp dried chamomile flowers
- 1 tbsp dried lavender flowers
- 1 tsp dried lemon balm
- 1 cup filtered water
- ½ cup raw honey

DIRECTIONS

1. Add all herbs and water to a saucepan.
2. Simmer on low heat for 20 minutes. Reduce liquid by half.
3. Strain and stir in raw honey.
4. Store in a glass jar in the refrigerator for up to 2 weeks.
5. Take 1 tsp before bed.

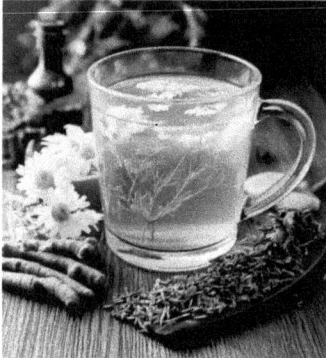

Soothing Sleep Decoction

Purpose: Reducess nighttime restlessness and promotes sustained sleep.

INGREDIENTS

- 1 tbsp dried valerian root
- 1 tbsp dried ashwagandha root
- 1 tsp dried chamomile flowers
- 1 tsp dried licorice root
- 3 cups filtered water

DIRECTIONS

1. Add all herbs and water to a small saucepan.
2. Bring to a gentle simmer and let it steep for 20 minutes.
3. Strain and sip warm, 30 minutes before bed to encourage deep sleep.

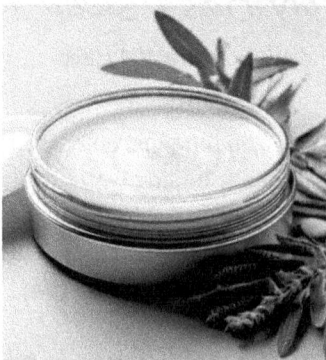

Sleepy-Time Herbal Foot Balm

Purpose: Relaxes the nervous system, relieves tension, and aids restful sleep.

INGREDIENTS

- 2 tbsp coconut oil
- 1 tbsp shea butter
- 1 tbsp beeswax
- 5 drops clary sage essential oil
- 5 drops cedarwood essential oil
- 5 drops vetiver essential oil

DIRECTIONS

1. Melt coconut oil, shea butter, and beeswax in a double boiler.
2. Remove from heat and stir in essential oils.
3. Pour into a small glass jar and let cool until solid.
4. Massage onto feet, temples, and wrists before bed for deep sleep.

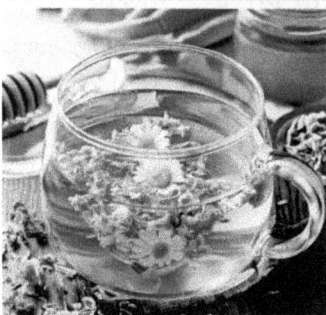

Dreamy Nighttime Infusion

Purpose: Relaxes the mind, reduces stress, and promotes deep sleep.

INGREDIENTS

- 1 tsp dried chamomile flowers
- 1 tsp dried lemon balm
- ½ tsp dried passionflower
- ½ tsp dried lavender
- 1 cup hot filtered water
- 1 tsp raw honey

DIRECTIONS

1. Add all herbs to a tea infuser or mug.
2. Pour hot (not boiling) water over the herbs; steep for 10–15 minutes.
3. Strain and stir in honey.
4. Sip 30–60 minutes before bed.

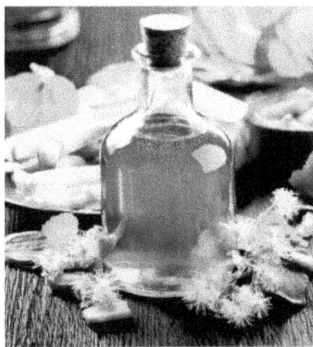

Licorice Root & Linden Calming Syrup

Purpose: Reduces stress and soothes the nervous system.

INGREDIENTS
- 1 tablespoon dried licorice root
- 1 tablespoon dried linden flowers
- 2 cups water
- 1/4 cup honey

DIRECTIONS
1. Simmer licorice root and linden flowers in water for 15 minutes.
2. Strain and mix the liquid with honey.
3. Store in a glass jar in the refrigerator and take 1-2 teaspoons as needed to relax.

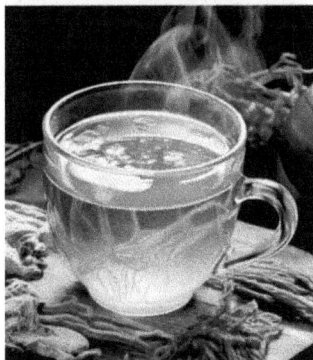

Lion's Mane & Reishi Stress-Relief Decoction

Purpose: Reduces stress, promotes relaxation, and supports overall health.

INGREDIENTS
- 1 tablespoon dried lion's mane mushroom pieces
- 1 tablespoon dried reishi mushroom slices
- 2 cups water

DIRECTIONS
1. Add lion's mane and reishi mushrooms to a pot with water.
2. Simmer on low heat for 30-40 minutes.
3. Strain and drink warm.

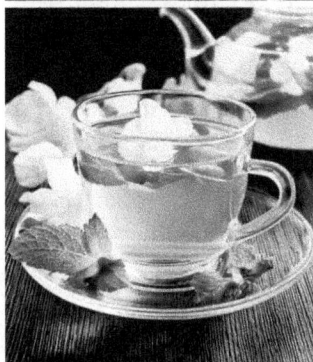

Evening Primrose & Lemon Relaxing Tea

Purpose: Promotes relaxation, eases anxiety, and supports emotional well-being.

INGREDIENTS
- 1 teaspoon dried evening primrose leaves
- 1 teaspoon dried lemon balm leaves
- 1 cup boiling water

DIRECTIONS
1. Combine evening primrose and lemon balm in a teapot or mug.
2. Pour boiling water over the herbs and steep for 10 minutes.
3. Strain and drink warm.

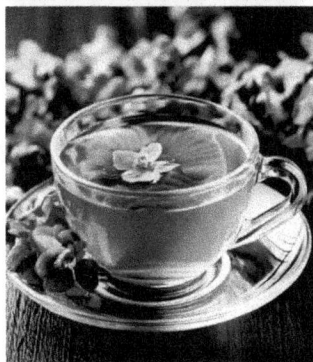

Violet & Skullcap Nervous System Tea

Purpose: Calms the nervous system, reduces tension, and supports balance.

INGREDIENTS
- 1 teaspoon dried Skullcap leaves
- 1 teaspoon dried Violet leaves
- 1 cup boiling water

DIRECTIONS
1. Combine skullcap and violet leaves in a mug.
2. Pour boiling water over the herbs and steep for 8–10 minutes.
3. Strain and sip slowly to ease stress and calm the nerves.

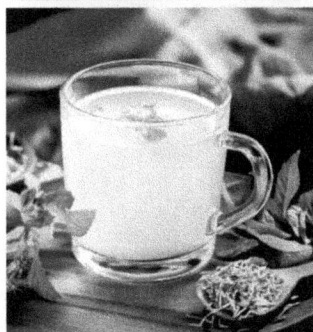

Valerian & Ashwagandha Sleep Tonic

Purpose: Promotes deep sleep, calms the nervous system, and reduces stress.

INGREDIENTS
- 1 teaspoon dried Valerian root
- 1 teaspoon dried Ashwagandha
- 1 cup boiling water
- 1 teaspoon honey

DIRECTIONS
1. Combine valerian root and ashwagandha in a mug.
2. Pour boiling water over the herbs. Steep for 10–12 minutes.
3. Strain the tea and add honey.
4. Drink 30 minutes before bed.

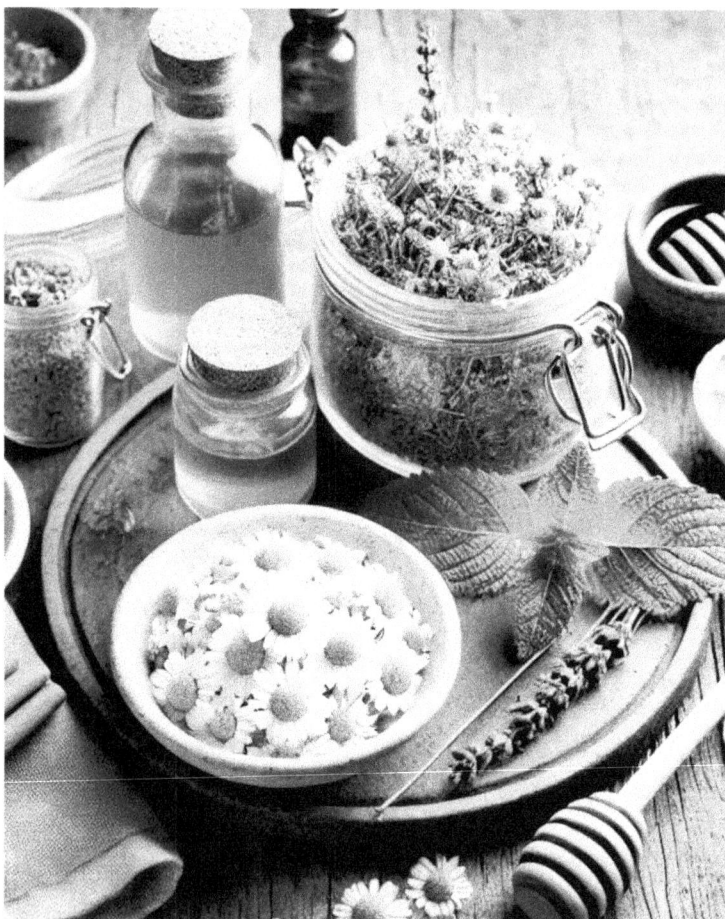

Chamomile Calming Elixir

Purpose: Promotes restful sleep and calms anxiety.

INGREDIENTS

- 2 cups water
- 1 tablespoon dried chamomile flowers
- 1 teaspoon dried lavender flowers
- 1 teaspoon lemon balm leaves
- 1-2 teaspoons raw honey
- 1/2 teaspoon vanilla extract
- A pinch of cinnamon or nutmeg

DIRECTIONS

1. Bring 2 cups of water to a gentle boil.
2. Place chamomile, lavender, and lemon balm in a teapot or heatproof jar. Pour the hot water over the herbs, cover, and let steep for 10-15 minutes.
3. Strain the liquid into a mug or jar, discarding the herbs.
4. Stir in honey, vanilla extract, and a pinch of cinnamon or nutmeg, if desired, for additional flavor and relaxation.
5. Sip slowly, preferably 30 minutes before bedtime, to help unwind and prepare for a peaceful night's sleep.

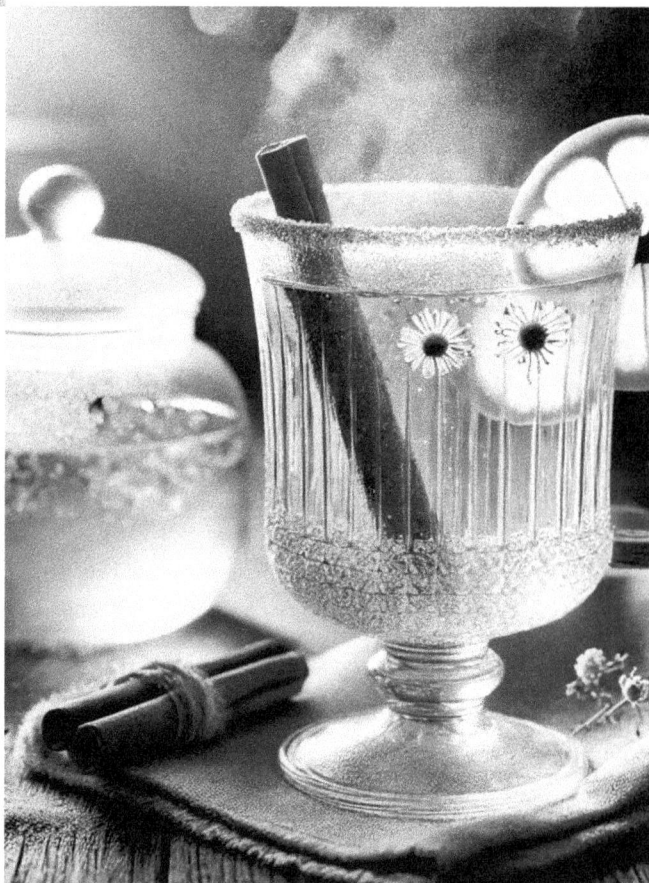

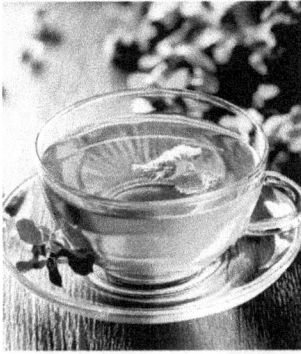

Violet & Catnip Calming Tea

Purpose: Reduces anxiety and promotes relaxation.

INGREDIENTS

- 1 teaspoon dried violet leaves
- 1 teaspoon dried catnip leaves
- 1 cup boiling water

DIRECTIONS

1. Add violet and catnip leaves to a teapot or mug.
2. Pour boiling water over the herbs and steep for 8-10 minutes.
3. Strain and enjoy warm to promote calmness and relaxation.

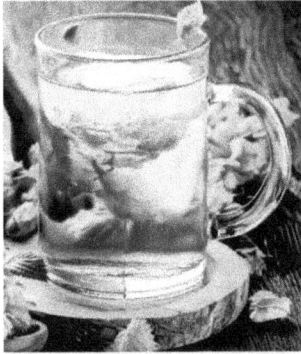

Hops & Skullcap Anxiety-Relief Infusion

Purpose: Relaxes the nervous system and reduces stress and anxiety.

INGREDIENTS

- 1 tablespoon dried hops flowers
- 1 teaspoon dried skullcap leaves
- 1 teaspoon valerian root
- 2 cups hot water

DIRECTIONS

1. Add hops, skullcap, and valerian root to a heatproof jar or mug.
2. Pour hot water over the herbs, cover, and steep for 10-15 minutes.
3. Strain and drink 30 minutes before bedtime for optimal results.

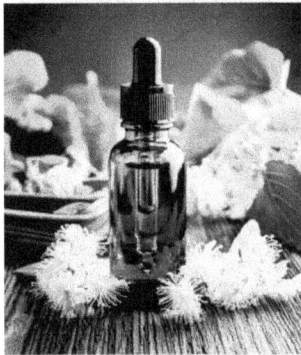

LindenStress-Relief Tincture

Purpose: Calms the mind, eases muscle tension, and supports relaxation.

INGREDIENTS

- 1 tablespoon dried linden flowers
- 1 tablespoon dried meadowsweet flowers
- 1/2 cup vodka or food-grade alcohol

DIRECTIONS

1. Add ingredients to a clean glass jar and cover with vodka.
2. Seal the jar tightly and store in a cool, dark place for 4-6 weeks, shaking occasionally.
3. Strain the mixture into a dark glass bottle with a dropper.
4. Take 1-2 droppers (30-60 drops) diluted in water before bedtime.

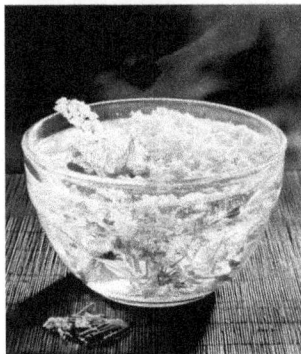

Meadowsweet Relaxation Bath

Purpose: Relaxes muscles, calms the mind, and relieves stress-related tension.

INGREDIENTS

- 1/4 cup dried goldenrod flowers
- 1/4 cup dried meadowsweet leaves
- 4 cups boiling water

DIRECTIONS

1. Add ingredients to a large bowl and pour boiling water over them.
2. Let steep for 15 minutes, then strain the liquid into your bathwater.
3. Soak for 20-30 minutes to relieve stress and relax your body.

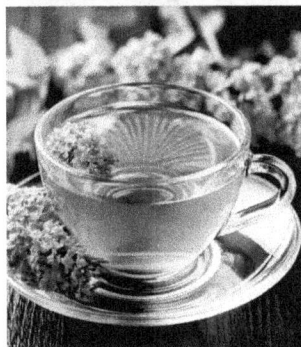

Blue Vervain Stress-Relief Tea

Purpose: Reduces stress, eases nervous tension, and promotes relaxation.

INGREDIENTS

- 1 teaspoon dried kava kava root
- 1 teaspoon dried blue vervain leaves
- 1 teaspoon dried skullcap leaves
- 1 cup hot water

DIRECTIONS

1. Combine all ingredients in a teapot or mug.
2. Pour hot water over the herbs and steep for 10-15 minutes.
3. Strain and drink warm.

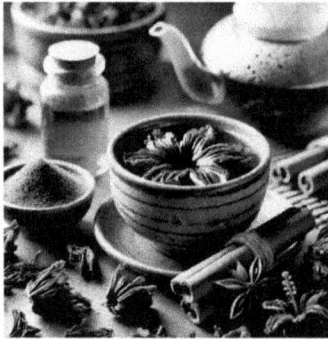

Hibiscus & Cinnamon Slimming Tea

Purpose: Reduces bloating and supports weight management.

INGREDIENTS
- 1 tsp dried hibiscus flowers
- ½ tsp cinnamon powder
- 1 cup boiling water

DIRECTIONS
1. Steep hibiscus flowers and cinnamon in boiling water for 5 minutes.
2. Strain and drink warm after meals.

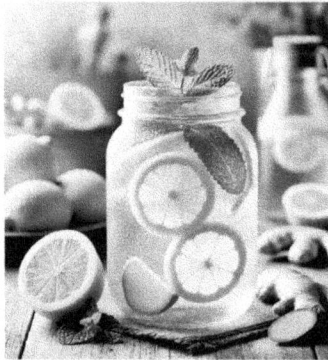

Lemon Ginger Detox Water

Purpose: Aids in digestion, fat metabolism, and detoxification.

INGREDIENTS
- 1 liter water
- 1 lemon, sliced
- 1-inch piece of ginger, sliced
- A few mint leaves

DIRECTIONS
1. Combine all ingredients in a jar and let infuse overnight in the refrigerator.
2. Drink throughout the day.

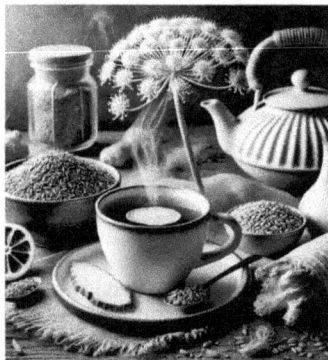

Chicory Root & Fennel Tea Blend

Purpose: Supports digestion, reduces bloating, and curbs appetite naturally.

INGREDIENTS
- 1 tablespoon dried chicory root
- 1 teaspoon fennel seeds
- 1 slice of fresh ginger
- 2 cups water

DIRECTIONS
1. Add chicory root, fennel seeds, and ginger to a small pot.
2. Pour in the water and bring to a gentle boil.
3. Reduce the heat and let simmer for 10 minutes.
4. Strain the tea into a cup and enjoy warm.

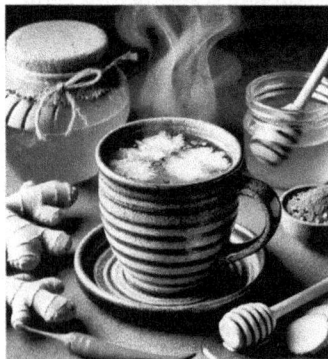

Ginger & Cayenne Energy Booster

Purpose: Increases calorie burning and reduces cravings.

INGREDIENTS
- 1 cup hot water
- 1 tsp grated ginger
- A pinch of cayenne pepper
- 1 tsp honey

DIRECTIONS
1. Steep ginger in hot water for 5 minutes.
2. Add cayenne and honey, then drink warm.

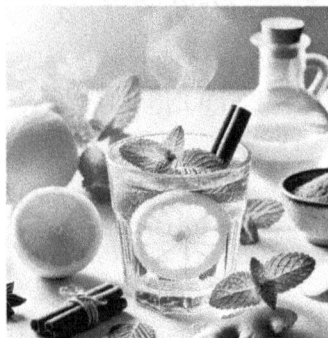

Cinnamon & Mint Metabolism Booster

Purpose: Supports digestion, boosts metabolism, and helps reduce cravings.

INGREDIENTS
- 1 cup warm water
- 1 slice of lemon
- 4-5 fresh mint leaves
- 1 cinnamon stick
- 1 teaspoon grated ginger

DIRECTIONS
1. Heat the water but not boiling.
2. Add the ingredients to the water.
3. Let the mixture steep for 5-7 minutes to infuse the flavors.
4. Strain if desired and drink warm.

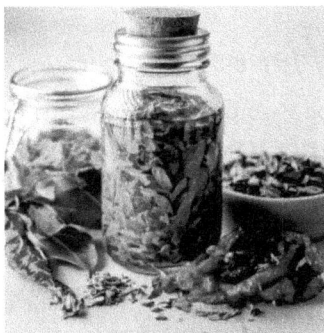

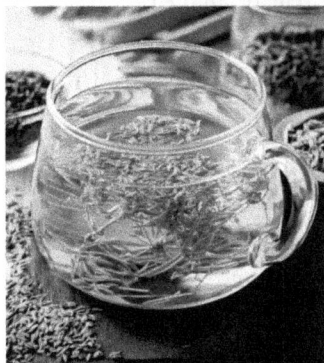

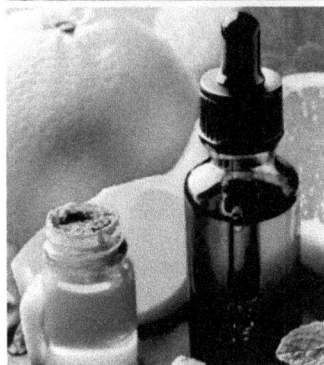

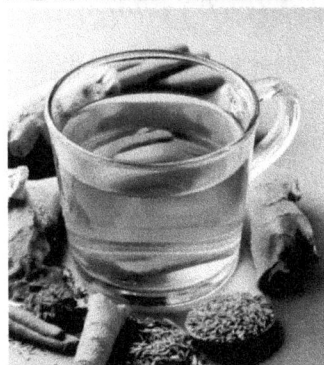

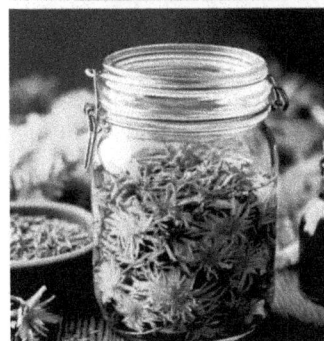

Fat-Burning Herbal Tincture

Purpose: Boosts metabolism, curbs cravings, and enhances digestion.

INGREDIENTS

- 1 tbsp dried cayenne pepper
- 1 tbsp dried ginger root
- 1 tbsp dried green tea leaves
- ½ cup vodka or apple cider vinegar
- 1 glass jar with a lid

DIRECTIONS

1. Add all dried herbs to a glass jar.
2. Submerge herbs with vodka or apple cider vinegar,
3. Seal and store in a cool, dark place for 4–6 weeks, shaking every few days.
4. Strain and store in a dark glass bottle.
5. Take ½ teaspoon diluted in water before meals.

Digestive Harmony Decoction

Purpose: Reduces bloating, aids digestion, and regulates appetite.

INGREDIENTS

- 1 tbsp fennel seeds
- 1 tbsp dried burdock root
- 1 tsp cumin seeds
- 1 tsp dried licorice root
- 3 cups filtered water

DIRECTIONS

1. Add all herbs and water to a small saucepan.
2. Bring to a gentle simmer, then reduce heat and let simmer for 20 minutes.
3. Strain and drink ½ cup before meals to support digestion and appetite regulation.

Metabolism-Boosting Aromatherapy Blend

Purpose: Energizes the body, curbs cravings, and stimulates fat-burning with aromatic herbs.

INGREDIENTS

- 5 drops grapefruit essential oil
- 5 drops peppermint essential oil
- 5 drops ginger essential oil
- 2 tbsp carrier oil (jojoba or coconut oil)

DIRECTIONS

1. Mix all oils in a small glass bottle.
2. Apply to wrists, neck, or inhale deeply before meals to reduce cravings and energize metabolism.

Fire & Flow Digestive Decoction

Purpose: Stimulates digestion, supports fat metabolism, and reduces bloating.

INGREDIENTS

- 1 tbsp dried ginger root
- 1 tsp dried cayenne pepper
- 1 tsp dried cinnamon chips
- ½ tsp dried fennel seeds
- 3 cups filtered water

DIRECTIONS

1. Add all herbs to a saucepan with 3 cups of water.
2. Bring to a gentle simmer and let steep for 15–20 minutes.
3. Strain and drink ½ cup before meals to boost digestion and metabolism.

Lunar Dandelion Metabolism Tincture

Purpose: Supports the liver, reduces water retention, and balances metabolism.

INGREDIENTS

- 1 tbsp dried dandelion root
- 1 tbsp dried nettle leaf
- 1 tbsp dried fennel seeds
- ½ cup vodka or apple cider vinegar (non-alcoholic version)
- 1 glass jar with lid

DIRECTIONS

1. Place all herbs in a clean glass jar.
2. Pour vodka or apple cider vinegar over the herbs, fully submerged.
3. Seal and store under the full moon for 4–6 weeks. Shake occasionally.
4. Strain and store in a dark glass bottle.
5. Take ½ teaspoon before bed.

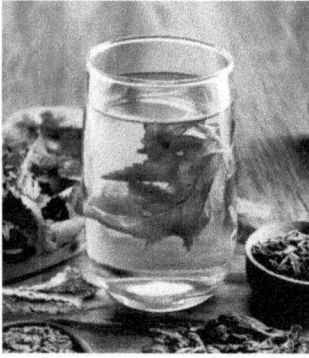

Iron-Boosting Herbal Tonic

Purpose: Enhances energy levels and iron absorption to prevent anemia.

INGREDIENTS

- 1 tablespoon dried nettles
- 1 tablespoon dried yellow dock root
- 1 teaspoon dried hibiscus
- 1 teaspoon dried rose hips
- 2 cups water

DIRECTIONS

1. Bring water to a gentle simmer and add all herbs.
2. Let simmer for 15-20 minutes, then remove from heat.
3. Strain and drink 1 cup daily to replenish iron and boost circulation.
4. Store extra in the refrigerator for up to 2 days.

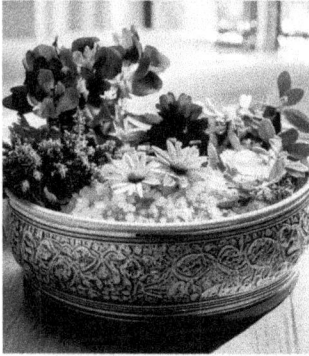

Relaxing Herbal Bath Soak

Purpose: Soothes cramps, reduces stress, and promotes deep relaxation.

INGREDIENTS

- ½ cup dried violet flowers
- ½ cup dried chamomile
- ½ cup dried rose petals
- ¼ cup Epsom salts
- 10 drops clary sage essential oil

DIRECTIONS

1. Mix all dried herbs and place in a muslin bag or cheesecloth.
2. Fill the bathtub with warm water and add the herb bag.
3. Let the herbs steep for 10 minutes before getting in.
4. Soak for at least 20 minutes.

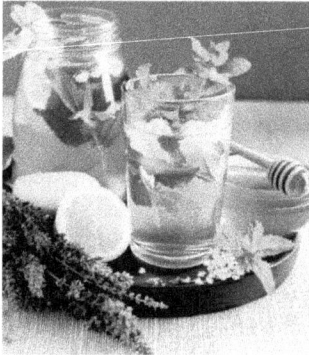

Mood-Boosting Herbal Elixir

Purpose: Helps alleviate mood swings, anxiety, and emotional stress.

INGREDIENTS

- 1 teaspoon dried lemon balm
- 1 teaspoon dried St. John's Wort
- 1 teaspoon dried holy basil
- 1 teaspoon dried lavender
- 1 teaspoon raw honey
- 2 cups boiling water

DIRECTIONS

1. Add dried herbs to a teapot or heat-proof jar.
2. Pour boiling water over the herbs; steep for 10-15 minutes.
3. Strain and sweeten with honey.
4. Drink warm to calm the mind and stabilize mood fluctuations.

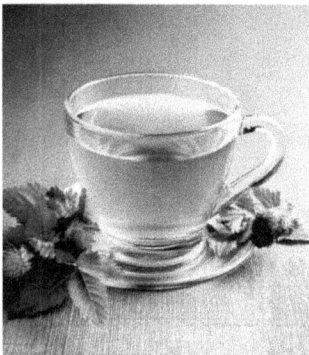

Fertility-Boosting Herbal Infusion

Purpose: Supports reproductive health and hormones to enhance fertility naturally.

INGREDIENTS

- 1 teaspoon dried red clover
- 1 teaspoon dried red raspberry leaf
- 1 teaspoon dried nettle leaf
- 1 teaspoon dried maca root powder
- 2 cups boiling water

DIRECTIONS

1. Combine dried herbs in a teapot or heat-proof container.
2. Pour boiling water over the herbs, cover, and steep for 15-20 minutes.
3. Strain and drink 1 cup daily.

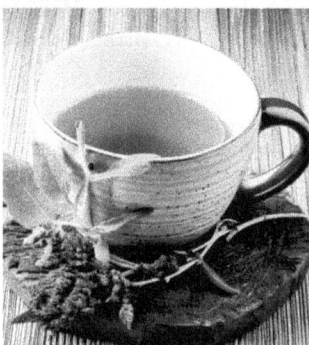

Menopause Support Herbal Tea

Purpose: Helps ease hot flashes, mood swings, and hormonal imbalances.

INGREDIENTS

- 1 teaspoon dried black cohosh
- 1 teaspoon dried sage
- 1 teaspoon dried red clover
- 1 teaspoon dried licorice root
- 2 cups boiling water

DIRECTIONS

1. Combine all dried herbs in a teapot or heat-proof container.
2. Pour boiling water over the herbs, cover, and let steep for 15 minutes.
3. Strain and drink 1-2 cups daily to support hormonal balance during menopause.
4. Store any extra in the fridge for up to 24 hours.

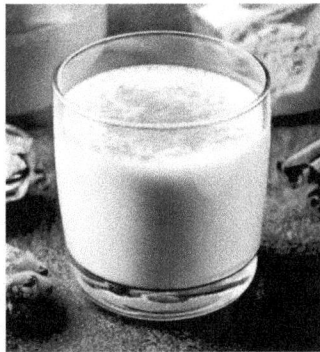

Hormone-Balancing Moon Milk

Purpose: Supports hormonal balance, reduces stress, and promotes restful sleep.

INGREDIENTS

- 1 cup warm almond or oat milk
- ½ tsp ashwagandha powder
- ½ tsp maca root powder
- ¼ tsp cinnamon
- 1 tsp honey

DIRECTIONS

1. Heat the milk until warm but not boiling.
2. Stir in ashwagandha, maca, and cinnamon until well combined.
3. Sweeten with honey if desired.
4. Enjoy before bedtime.

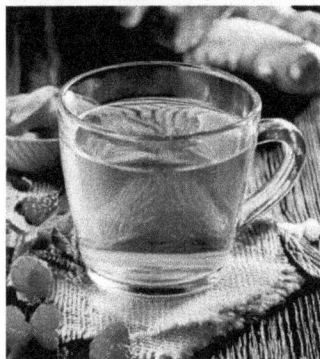

Soothing Raspberry Leaf Tea

Purpose: Relieves menstrual cramps and eases PMS symptoms.

INGREDIENTS

- 1 tbsp dried raspberry leaf
- 1 tsp dried peppermint
- ½ tsp grated fresh ginger
- 2 cups hot water
- Honey or lemon

DIRECTIONS

1. Add all herbs to a teapot or strainer.
2. Pour hot water over the herbs and steep for 10-15 minutes.
3. Strain and sweeten with honey or lemon if desired.
4. Drink 1-2 cups daily for relief.

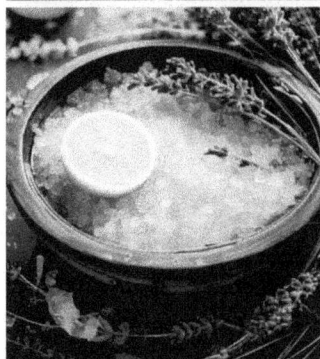

Stress-Relief Lemon Balm Bath Soak

Purpose: Eases stress, relaxes muscles, and promotes deep relaxation.

INGREDIENTS

- ½ cup Epsom salt
- ¼ cup dried lavender flowers
- ¼ cup dried lemon balm
- 10 drops lavender essential oil

DIRECTIONS

1. Mix Epsom salt, lavender, and lemon balm in a bowl.
2. Add lavender essential oil and stir.
3. Store in a jar and use ½ cup per bath.
4. Soak for 20 minutes to ease stress.

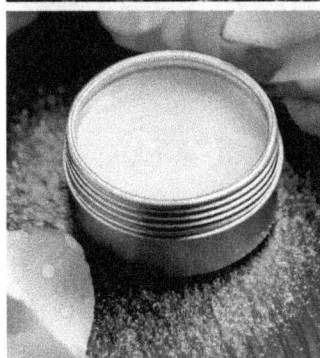

Rose & Honey Lip Balm

Purpose: Hydrates and softens lips while offering gentle antioxidant protection.

INGREDIENTS

- 1 tbsp coconut oil
- 1 tbsp beeswax pellets
- 1 tsp honey
- ½ tsp dried rose petals

DIRECTIONS

1. Melt coconut oil and beeswax in a double boiler.
2. Stir in honey and crushed dried rose petals until well combined.
3. Pour into small containers and let cool until solid.
4. Apply as needed for hydrated lips.

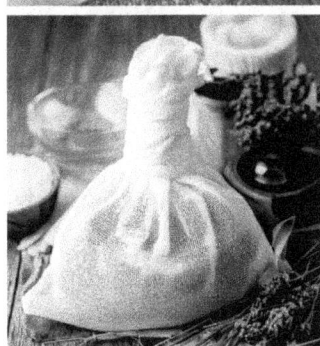

Soothing Poultice for Cramp Relief

Purpose: Eases cramps, promotes relaxation, and provides natural pain relief.

INGREDIENTS

- 2 tbsp grated fresh ginger
- 1 tbsp dried chamomile flowers
- 1 tbsp dried lavender flowers
- 1 tbsp coconut oil or olive oil
- A small cotton cloth or muslin bag

DIRECTIONS

1. Mix flowers in a bowl.
2. Add coconut oil and stir.
3. Spread the mixture onto a clean cotton cloth or place in a muslin bag.
4. Warm the poultice by holding it over a bowl of steaming water.
5. Apply to the lower abdomen and cover with a warm towel.
6. Relax for 15-20 minutes.

WOUND CARE

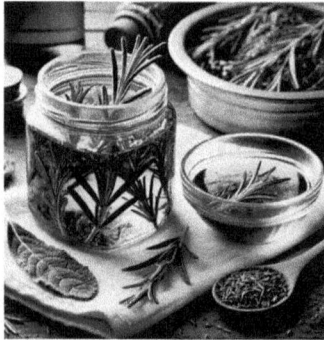

Rosemary & Plantain Antiseptic Wash

Purpose: Cleans wounds, prevents infection, and soothes irritated skin.

INGREDIENTS

- 1 teaspoon dried rosemary
- 1 teaspoon dried plantain leaves
- 2 cups boiling water

DIRECTIONS

1. Add rosemary and plantain to a teapot or bowl.
2. Pour boiling water over the herbs and steep for 15 minutes.
3. Strain and use the infusion to gently clean wounds or inflamed skin.

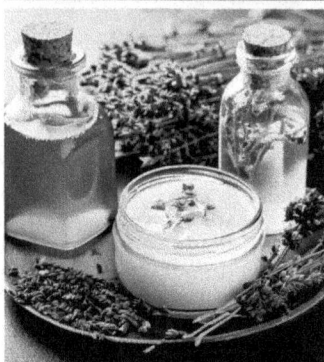

Calendula & Thyme Antimicrobial Salve

Purpose: Fights infection and promotes faster wound healing.

INGREDIENTS

- 1/4 cup dried calendula flowers
- 1 teaspoon dried thyme leaves
- 1/2 cup olive oil or coconut oil
- 2 tablespoons beeswax pellets

DIRECTIONS

1. Infuse all ingredients - heat them together for 1-2 hours.
2. Strain the oil and mix it with melted beeswax in a double boiler.
3. Pour the mixture into a clean jar to cool.
4. Apply to wounds or cuts.

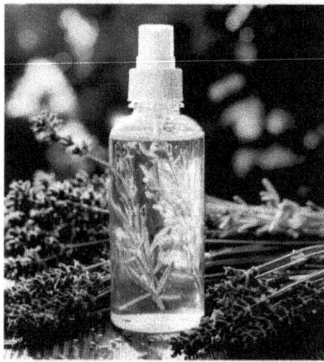

Lavender and Tea Tree Antiseptic Spray

Purpose: Cleans and disinfects minor cuts, scrapes, and wounds.

INGREDIENTS

- 1/2 cup distilled water
- 1 tbsp witch hazel
- 5 drops lavender essential oil
- 5 drops tea tree essential oil

DIRECTIONS

1. Mix all ingredients in a spray bottle.
2. Shake well before use.
3. Spray directly onto wounds or use with a clean cotton pad to cleanse the area.

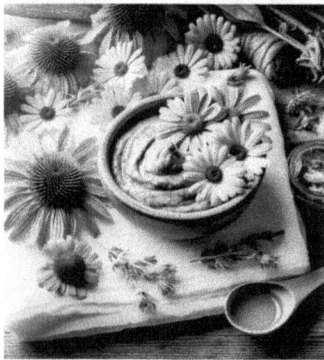

Echinacea & Calendula Healing Poultice

Purpose: Supports immune response and tissue repair.

INGREDIENTS

- 1 tablespoon dried echinacea root or flowers
- 1 tablespoon dried calendula flowers
- Warm water (enough to make a paste)

DIRECTIONS

1. Grind or crush echinacea and calendula into a powder if needed.
2. Mix the herbs with enough warm water to form a paste.
3. Apply the paste directly to the wound and cover with a clean cloth or gauze.

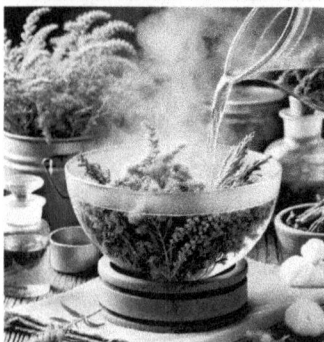

Witch Hazel Antiseptic Wash

Purpose: Cleans wounds, reduces inflammation, and promotes healing.

INGREDIENTS

- 1 tablespoon dried goldenrod flowers
- 1 tablespoon dried witch hazel bark or leaves
- 2 cups boiling water

DIRECTIONS

1. Add ingredients to a heatproof bowl.
2. Pour boiling water over the herbs and cover.
3. Let steep for 15-20 minutes, then strain into a clean container.
4. Use a clean cloth or cotton pad to gently cleanse wounds or inflamed skin.

CONCLUSION

"The power of nature is beyond human imagination. The greatest truths are found in the smallest plants."

— Nicholas Culpeper, Herbalist and Physician

As you reach the end of *Herbal Home Apothecary*, consider it not a conclusion but an opening chapter in your journey into natural healing. Herbalism and essential oil therapy are far more than tools for wellness—they are gateways to reconnecting with the wisdom of nature. In this ancient practice, healing extends beyond the physical, fostering a deeper relationship with the world around you. Let this book guide you to explore, experiment, and personalize your herbal remedies.

Holistic health is a journey of balance—mind, body, and spirit working in harmony to achieve a state of well-being. By integrating healthy behaviors such as mindful eating, regular movement, and stress management with the timeless practice of herbal healing, you create a comprehensive approach to wellness. Herbal remedies complement these habits by addressing physical ailments and emotional resilience. Together, these practices cultivate a lifestyle rooted in vitality and intention, empowering you to live with energy, clarity, and connection to the natural rhythms of life.

The natural world is a treasure trove of possibilities waiting for you to unlock its potential. Approach this path with curiosity and reverence, trusting that the answers you seek are already present in the plants, flowers, and roots around you. May you find wellness, peace, and inspiration as you blend your remedies. Nature has always provided the answers—it's up to you to ask the right questions and uncover its wisdom.

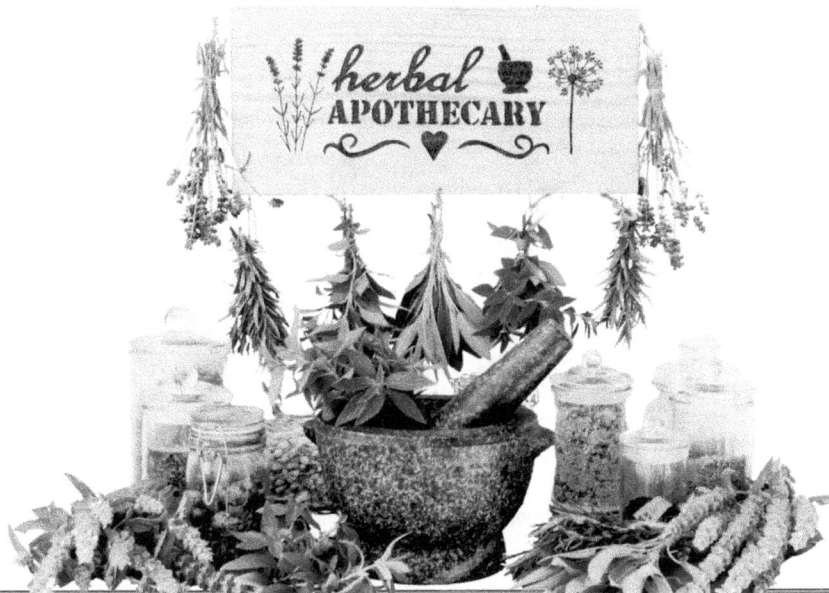

REFERENCES

Balkrishna, A., Sharma, N., Srivastava, D., Kukreti, A., Srivastava, S., & Arya, V. (2024). Exploring the safety, efficacy, and bioactivity of herbal medicines: Bridging traditional wisdom and modern science in healthcare. Future Integrative Medicine, 3(1), 35–49.

Battu, H., & Madhavi, N. (2023). A short concise note of current trends and future prospects on herbal medicine. Pharmacognosy Research, 15(4), 615–622.

Brown, D. (2001). Encyclopedia of herbs and their medicinal uses. DK Publishing.

Chaughule, R. S., & Barve, R. S. (2024). Role of herbal medicines in the treatment of infectious diseases. Vegetos, 37, 41–51.

Cohen, M. M. (2014). Tulsi - Ocimum sanctum: A herb for all reasons. Journal of Ayurveda and Integrative Medicine, 5(4), 251–259.

Culpeper, N. (1952). The Complete Herbal and English Physician. London; A. Cross Printer 89, Paul Street, Finsbury.

Dai, Y. K., Wu, Y. B., Wen, H., Li, R. L., Chen, W. J., Tang, C., Lu, L., & Hu, L. (2020). Different traditional herbal medicines for the treatment of gastroesophageal reflux disease in adults. Frontiers in Pharmacology.

David, S., & Cunningham, R. (2019). Echinacea for the prevention and treatment of upper respiratory tract infections: A systematic review and meta-analysis. Complementary Therapies in Medicine, 44, 18–26.

Duke, J. A. (2002). Handbook of medicinal herbs (2nd ed.). CRC Press.

Gagnier, J. J., Oltean, H., Van Tulder, M. W., & Berman, B. (2016). Herbal medicine for low back pain: A Cochrane review. Spine, 41(2), 116–133.

Harris, D. J., & Harris, J. S. (2013). Plant lore, legends, and lyrics. Dover Publications.

Houghton, P. J., & Houghton, R. A. (2007). Herbal medicine: Current trends and future directions. The Pharmaceutical Press.

Jin, L., Zheng, J., Honarvar, N., & Chen, X. (2020). Traditional Chinese Medicine in the United States: Current state, regulations, challenges, and the way forward. Traditional Medicine and Modern Medicine, 3(2), 77-84.

Mabberley, D. J. (2008). Mabberley's plant-book: A portable dictionary of plants, their classification, and uses (3rd ed.). Cambridge University Press.

Martins, A., Maia, E., & Praça, I. (2023). Herb-drug interactions: A holistic decision support system in healthcare.

Newall, C. A., Anderson, L. A., & Phillipson, J. D. (1996). Herbal medicines: A guide for health-care professionals. Pharmaceutical Press.

Musa, H. H., Musa, T. H., Oderinde, O., Musa, I. H., Shonekan, O. O., Akintunde, T. Y., & Onasanya, A. K. (2022). Traditional herbal medicine: Overview of research indexed in the Scopus database. Advances in Traditional Medicine, 1–11.

Parvin, K., Srivastava, A., Hidangmayum, N., Bansal, S., Meher, R., & Awasthi, R. (2023). Exploring the evolving role of herbal and alternative medicine in modern healthcare. Acta Traditional Medicine, 2(1), 35–42.

Petrovska, B. B. (2012). Historical review of medicinal plants' usage. Pharmacognosy Reviews, 6(11), 1–5.

Salm, S., Rutz, J., van den Akker, M., Blaheta, R. A., & Bachmeier, B. E. (2023). Current state of research on the clinical benefits of herbal medicines for non-life-threatening ailments. Frontiers in Pharmacology, 14, Article 1234701.

Šantić, Ž., Pravdić, N., & Bevanda, M. (2017). The historical use of medicinal plants in traditional and scientific medicine. Psychiatria Danubina, 29, 787–792.

Shi, A., Long, Y., Ma, Y., Yu, S., Li, D., Deng, J., et al. (2023). Natural essential oils derived from herbal medicines: A promising therapy strategy for treating cognitive impairment. Frontiers in Aging Neuroscience, 15, Article 1104269.

Walker, A. F. (2006). Herbal medicine: The science of the art. The Proceedings of the Nutrition Society, 65(2), 145–152.

Wang, H., Chen, Y., Wang, L., Liu, Q., Yang, S., & Wang, C. (2023). Advancing herbal medicine: Enhancing product quality and safety through robust quality control practices. Frontiers in Pharmacology, 14, Article 1265178.

Wei, X., & Others. (2023). Efficacy and mechanism of herbal medicines and their active compounds in treating cardiovascular diseases. Frontiers in Pharmacology, 14, Article 1236821.

World Health Organization. (2019). WHO global report on traditional and complementary medicine 2019. World Health Organization.

Wu, S., Wang, C., Bai, D., Chen, N., Hu, J., & Zhang, J. (2023). Perspectives of international multi-center clinical trials on traditional Chinese herbal medicine. Frontiers in Pharmacology, 14, Article 1195364.

ABOUT THE AUTHOR

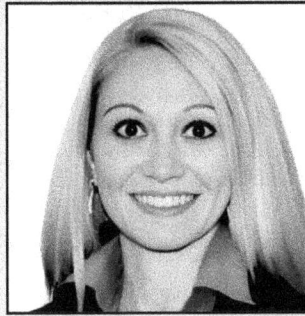

Tina M. Penhollow, Ph.D., MCHES is a health behavior scientist, educator, and best-selling author specializing in holistic wellness, herbal medicine, and natural healing. With over two decades of expertise in health science, aging, and alternative medicine, she blends cutting-edge research with time-honored healing traditions, offering a unique and practical approach to well-being.

As a professor of health science, Dr. Penhollow is dedicated to empowering individuals with science-backed, actionable strategies to enhance their health naturally. Her work bridges modern scientific research with ancient herbal wisdom, making natural remedies and holistic wellness accessible to those seeking a more balanced, vibrant life.

Beyond the classroom and writing, Dr. Penhollow enjoys spending time with her family and her beloved dog, Maverick. She is also an avid explorer of nature, continuously researching plant-based healing and integrating her findings into her work. When she's not delving into herbal medicine, she enjoys perfecting her golf game and embracing the restorative power of the outdoors.

Thank You!

Dear Fellow Herbalist,

Thank You for Exploring *Herbal Home Apothecary Book!*

I am truly honored that you've taken the time to embark on this journey into the transformative power of herbal healing. This book was created with a deep passion for nature's timeless wisdom, and I hope it has inspired and empowered you to embrace the benefits of natural remedies for gut health and overall wellness.

If you found value in these pages, I would be incredibly grateful if you could take a moment to leave a review on the platform where you purchased this book. Your feedback not only supports independent authors but also helps others discover the beauty and benefits of herbal healing. Your words have the power to inspire future herbalists, wellness seekers, and nature enthusiasts to continue this rich tradition of healing.

Together, we can preserve and share this knowledge, ensuring it continues to thrive for generations to come.

Wishing you vibrant health, joy, and an abundance of herbal wisdom as you continue your journey!

With gratitude,
 Dr. Tina M. Penhollow

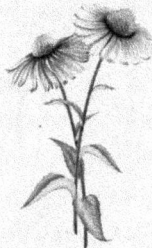